Heart & Hands

THIRD EDITION

Heart & Hands

A Midwife's Guide to Pregnancy & Birth

Elizabeth Davis

Photographs by Suzanne Arms • *Illustrations by Linda Harrison*

CELESTIAL ARTS
BERKELEY, CALIFORNIA

CELESTIAL ARTS
P.O. Box 7123
Berkeley, CA 94707

Cover photograph by Suzanne Arms
Cover design by Toni Tajima
Interior design by Shelley Firth
Illustrations by Linda Harrison

THIRD EDITION 1997
UPDATED EDITION 1992
SECOND EDITION 1987

First published as *A Guide to Midwifery: Heart & Hands*
by John Muir Publications, 1981

Library of Congress Cataloging-in-Publication Data
Davis, Elizabeth, 1950-
Heart & hands: a midwife's guide to pregnancy & birth/by
Elizabeth Davis. — 3rd ed.
p.   cm.
Includes bibliographical references and index.
ISBN 0-89087-838-2 (pbk.)
1. Midwifery.   2.Obstetrics.   I. Title.
RG950. D38   1997
618.2—dc21   97-40593
CIP

Printed in Canada

1 2 3 4 5 6 7 — 01 00 99 98 97

Acknowledgments

I begin by thanking my teacher, Tina Garzero, for her patience and love in teaching me this great art and way of being. To John Walsh, I will always remember your humor and guidance.

To Janice Kalman, dear friend and companion in all walks of midwifery life, my deepest thanks for expert technical review of the manuscript.

Once again, I must acknowledge Linda Harrison for her stunning illustrations. And to Suzanne Arms, for the cover photo and new photos throughout, my love and gratitude.

To Shannon Anton, little sister/wise one, thank you for your excellent sections on homeopathy and herbs in pregnancy, birth and postpartum, as well as the powerful account of Liam Andrew.

For the use of photos from the first and second editions, I wish to thank the following:

Ed Buryn, pages 93, 97, 115, copyright © 1981.
Gary Yost, pages 129, 131, 186, copyright © 1981.
Katy Raddatz, pages 81, 107, copyright © 1981.

A very special thanks and tribute to all the midwives who appear in the book, or who have assisted the families pictured. The intimate portrayal of your care is a precious addition to this work. Likewise, to the parents and children pictured herein—your contribution to better birth experiences is of great value, and I thank you!

To the staff at Celestial Arts—my editor Heather Garnos, who was cheerful and enduring to the end; managing editor Veronica Randall, who got the project on track; Mary Ann Anderson, for book production, Toni Tajima for cover design; and Shelley Firth for book design and typesetting, heartfelt thanks for your thoroughness, patience, and good humor.

A special thanks to David Hinds, my publisher, for his long-standing friendship and commitment to this project.

Finally, deep appreciation to my children at home, John and Celeste, for enduring the deprivations associated with this revision, and to my darling husband Jim, for seeing me through.

Contents

Reader Please Note

The medical and health procedures in this book are based on the training, personal experiences, and research of the author and on recommendations of responsible medical sources. But because each person and situation is unique, the author and publisher urge the reader to check with a qualified health professional before using any procedure where there is any question as to its appropriateness. The publisher does not advocate the use of any particular birth-related technique, but believes this information should be available to the public. Because there are risks involved, the author and publisher are not responsible for any adverse effects or consequences resulting from the use of any of the suggestions, preparations, or procedures in this book. Please do not use these unless you are willing to assume these risks. Feel free to consult a physician or other qualified health professional. It is a sign of wisdom, not cowardice, to seek a second or third opinion.

About the Author

Elizabeth Davis, C.P.M., is a renowned expert on women's issues and has been a midwife, women's health care specialist, educator, and consultant for over 20 years. She is active in the international women's rights movement, and lectures widely on midwifery, sexuality, and women's spirituality.

She has served as a representative to the Midwives Alliance of North America, and as president of the Midwifery Education Accreditation Council for the United States. She is co-founder of the Midwifery Institute of California, a three-year, apprenticeship-based midwifery program. She holds a degree in Holistic Maternity Care from Antioch University, and is certified by the North American Registry of Midwives.

Davis is also the author of *Energetic Pregnancy: A Guide to Achieving Balance, Vitality & Well Being from Conception to Birth and Beyond, Women's Intuition, Women, Sex & Desire: Exploring Your Sexuality at Every Stage of Life*, and (with co-author Carol Leonard), *The Women's Wheel of Life: Thirteen Archetypes of Woman at Her Fullest Power*. She lives in Windsor, California and is the mother of three children.

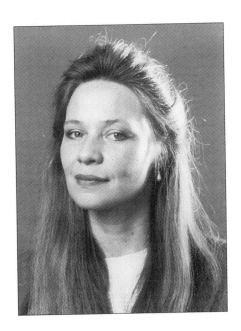

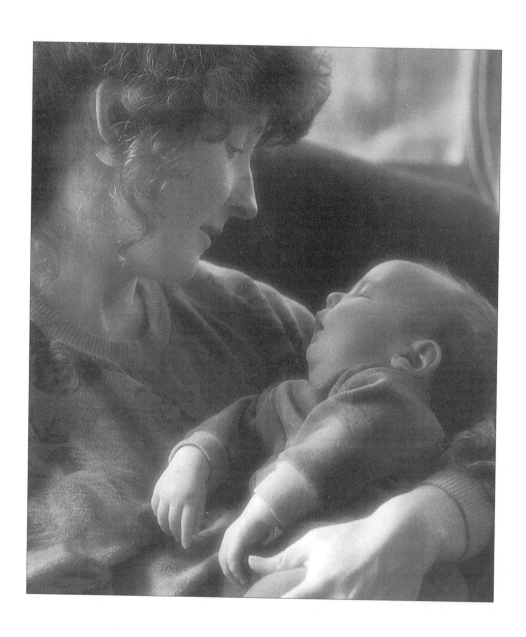

Preface to the Third Edition

More than a revision, this third edition has been completely rewritten to include 40% new material. Like its predecessors, it is both a text for beginning midwives and a reference for parents interested in understanding the nuts and bolts of midwifery care. It features new sections on homeopathy and herbs for the childbearing cycle, VBAC, sexual abuse, water birth, and adoption. Boxed sections for parents have been updated and expanded. For aspiring midwives, great pains have been taken to clarify existing material, and to highlight and better define crucial terminology. New sections on fetal development, cardinal movements of the fetus during labor, and the physiology of breastfeeding make this a more complete beginner's text. Experienced midwives will find updated information on hepatitis, HIV, and GBS screening, group midwifery practice, malpractice concerns, and guidelines for structuring apprenticeship, plus new prenatal and intrapartum case histories.

Sales of *Heart & Hands* passed the 100,000 mark this year. This pleases me more than words can say. I wrote the original edition in 1979, with no greater intent than to organize and deliver myself of knowledge and experience accumulated in my first few years of practice. Before long, *Heart & Hands* acquired a life of its own, which carried me along in its wake and set my own life on course.

Shortly after the first edition was published in 1981, I was asked to serve on the initial board of the Midwives Alliance of North America (MANA) as regional representative for the Pacific states. The big shocker of my burgeoning political career came when I was cornered by two midwives I greatly admired, Tish Demmin and Carol Leonard, who, having already passed progressive midwifery legislation in their respective states, asked me point-blank, "So, Liz, what are you going to do to organize California?" I must admit the thought had never crossed my mind, and the prospect was more than daunting, in light of the number of midwives then under investigation for illegal practice, and the general climate of fear and denial.

I asked for help, and was advised to work with midwives in my state to devise a process of self-regulation, i.e., put together a competency-based certification process. When I questioned the necessity of this obviously huge undertaking, they pointed out that if we didn't make moves to regulate ourselves soon, someone else—the medical profession—would do it for us. With the help of my students and colleagues, this dream became a reality in 1986.

That year was a busy one. I served as a consultant to a statewide Alternative Birthing Methods Study, as chairwoman of the annual MANA convention in San Francisco, and as legislative co-chair for the California Association of Midwives. I also revised *Heart & Hands* for the first time, expanding it to reflect midwifery's growing sophistication. Midwives were out from the underground, and consumers were articulating their love of birthing with midwives as never before.

Then, when national certification became politically viable in 1993, I called the first national planning and development meeting and, with the help of NARM, invited midwives from all 50 states who had been instrumental in passing legislation or founding certification in their jurisdictions. Forty attended, and it was from this pool of midwife representatives that our national process was formulated. I also served as president of the Midwifery Education Accreditation Council (MEAC) at this time, and helped develop an accreditation process for direct-entry midwifery programs. And in 1995, Shannon Anton and I founded the Midwifery Institute of California, dedicated to preserving midwifery apprenticeship.

In all of this, and through speaking engagements in countries as diverse as Thailand and Australia, I have had opportunity to meet so many dedicated and inspiring women—midwives who know their strength, own their vision, and are in for the long haul. I cannot tell you how much difference this has made to me, to have "sisters on a journey" at my side, ever ready for hard work or good times! This fulfills my maidenhood vision of being with women in a loving, non-competitive, wildly empowering way—a vision that isolated me in the '50s but brings me nothing but joy and affirmation at the dawn of the millenium.

If I may, a few words of advice. Mothers, believe in yourselves, claim the authority of intuitive knowing and women's mysteries, and use this to make the experience of giving birth ever more free and fulfilling for your daughters. Midwifery students, go for your dreams, aim high, and don't be afraid to take risks for what you believe in. Experienced midwives, reanimate yourselves in the Womb of the Mother, extend the weaving of the web, and speak the truth with grace and conviction.

To all of you, great gratitude for your presence in *Heart & Hands*.

Preface to the Original Edition

The purpose of this book is to offer a practical guide to midwifery—to instruct those women interested in becoming midwives, and to convey the realities of practice. Midwifery is a lost and found art, finding its place in our time via its links to feminism and expanding consciousness. It also appeals to a growing do-it-yourself resourcefulness. Women who want to be midwives have usually experienced birth firsthand and want to share and facilitate a new awareness of the power of being female. Most are seeking to extend their relationships with other mothers and babies. Many women who think that midwifery is their calling will read this book and realize that there are many other related areas that need development, such as birth education, postpartum support, and family counseling.

This book is intended to demystify the medical elitism surrounding a very basic, natural body process. There are other books which give more detailed information on obstetrics, but none explains how to adapt this information to individual women and how to bend the rules to fit each situation. This is a book on *practical midwifery*, with a special focus on creative management of complications. Thus it provides some answers for parents who want more than just good quality care and are seeking to understand the various alternative solutions to problems which may arise in pregnancy and birthing. This information is also intended for midwives practicing in remote areas with little or no medical consultation.

However, this manual is only a partial guide to midwifery practice, as nothing can substitute for experience—the educated intuition which comes from attending many birthings. But at least the suggested practices and procedures may stimulate the aspiring midwife to question and study, and may also inspire dedicated practitioners to break ground with new, responsible methods. If this book moves parents and health professionals alike to innovative thought and humanistic understanding, the heart of its purpose will be realized.

Thanks be to the midwives—a positive, loving, bright, and pioneering bunch of women—for freely sharing skills and information without which this book would not have been written.

Also by Elizabeth Davis

The Women's Wheel of Life:
Thirteen Archetypes of Woman at Her Fullest Power

Women, Sex & Desire:
Exploring Your Sexuality at Every Stage of Life

Women's Intuition

Energetic Pregnancy:
A Guide to Achieving Balance, Vitality & Well Being
from Conception to Birth and Beyond

CHAPTER 1

The Midwife: A Profile

From the very beginning, women have helped one another give birth. One particularly attuned to this task emerged as town or village midwife, wielding the healing skills of her time and culture. It is the midwife, not the physician, who has attended birth for most of human existence, certainly in indigenous societies. And in modern-day cultures of Denmark, Holland, and Sweden, midwife-assisted birth remains the norm. In fact, the six countries with the lowest perinatal mortality rates in the world all make generous use of midwives, who attend 70 percent of all births. In the United States, where midwives assist only 5 percent of births due to political constraints, perinatal mortality is alarmingly high: *we rank number 24 worldwide.*

However, despite the efficacy of the midwifery model, midwives have been persecuted throughout history, particularly in western nations. During the Inquisition, and the subsequent period known as the "burning times," the main targets for persecution were midwives. Healing by way of nature and aligned with the wisdom of the body, midwives inadvertently opposed the most basic tenet of Christianity—original sin—and were therefore threatening to the Church. No wonder that the *Malleus Maleficarum*, handbook of the Inquisition, declared, "No one does more harm to the Catholic faith than midwives."

In the United States, attacks against midwifery accelerated at the turn of the century when medicine became a profession for profit, and the newly-emerging male physician became eager for the revenues of childbirth. Women were barred from university, thus those wanting to attend childbirth could not acquire the requisite credentials.

Midwifery was nearly eradicated at this point, so vehement was the campaign of male physicians to discredit midwife practitioners, who were portrayed as slovenly, immoral, drunken, promiscuous, and perverse, "whores with dirty fingers." In medieval times, midwives were branded consorts of the Devil; now they became "loose women" intent on their own ways of healing, in contrast to "good girls" who pursued nursing and accepted roles subservient to the physician and his methods.

Predictably, physician-attended birth proved to be both expensive and unsafe. For example, the high incidence of childbed fever associated with hospital birth in the early 1900s not only cost women their lives, but cost their surviving families a tidy sum. On the other hand, women who could not afford to be in hospital continued to rely on the midwife's skill in preventative medicine: her emphasis on cleanliness, good nutrition, and the use of herbs. Thus midwives of the past fostered their client's strength while providing education and counseling on a variety of health and family issues, much as they do today. The midwife's scope of practice has traditionally been care "from womb to tomb," employing a community health approach in treating a spectrum of women's diseases and afflictions.

For midwives to continue to assert their time-honored scope of practice meant war with the increasingly powerful medical profession—a war that continues to this day. Left to themselves, midwives would never have survived; they were poor, politically powerless, and disorganized. Midwifery is alive in our society today for one reason only, and that is women's insistence on midwifery care. Midwifery is simply a fact of life, perpetuated by the needs and desires of birthing women and their supporters.

Although traditional midwives trained by apprenticeship have practiced almost continuously in the United States, the development of nurse-midwifery is fairly recent. The Frontier Nursing Service began training midwives in 1939, using a model developed in England. There are now over 30 programs preparing nurse-midwives, although barriers to practice are considerable. Physicians have mixed reactions to the nurse-midwife—on the one hand, they find her a valuable adjunct to a busy practice, but on the other hand, if she seeks to practice independently with her own case load, she is little more than a threat, an economic competitor. That the physician expects the nurse to play a subordinate role is rooted in our cultural oppression of women healers, and is likewise endemic to our technocratic model of medicine. In contrast, the midwife's responsibilities require that she have the autonomy to make her own decisions in case of crisis, and to use interventions, maneuvers, and procedures in case of emergency that inadvertently cross into the physician's self-proclaimed scope of practice.

The question of how to establish and maintain legitimacy within the current medical system has caused sharp divisions among nurse-midwives. The American College of Nurse-Midwives (ACNM) is almost evenly divided between those who align more strongly with nursing than midwifery, and vice versa. The debate continues as to whether training as a nurse is of benefit to the aspiring midwife. It is noteworthy that in the Netherlands (where midwifery is long-established), midwifery applicants lose points for having a nursing background, for it is well understood that the nurse must follow orders, whereas the midwife must be able to think and act independently. The United States is the only country in the world that utilizes the title nurse-midwife—everywhere else, a midwife is simply a midwife!

Nurse-midwifery does enjoy fully secure legal status in the U.S., whereas traditional midwifery remains illegal in many states. Although traditional midwives have struggled to reanimate old midwifery laws and/or forge new ones, they continue to meet with bitter opposition from the richest and most powerful legislative lobby in the country, the American Medical Association. In California alone,

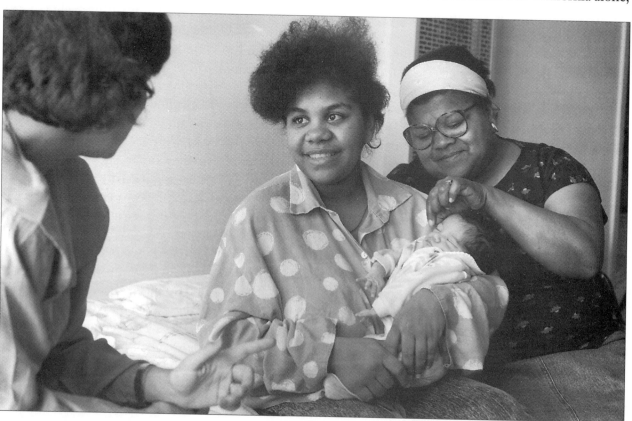

seven attempts at legalization were made over a ten-year period, during which more than 50 midwives were investigated, arrested, and prosecuted. Some 350 traditional midwives once practiced in the "golden state," but a decade later, their ranks had dwindled to 60 or so. How, and why, did this happen?

In 1976, midwife Kate Boland was visited by a pregnant agent wired for sound, who garnered evidence that resulted in Kate being found guilty of practicing medicine without a license. Thus in California, as in numerous other states, the practice of midwifery was defined by case law as an automatic misdemeanor. The law further directs that any misdemeanor associated with death or injury, regardless of whether death/injury was unpreventible or accidental, shall be subject to felony charges of manslaughter or murder. It has cost midwives a tremendous sum—tens of thousands of dollars—to defend themselves and their colleagues against counts of murder. This money has been hard to come by, and would have been better used for political organization, or to educate the public regarding midwifery. We do not exaggerate in terming this modern-day war against midwives a "witch hunt."

And yet, the continued threats of criminal prosecution in combination with dwindling ranks and resources have been undeniably strong motivators of the effort to legalize midwifery practice. It is a testament to the fortitude and vision of traditional midwives that they have been able to survive the costs—not just financial, but personal—of such difficult and seemingly endless legal battles!

We owe the evolution of midwifery's legitimacy to the vision and persistence of these, our contemporary founding mothers, who encouraged the next generation to take up the banner of self-regulation. By the early '80s, traditional midwives began creating their own standards of practice and mechanisms for certification state by state, even in jurisdictions where legislative efforts appeared futile. Then, in 1982, the Midwives Alliance of North America (MANA) was founded to enable midwives "of every stripe" to articulate their goals and visions, and find support in their struggle for legitimization. Licensing or legal certification for

traditional midwives is now available in 15 states, the practice is legal but unregulated in 14 states, and in 4 more, legal status remains undefined. This has led to a somewhat confusing barrage of professional titles: LM/licensed midwife, CM/certified midwife, DEM/direct-entry midwife. (The latter pertains more to educational preparation than professional status, denoting a midwife who has been trained to the profession directly, without nursing background.)

Several historic events bear mentioning at this juncture. At their annual convention in 1985, MANA members first considered the possibility of national midwifery certification. However, the notion was shelved indefinitely, for fear that setting national standards for midwifery competency might negatively impact states just beginning to develop their own grassroots processes of self-regulation. Then, in 1991, the Carnegie Foundation funded a task force of midwives from diverse educational backgrounds to address the future of midwifery education. This group produced a document entitled *Midwifery Certification in the United States*, historic in that it established *identical competencies and scope of practice for all midwives, regardless of training route and/or nursing background*. Before long, there was renewed discussion of national certification for direct-entry midwives.

Some years earlier, MANA established the North American Registry of Midwives (NARM) to administer a national registry exam. This group now began to consider the possibility of administering a national certification process. Then a core group of state leaders, many of whom had formulated and passed midwifery legislation in their respective jurisdictions, were told of these developments and organized to form the certification task force (CTF), with dual purposes of developing a prototype certification process and providing technical assistance to NARM. After numerous meetings at both state and national levels, a process was approved by the MANA membership, and in 1995, the first Certified Professional Midwife (CPM) was recognized by NARM.

NARM Certification is a *competency-based assessment process*. No specific educational pathway is delineated, but the candidate must be able to demonstrate entry-level midwifery knowledge and skill. The process is comprised of certain components commonly found in midwifery licensing and certification mechanisms. These are: 1) verification of requisite clinical experience; 2) verification of requisite skills and caregiving abilities; 3) verification of character/letters of recommendation; 4) verification of knowledge through comprehensive written exam. Once certified, the midwife must agree to fulfill continuing educational requirements, keep CPR and neonatal resuscitation training updated, work within the confines of MANA's core competencies, and uphold professional standards and ethics of practice.

In contrast, the ACNM offers certification only to those who have passed the national exam and *have completed an accredited program*. Barriers to accreditation are formidable for direct-entry programs, particularly as regards the apprenticeship model of midwifery education. This is why both the CTF and NARM focused on constructing a certification process that would incorporate a variety of educational routes to practice.

How does national midwifery certification interface with state licensure or certification? Although relatively new, it seems likely that national certification will eventually be adopted state by state as the universal process for assessing midwifery competence. States with unduly restrictive practice provisions could use national certification as rationale for legal amendment, or other regulatory changes. Many states already utilize the NARM test as their licensing or certification board exam. As more and more states adopt the national process in its entirety, reciprocity will be increasingly available for midwives wishing to relocate, and the entire profession will benefit from self-regulation.

Self-regulation is certainly the point where battle lines are drawn between midwives and the medical profession. Many nurse-midwives believe that higher education, i.e., masters-level midwifery, is the key to greater professional autonomy. Conversely, most direct-entry midwives believe that no credential will be enough as long as physicians are the ruling class, and that midwives must define midwifery on its own terms, rather than

continue to jump through a seemingly endless series of legitimacy hoops.

In spite of these differences, leaders of the midwifery movement predict that midwives will one day unite behind the issue of independent practice. This day may come sooner rather than later, as the fight for autonomous midwifery has become an international battle; there is not a single culture in the world where midwives are not somehow restricted in caregiving. German midwives may assist deliveries but cannot give prenatal care; Italian midwives can give prenatal care but must call the physician when delivery is imminent. In order to address the worldwide struggle of midwives to meet their communities' needs and take their rightful place in the healthcare system, the World Health Organization drafted the *International Definition of a Midwife*, which was adopted in 1972 by both the International Confederation of Midwives (ICM) and the International Federation of Gynecologists and Obstetricians (FIGO):

A midwife is a person who, having been regularly admitted to a midwifery educational program duly recognized in the jurisdiction in which it is located, has successfully completed the prescribed course of studies in midwifery and has acquired the requisite qualifications to be registered and/or legally licensed to practice midwifery.

The sphere of practice: She must be able to give the necessary supervision, care and advice to women during pregnancy, labor and postpartum period, to conduct deliveries on her own responsibility, and to care for the newborn and the infant. This care includes preventive measures, the detection of abnormal conditions in mother and child, the procurement of medical assistance, and the execution of emergency measures in the absence of medical help.

She has an important task in counseling and education-not only for patients, but also within the family and community. The work should involve antenatal education and preparation for parenthood and extends to certain areas of gynecology, family planning and child care.

She may practice in hospitals, clinics, health units, domiciliary conditions or any other service."

Particularly powerful in this statement are the assertions that the midwife may "conduct deliveries on her own responsibility," and "execute emergency measures in the absence of medical help." This definition is remarkable not only for what it says, but for what it leaves unspoken. Nowhere do we find any stricture regarding the "risk status" of our clients, nor any attempt to limit our practice to "childbearing women," "well women," or "interconceptional care"—terms commonly used in midwifery statutes to restrict scope of practice. It is a perfect expression of the midwife's role.

Other pivotal documents have been generated by the membership of MANA, including *MANA Standards and Qualifications for the Art and Practice of Midwifery, MANA Statement of Values and Ethics,* and *MANA Core Competencies for Midwifery Practice.* (See Appendix A.)

Yet another organization that has contributed to the professionalization of midwifery is the Midwifery Education Accreditation Council. MEAC was founded by a group of midwifery educators who wanted to promote better learning experiences for students by linking their educational programs to the accountability mechanisms and funding opportunities inherent in accreditation. MEAC's primary goal is to preserve a variety of educational routes to midwifery practice, particularly that of apprenticeship. (Addresses for MEAC, MANA, ACNM, and NARM may be found in Appendix B.)

*   *   *

Considering the troubled past and challenging present of midwifery, we can hardly help but pose the question: What makes midwifery such a deeply desired birthing option? Simply put, midwifery promotes well-being. It is an art of service, in that the midwife recognizes, responds to, and cooperates with natural forces. In this sense, midwifery is ecologically attuned, involving the wise utilization of resources and respect for the balance of nature. This is an exhilarating and important aspect of the work, i.e., supporting life in a way that sustains global community.

Above all, true midwifery care is personalized care. Despite parameters of safety the midwife must uphold, she knows that wellness is an amorphous state, with periodic deviations from normal.

Her task is to decipher the unique and ever-changing patterns of her client's well-being. The more thorough and continuous her care, the more likely she is to detect a complication at its inception. And the better she and her client communicate, the more readily they will be able to develop and implement a prompt solution. She and her client are a team, but the locus of responsibility rests with the expectant mother, who is at the helm of her healthcare experience.

Birth is indeed a pinnacle event, but is merely the finishing touch to pre-established intimacy between midwife, mother, and her supporters. Every birth has some potential for complications, but with continuity of care, the midwife's competence in handling these is facilitated both by foreknowledge of the mother's condition and by the mother's trust in her abilities.

The essence of midwifery is staying in the moment, being humble, and paying attention. But this seemingly simple approach is not easy to maintain, as it is the antithesis of control. And control is king in our culture, particularly in medical practice. Early in their training, physicians learn to seek control of their patients, control of their own emotions, control of outcomes via standardized procedures. They learn virtually nothing of the art of caregiving, but are taught instead to bypass personal involvement, to mistrust their intuition, to rely only on hard evidence, to seek pathology, and to fear death. Obstetrical students learn not only to identify, but to expect medical disasters. Accordingly, they are anxious to control pregnancy and birth at all costs, which precludes letting nature take its course.

But standardized, fear-based care has never appealed to women. What we really want is competent, sensitive attention to our entire condition. We define our health as more than physical; we expect care that will enable us to be fully ourselves, at our greatest potential. This is precisely what midwives have to offer. Midwifery has been dubbed an art of invisibility because it is non-interventive, except to render that which is needed to promote balance or restore harmony.

Let's take a closer look at today's midwife: what is she like as a person, and what role does she play in society? Midwives are found in every class and ethnic group in our culture, but the main thing they have in common is *persistence*. Whether she is a nurse or empirically trained, working openly or underground, doing hospital or home births, a midwife in these times faces tremendous obstacles in establishing and maintaining a practice. Engaging in illegal practice is especially difficult, for the midwife must risk her personal freedom in order to maintain responsibility for her clients. This takes strong, independent character, and a willingness to go against society's mores. And herein lies the secret to the midwife's notoriety: she is a rebel, and a female one at that!

It is ironic that the feminist movement has not aligned itself with the midwifery issue, especially since reproductive self-determination is otherwise a central tenet of feminist policy. Truly, what could be more feminist than the practice of midwifery? The most potent lesson of childbirth is the revelation of essential feminine force. Giving birth calls on a woman to shed her social skin and discover unique abilities to cooperate with and surrender to natural forces. Birth can profoundly transform and renew a woman, strengthen her faith, and deepen her identity. Hence the midwife, guardian and facilitator of this process, is intrinsically feminist by the very nature of her work!

Remember, midwifery is a tradition of care "from womb to tomb," in which midwives revere and facilitate all the physiologic milestones of women's lives: menarche, childbirth, and menopause. These times of transition are more than biological, and are traditionally known as Blood Mysteries. This is because women gain wisdom in these life passages that transcends reason and is mysteriously borne on the body. Many indigenous cultures have deliberately created rites of passage for men involving self-immolation and suffering, such as the Native American Sundance or vision-quest, in order to replicate the growth and transformation rendered naturally to women through their Blood Mysteries.

In their true capacity, midwives are concerned with women's well-being in a whole life context. Clearly, the transition of childbirth is more than having a baby; it is a pivotal event in a woman's

personal development. Midwives not only care about what happens to women during birth, but after. They know that those who labor on their own terms and triumph in spontaneous birthing will mother in a fiercely independent fashion, with newfound inner certainty.

Happy mothers also reach out confidently for whatever assistance they need. The evolutionary social aspect of midwifery is that it motivates women to extend to one another the power and responsibility found in giving birth, to go beyond the isolation of the nuclear family, to network and share their resources, to raise their children cooperatively. Thus midwifery is linked to social innovations in childcare, renewed emphasis on extended family, and holistic health care that acknowledges factors of nutrition, lifestyle, rest, and support as crucial to women's well-being. Women who choose midwifery—client and practitioner alike—seek connection, long to rise above divisiveness and competition, and yearn to create community.

Above all else, midwives are advocates of choice. They vigorously defend the right of parents to choose the place of birth, as they likewise fight for their own right to practice in various settings. Hospital privileges are frequently denied midwives and the physicians who support them. And despite a veritable glut of studies showing home birth to be as safe or safer than hospital birth, the controversy surrounding domiciliary midwifery persists.

*　　*　　*

To reiterate, the locus of responsibility in midwifery care is with the mother and her supporters. It is nearly impossible to realize woman-centered childbirth in the hospital setting, where practice is circumscribed by protocol, and protocol is designed to cover liability bases that have little to do with good care, let alone common sense. We have lost some of our finest obstetricians since the advent of the malpractice crisis: those who could not, in good conscience, perform a requisite battery of tests or procedures at odds with their patients' well-being. It is more than unfortunate that our malpractice system fails to differentiate between acts of fate and those of misconduct; our trial

CHOOSING A MIDWIFE

1. How was she trained? In a home or hospital setting? Is she licensed/certified? If not, are former clients/community members available that can vouch for her?

2. What is her experience? How many births has she attended since completing her training? Has she worked in a variety of settings/ practices?

3. What do her services include? Complete prenatal care? Home visits (how many)? Sibling preparation? Postpartum follow-up (how much)? Lab work? Prepared childbirth classes?

4. Does she work alone or with assistants? How many? If there are several, can you choose one to be at your birth? How often will you see this assistant during pregnancy? What, exactly, is the assistant's role?

5. Does she have a ceiling on the number of births she attends per month? Is this in keeping with the amount of assistance she has? What would happen if two births were running simultaneously? Has she ever missed a birth? If so, what were the circumstances?

6. Who would back her up in case of emergency? Another midwife? Will you have a chance to meet her before the birth?

7. What is her communications system like? Does she have a beeper? If not, how do you reach her? Is she available 24 hours a day at all times? What if she goes on vacation at some point in the pregnancy? Who takes calls, and how do you reach them?

8. What experience has she had with complications? Which ones? Has she ever had to resuscitate a baby? How would she handle a hemorrhage?

9. What equipment does she bring to births? Oxygen, IV fluids, ambu-bag for baby? Medications for hemorrhage?

10. What is her medical backup like? Does she have a particular backup physician/hospital? Is this covered by your insurance? If so, what are her privileges in this hospital setting? If not, can she work with physician/hospital under your insurance plan? What about pediatric backup?

11. What are her fees? What is included? What if you move or change your mind during the pregnancy? Is the fee competitive? How does she want it to be paid?

12. What other costs might you incur? Lab, birth classes? In the event of transport, how much does her backup physician charge? Does he/she charge for routine prenatal consultation and if so, how much? What are basic hospital charges? If you do not have insurance, is there any type of retroactive coverage (state aid) available?

13. What is her philosophy of care? Why is she a midwife? What are her basic beliefs about birth? Does she encourage family participation? Father participation? How? What are her expectations of you regarding self-care in pregnancy? Do you like her? Feel comfortable in her presence? Can you be honest with her? Will she be honest with you? Can you trust her, and yet feel free to make your own decisions? Do you want her at your birth?

lawyers, posing yet another threat to midwifery and choice, stand to profit whenever there is unhappy outcome in childbirth, regardless of fault. For midwives, this has meant a dearth of good backup, and more urgency than ever to advance a woman-centered model of maternity care.

No wonder most women who choose care with a midwife also choose to give birth at home. They instinctively seek the comfort, privacy, and opportunity for family participation found in their own environment, as well as the decreased likelihood of interventions. Research has repeatedly shown that the more relaxed and at ease a laboring woman feels, the more efficiently her body will function. If she becomes stressed or frightened, she will release hormones (catecholamines) which inhibit cervical dilation. In fact, research shows that whenever a birthing mammal is moved, threatened, denied privacy, or otherwise disturbed in labor, an arrest of progress will occur.

This is why pitocin—a synthetic form of oxytocin, the hormone that causes uterine contractions—is so commonly used in hospital birth. Unfortunately, pitocin also causes contractions to be so unnaturally strong and painful that many women hoping for natural childbirth end up requesting pain relief. What is worse is that most pain medications interfere with labor, and further increase the use of pitocin. And there is a limit—if the uterus is pushed too hard, it will not relax enough between contractions for healthy circulation and the fetus may go into distress, with cesarean section the only solution. The cesarean rate in most hospitals is over 25 percent, whereas midwifery practices boast less than 5 percent. *When women are in charge of their environment, when they have the privacy to labor undisturbed, when they feel completely at ease and supported, outcomes are always superior.*

Thus the midwife's most basic responsibility to her clients is to do everything she can to promote their relaxation and peace of mind. Beyond her repertoire of medical techniques, her skills encompass less concrete abilities to intuit, evoke and channel vital energy. Her hands are her most precious tools, as she senses, heals and blesses with her touch. She is infinitely patient—she waits, and waits, and waits some more. Yet she is ever attentive to the mother's condition, the baby's needs. Quietly aware, she serves as a mirror, and offers suggestions in timely fashion. She continually strives to reserve judgement, but is willing to speak the truth as the need arises.

Above all else, she keeps the following dictum in mind: "It's not my birth." Upholding this tenet of woman-centered midwifery means replacing one's personal biases and expectations of birth with whatever the mother and her supporters need or desire. Experienced midwives often speak of women's extraordinary ability for self-determination in giving birth. We must never forget to ask laboring women their opinions in crisis situations, or their perceptions of how to facilitate progress if it is lagging. Put simply, miracles happen in childbirth. The midwife must keep her senses ever alert, the parameters of safety ever in mind, and then stand back, let birth happen, and gratefully bear witness.

We must do all we can to advance the truth of midwifery's many benefits. Ultimately, the decision of where and with whom she gives birth belongs to the expectant mother. She must have better access to unbiased information in order to freely choose both place of birth and an assistant with the personal qualities and competence to suit her. Midwives have an urgent obligation to educate the public, and to stand firm in their support of woman-centered birth. Why? Because whenever a woman reclaims her right to experience childbirth exactly as she desires, she opens the door to unprecedented joy and fulfillment for herself and her intimates, and firmly reestablishes the primacy of motherhood in our culture. We can afford to wait no longer to heed society's call for midwifery care!

CHAPTER 2

Prenatal Care

Most midwives routinely provide comprehensive prenatal care, personally seeing their expectant clients at nearly every visit. Only by giving continuous care can the midwife get to know a woman well enough to have some sense of what to anticipate at her birth. Prenatal assessment is the cornerstone of midwifery care; the better we do our work prenatally, the less we are surprised by long, drawn-out labors. Every expectant mother's physical and emotional condition is unique, and can only be appreciated by repeated, regular contact. This helps us build rapport and a solid working relationship, and is what we call *continuity of care*.

Careful assessment is important throughout pregnancy, but becomes particularly crucial during the last six weeks. At this point, the midwife can identify certain factors regarding the baby's position, growth rate, and size, and relate these to the mother's condition. On this basis, she may realistically prepare both the mother and herself for a short or long labor, and make suggestions to help make the birth easier or to forestall complications. On a technical level, knowing the baby's and mother's prenatal norms enables the midwife to make appropriate determinations of acceptable range during the birth itself. For everyone concerned, prenatal care definitely proves its worth in terms of time, energy, and anxiety spared at deliveries.

Prenatal care really means wellness care, and as such involves nutritional counseling, exercise recommendations, non-allopathic healing options of herbology or homeopathy, and mind-body integration techniques like yoga and meditation. It also includes essential tests and procedures for screening any complications of pregnancy. Routine urinalysis, blood pressure evaluation, uterine/fetal palpation, fetal heart ausculation, and assessment of fundal height/fetal growth are detailed later in this chapter, as is lab work and its interpretation. If any significant abnormality arises, medical consultation should be sought for guidance and prognosis.

Your first contact with a woman seeking your services may be by phone. If the two of you are already familiar, your task will be to put aside preconceived notions and be open to new perceptions during this preliminary discussion of her pregnancy. Ask the expectant mother specifically how she became interested in having her baby with you.

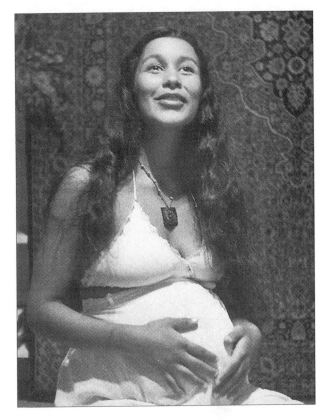

This will help you see how well founded her interest is and whether it is worth pursuing further.

If the initial information checks out well, go ahead with questions about her general health, relationship with partner (if applicable), previous pregnancies, or history of medical problems. Hopefully, she will ask you questions regarding your philosophy, experience, backup, etc. If you decide to meet, an initial visit should be scheduled within the next week or so, preferably at a time when her partner can also attend. Plan to spend at least two hours on this visit, as there will be plenty to discuss, and physical examinations to perform.

Never try to talk a woman into giving birth at home or selecting your practice. Let it be her decision to come to you. To uphold principles of woman-centered caregiving, it is crucial that the expectant mother's responsibility for her childbirth experience be established from the beginning.

THE INITIAL INTERVIEW

This very personal, in-depth meeting with the mother is your opportunity to understand her ideals surrounding birth and parenting, and to provide her with appropriate information. If she has had other children, she will share her previous experience. If this is her first, she will be full of questions. Elicit reasons for choosing home birth from both the woman and her partner. Notice priorities. Expectant parents primarily concerned with saving money must be made to see the commitment involved in birthing at home. And beware of those who say they " hate hospitals"—parents stuck in a negative, reactionary vein need more insight.

Just remember that your most basic task in the initial interview is to determine whether you, the mother, and her partner are suited to work together. The best way to do this is to relax and be as open as possible. Follow the energetic leads and physical pacing of your interviewees, matching their timing and style of conversation so they will feel sufficiently relaxed to disclose their true beliefs and concerns. Unless the expectant mother feels fully in charge, even your most sage advice will fall on deaf ears. On the other hand, if you gain her trust, your every hint is apt to be taken seriously.

In other words, use the initial visit to receive the expectant mother and her partner body and soul, then notice how contact with them affects you. If you later feel uneasy, apprehensive, or distracted, you may not be a match. In 20 years' practice, I've had ample opportunity to listen to midwives recount their unhappy outcomes, and in each and every case, they ruefully remember feeling uncomfortable at the initial visit with clients who later turned out to be troublesome. Do pay attention to your first impressions!

Who will be at the birth? The expectant mother's answer will give you some insight into her emotional aspect: is she private or more social in nature? Ask to meet her birth team as soon as possible, in order to identify any gaps in her support system. Many women initially plan on having quite a party of friends and relatives at the birth, then whittle down participants as pregnancy advances. And you can certainly help her choreograph the event as it draws near. But each and every person interested in being at the birth should also be directed to the expectant mother's needs for postpartum assistance! It is never to early to start lining up dinner service, or help with laundry, housework, etc. for the first few weeks after the baby comes.

How does the expectant mother define your role in pregnancy, labor, and postpartum? Does she want lots of guidance and participation, or will her partner be her main support? If she wants help from her partner, do her expectations of his/her involvement seem realistic? Does he/she want to help with the delivery? If they want to do most of it themselves, do they understand the necessity of routine checks from time to time? As the mother and her partner express their hopes and desires, it becomes easier for you to anticipate their needs and tailor your level of participation.

Throughout this discussion, there may be appropriate moments for passing along information, suggesting resources for further study, or providing referrals to groups or individuals. Help the expectant parents realize that there is a lot to learn, and that it's up to each of them to do some exploring. Recommend specific books, magazines or newsletters, video presentations, or prenatal exercise/support groups. Generate a reading list to provide at this first meeting, including referrals to local chapters of organizations like La Leche League, International, or Informed Birth and Parenting (see Appendix B).

Other topics essential to broach include your training and background, philosophy, and style of practice. The easiest way to present this information is to formulate a *Professional Disclosure/ Consent to Care* document for expectant parents to take home, read thoroughly, and bring back to sign in your presence. In addition to the above items, outline your expectations of clients, your limitations and how you work with them, and the nature of your relationship to the medical community. Make some statement regarding complications, particularly emergency complications which might result in injury or death to mother or baby. Of course you should stress that thorough prenatal care and careful monitoring of mother and baby will go a long way towards preventing these, but make clear that some complications are unforeseeable. The consent to care language should state that clients voluntarily agree to work with you in full knowledge of your limitations, and with their signature, further release you and your associates from all liability. It is also wise to include a statement that in the event of a dispute, parents agree to seek arbitration before taking legal action.

As you review and discuss this form with parents, watch for any nervous or negative reactions. Note any resistance to hospital transport, or apprehension regarding life-threatening complications. If either parent seems unusually fearful, ask for his/ her worst nightmare. This is a great opportunity to reevaluate their commitment to home birth, as well as give thorough explanations of how certain complications occur. You can also point out the preventative role of prenatal care, impressing parents with the importance of keeping appointments and informing you of any unusual developments.

At some point early in caregiving, the two most serious emergencies—hemorrhage and fetal distress—require detailed discussion. Explain possible causes of hemorrhage and basic procedures for handling it. Also discuss your methods for dealing with a depressed baby, including tools and

techniques used for resuscitation. Most of the time, the midwife goes out of her way to inform parents of any unusual developments during labor, taking pains to thoroughly explain both standard and alternative approaches. In emergency situations you may not have time for this, so start teaching parents what they need to know right away.

MEDICAL HISTORY

Medical history can either be taken by interview, or provided by the expectant mother via take-home form (see Appendix C). It should include a review of all conditions and diseases that might impact this pregnancy. Diabetes, thyroid disease (hyperthyroidism), chronic lung disease, severe asthma, epilepsy, clotting abnormalities, congenital heart disease (grades 2 to 4), and kidney disease are definite contraindications for home birth. Conditions arising in pregnancy that rule out home birth are severe anemia, acute viral infection (e.g. rubella, cytomegalovirus, chicken pox), or initial herpes outbreak in the first trimester. Preexisting conditions of unresolved sexually transmitted disease, malnutrition, drug addiction, moderate-to-frequent alcohol use, and smoking (more than ten cigarettes daily) are also contraindications. Have handy a comprehensive obstetrical text to evaluate any irregularities in the medical history, and seek the consultation of peers or medical backup when in doubt.

Obstetrical history is of foremost importance. Note any history of transport and/or previous obstetrical emergencies such as postpartum hemorrhage, shoulder dystocia, or fetal hypoxia. Investigate thoroughly, and consider implications for the current pregnancy. A history of previous childbirth losses requires attention to the mother's emotional recovery. Perceived losses due to disappointing or less-than-ideal birth outcomes should also be discussed. Is there anything that the mother experienced with previous birthings that she wants to avoid this time? Or is there something she had hoped for previously that she would like to experience in this pregnancy? Don't forget the issue of child spacing; if she has had a child within the last two years, explore any impact of close-set childbearing on her physical or psychological health.

History of abortion should be thoroughly discussed. Did she have a problem with excessive or prolonged bleeding afterwards? Under what circumstances was the abortion performed? What kind of emotional side effects were experienced? Many women feel great loss with abortion ("It's like tearing your heart out," one woman said) and need to talk it over, either with you or with a specialist. The same is true of women with a history of repeated miscarriage (see section in Chapter Three), who may benefit from specialized treatment by an obstetrician. If the mother has had a saline or prostaglandin induced abortion, she experienced a version of labor and may have some very negative emotions associated with the sensation of uterine contractions. Do your best to forestall difficulties in labor by discussing this well in advance.

What about previous cesarean birth? Since research on **vaginal birth after cesarean (VBAC)** has shown no significant dangers to either mother or baby, many midwives assist VBAC at home, provided that the mother is in good health and the incision is bikini-line/horizontal (the classical/vertical incision may be inclined to rupture). Some midwives have their clients sign special consent forms for home birth, as definitive research on the safety of VBAC is relatively recent.

Psychological issues for mothers desiring VBAC are most significant. Frequently, women who have delivered by cesarean have been told surgery was required because their bones were too small, their hormone levels were off, or they somehow failed to progress. Comments like these leave devastating scars, and before vaginal birth is attempted, some healing must take place. Veterans of cesarean birth often need deep work, such as hypnotherapy, trance work, or other mind-body therapy, to reunite aspects of themselves torn asunder. And they need the support of other veterans, available through organizations such as the International Cesarean Awareness Network (ICAN—see Appendix B).

Assisting a woman with VBAC is a great privilege. The wise midwife encourages her to choose active, upright positions in labor. A standing delivery posture is both physiologically and psycho-logically efficacious; it is diametrically opposed to the passivity and helplessness women typically feel when having a cesarean (more on this in Chapter Four).

Gynecological history also has great significance in pregnancy. Check for history of **fibroids**, the prime symptom of which is painless bleeding with intercourse. Fibroids are benign uterine masses which vary in size, but tend to grow considerably during pregnancy. Depending on whether they are external or internal, pregnancy may be affected by reduced intrauterine space or disrupted placental implantation, and the immediate postpartum may be complicated by hemorrhage. A sonogram is definitely advisable to determine the exact size and location of fibroids.

Whenever there is history of gynecological surgery, consult with a backup physician. If the mother has had **cervical procedures** such as cauterization, cryosurgery, or cone biopsy, considerable scarring may have occurred, which could retard dilation. Scar tissue or adhesions may be softened by the use of evening primrose oil massaged gently onto the cervix toward the end of pregnancy. LEEP, a new procedure similar to cone biopsy, has been correlated to incompetent cervix and/or premature labor. Some midwives feel that any woman with a history of this procedure should be checked for cervical changes throughout pregnancy, or at least should be educated regarding signs of premature labor.

Contraceptive history is also important. If a woman used an IUD prior to conception, she may be anemic due to excessive menstruation and should have her hemoglobin levels checked as soon as possible. The IUD may also cause scarring of the uterine lining, which predisposes women to irregular implantation/ectopic pregnancy, or possible difficulty with placental separation. Pelvic inflammatory disease, or PID, has the same effect. Scar tissue may also form at the cervical os (see suggestions above re: evening primrose oil).

Family history is most important to determine the prevalence of hypertension, diabetes, cancer, or other genetically transmitted diseases that might impact pregnancy and/or require additional screening from a specialist.

Spend plenty of time reviewing any symptoms experienced with this pregnancy. Any incidence of bleeding or spotting is significant, and should be closely tracked by both mother and midwife. If bleeding becomes chronic or is combined with pain, consult immediately with backup to rule out ectopic pregnancy, missed abortion, molar pregnancy, or, if late in pregnancy, placental problems (see Chapter Three). A history of generalized edema experienced before conception or prior to twenty-four weeks should be medically evaluated; if occurring later in pregnancy, you must rule out preeclampsia (see Chapter Three). In either case, immediately ask the mother to eliminate heavily processed foods, and suggest she add plenty of high-quality protein, fresh vegetables, salt to taste, and ample fluids to her diet. Occasional headaches may be caused by hormones and circulatory changes, but a persistent headache, particularly if in combination with signs of preeclampsia, indicates a medical crisis and the need for immediate referral. Visual problems, or upper abdominal (epigastric) pain—especially on the right side—are also warning signs of preeclampsia (see Chapter Three).

Any history of flulike symptoms, such as swollen glands, extreme fatigue, or deep body aches, should be noted, although the most devastating viral infections of pregnancy are frequently asymptomatic. **Cytomegalovirus** is a fairly common infection—60 percent of the general population have antibodies—and is most damaging in the first trimester. **Toxoplasmosis** is known to cause severe neurological damage to the fetus, but only if contracted after ten weeks' gestation. Although there are no particular preventative measures for cytomegalovirus, a mother can minimize her chances of contracting toxoplasmosis by avoiding uncooked meat and any contact with cat feces (advise her to let someone else change the litter box). Even viral infections like chicken pox (varicella) can be extremely dangerous in pregnancy, so encourage all expectant mothers to avoid possible exposure.

Any report of painful vaginal sores combined with flulike malaise in early pregnancy may indicate an initial outbreak of **herpes**, particularly if the mother has no previous history. This can have serious consequences for the baby, and requires immediate consultation/referral to backup.

Barring an initial outbreak in the first trimester, protocol for managing preexisting herpes is everchanging, and has yet to catch up with the research. A Stanford study performed a decade ago on women with a history of herpes showed that the vast majority of those experiencing a reoccurrence while pregnant developed and passed on antibodies to their unborn fetuses. It has been speculated that these antibodies might serve to protect the fetus in the event of an outbreak near the onset of labor, when exposure to the virus might otherwise lead to central nervous system damage or death. Perhaps this is why transmission rates from mothers suffering a reoccurrence during labor are as low as 3 percent. Nevertheless, current medical management for women with history of herpes remains conservative—if active lesions are found as labor begins, a cesarean is performed. The standard of care during pregnancy is to culture the cervix with any outbreak, and if cervical shedding is noted, do a slide test (or at least a visual inspection) at the onset of labor to rule out cervical contamination. If the outbreak is vaginal only, and the lesion or lesions are crusted over and not in the immediate path of the baby, some midwives do permit vaginal birth.

Any history of vomiting with the current pregnancy should be carefully explored to rule out **hyperemesis gravidarium**. The expectant mother with this condition has more than occasional vomiting correlated to nausea in early pregnancy. Her vomiting is chronic and self-perpetuating; this so disrupts her electrolyte balance that she cannot retain either food or liquid and must be restabilized with intravenous replacement therapy before she can eat or drink again. It bears mentioning that hyperemesis gravidarium is one of the only conditions for which conventional medicine acknowledges emotional underpinnings, and some midwives do note a correlation between hyperemesis and psychological conflicts regarding pregnancy. Another theory is that elevated estrogen levels may sometimes cause liver irritation sufficient to engender the condition. With emotional factors outstanding, suggest counseling. Otherwise, have the mother immediately try dosing with ginger root, either freshly grated in tea or ground in capsules, taken three times daily, as you continue to monitor her condition.

Fatigue is certainly common in early pregnancy (due primarily to high levels of estrogen/progesterone), but fatigue combined with dizziness or nausea beyond the first trimester may indicate anemia (more on this condition in Chapter Three).

Any report of urinary tract problems must be addressed immediately. During pregnancy, characteristic signs of urinary tract infection (stinging, urgency, pain after urination) may be nearly absent, due to progesterone's softening effect upon the urethra. This can lead to kidney infection, or **pyelonephritis**, which in turn can lead to premature labor. Any woman with a history of bladder infection must be alerted to these facts, and should be told to call for screening with even the most subtle of symptoms.

Pay close attention, too, to any report of vaginal discharge or sign of infection. Depending on her symptoms, arrange for her to be screened for sexually transmitted diseases (STDs) that could negatively impact pregnancy (see Lab Work, this chapter).

It is also crucial to note the use of any prescription or over-the-counter medications (OTCs) with this pregnancy. Thirty percent of mental retardation is of unknown etiology. The fetus has an underdeveloped blood-brain barrier, which ordinarily protects the brain from harmful substances. Thus pregnant women should avoid OTCs with the same vigilance they do alcohol or recreational drugs.

The same is true of many household chemicals, substances used in the workplace, and environmentally-based chemicals found in drinking water or food. The midwife can research teratogenic side effects of medications in a current copy of *Physician's Desk Reference*, or may consult *Holistic Midwifery* (Frye) or *Will It Hurt the Baby?* (Abrams) to investigate risks of certain environmental or work-related chemical exposures. Regional phone numbers for teratogen information are also available toll free from the March of Dimes Birth Defects Foundation at (888) 663-4637.

A bonus in using the take-home medical history form is the final series of essay questions, which prompt parents to make definitive statements regarding their hopes, fears, and expectations. How they respond to the question of possible damage or death to mother or baby speaks to their level of emotional maturity, as well as their readiness to accept responsibility in the event of an unexpected outcome. Their responses regarding hospital transport are also important to review carefully, as anything less than full willingness to consider the midwife's directives may preclude establishing a healthy working relationship. Likewise, their responses regarding the midwife's role may indicate either compatibility or incompatibility with her style of practice.

Occasionally you'll encounter a woman unwilling to fill out take-home forms. She may profess enthusiasm for home birth (and act as if that's all she needs), yet in nearly every case, this stance bears out an inability to accept responsibility. If any part of the history is incomplete, send it home to be finished up before accepting her into your practice.

HIGH RISK FACTORS IN PREGNANCY

Medical/Health Factors

1. **Diabetes:** pre-existing diabetes is a definite contraindication to home birth.
   Dangers: fetal demise after 36 weeks, five times the normal incidence of fetal abnormalities, increased polyhydramnious, 30 to 50 percent higher incidence of preeclampsia, increased incidence of prematurity and newborn respiratory difficulties.

2. **Thyroid disease:** particularly hyperthroidism. Slight enlargement of the thyroid gland is normal in pregnancy, but persistent tachycardia or elevated levels of circulating thyroid hormone are symptoms of disease.
   Dangers: thyroid medication has potential for causing severe fetal complications. Hyperthyroidism can cause miscarriage, premature labor, and fetal anomalies. Untreated hypothyroidism can lead to cretinism in the newborn.

3. **Active tuberculosis:** refer to physician backup. If under treatment, prognosis for mother and baby is good, although the baby must be immediately separated from the mother if she is infectious.
   Dangers: slightly higher risk of miscarriage or premature labor.

4. **Chronic lung disease:** as diagnosed by medical history.
   Dangers: mother at risk for pulmonary complications, baby for fetal acidosis and hypoxia.

5. **Severe asthma:** as prediagnosed.
   Dangers: respiratory infections and stress may intensify attacks. Cardio-pulmonary function could be reduced, affecting fetal growth and well-being. Certain medications used to treat asthma are contraindicated for pregnancy.

6. **Epilepsy:** there is controversy over whether or not this condition is exacerbated by pregnancy.
   Dangers: anticonvulsant drugs may cause folic acid deficiency, which when treated with folic acid may cause seizures. The infant may develop deficiency of coagulation factors.

7. **Clotting abnormalities:** afibrinogenemia, hypofibrinogenemia, excessive fibrinalytic activity, or a combination of these.
   Dangers: can lead to maternal blood loss, shock, or death.

8. **Rh- with antibodies:** refer to physician backup.
   Dangers: hemolytic anemia, fetal or neonatal death (although intrauterine transfusion can avert this).

9. **Severe anemia:** hereditary anemias such as Thalassemia B or sickle-cell, as well as nutritional anemias (iron, B-12, and folic acid deficiencies) unresolved at term.
   Dangers: maternal infection, prolonged labor, hemorrhage, intrauterine growth retardation, fetal hypoxia during labor.

10. **Acute viral infection:** rubella, mumps, cytomegalovirus, herpes, coxsackie virus, pneumonia, hepatitis B or C, smallpox, severe influenza, polio.
    Dangers: possible birth defects, fetal or maternal death.

11. **Congenital heart disease:** refer to physician backup.
    Dangers: increased blood volume and weight put strain on impaired heart. Condition requires clinical, electrocardiographic, and radiologic surveillance.

12. **Renal disease:** impaired kidney function necessitates close medical surveillance in pregnancy. Signs of renal disease include protein in the urine, hypertension, edema, and elevated blood urea, all before the twentieth week.
    Dangers: acute renal failure.

13. **Extreme obesity:** pre-existing, with history of medical problems.
    Dangers: nearly two-thirds of extremely obese women have obstetrical complications, including diabetes, hypertension, pyelonephritis, uterine dysfunction, and hemorrhage.

HIGH RISK FACTORS IN PREGNANCY

Lifestyle and Personal Factors

1. **Tobacco use:** over ten cigarettes daily.
   Dangers: associated with intrauterine growth retardation, miscarriage, congenital heart disease, fetal hypoxia in labor.

2. **Malnutrition:** extreme dietary deficiencies (may be correlated to substance abuse, debilitating illness, eating disorders).
   Dangers: intrauterine growth retardation, preeclampsia, maternal or fetal infection, prematurity, stillbirth, dysfunctional labor, hemorrhage.

3. **Drug addiction:** chronic substance abuse.
   Dangers: intrauterine growth retardation, fetal hypoxia, respiratory distress syndrome (RDS), maternal malnutrition, infection, preeclampsia, dysfunctional labor, hemorrhage. Newborns whose mothers are addicted to cocaine, crack, crank, heroin, or barbituates will go through withdrawal within the first three days of delivery.

4. **Moderate-to-heavy alcohol use:** periodic bingeing, or more than two drinks per day of alcohol, may cause damage or defects.
   Dangers: fetal alcohol syndrome—fetus has 50 percent chance of mental retardation, 30 percent chance of anomaly, impaired eyesight, behavioral problems, stillbirth.

5. **Heavy caffeine use:** in excess of ten cups per day of moderately strong coffee, black tea, cola, or other caffeine-containing beverages.
   Dangers: maternal reproductive problems, fetal malformations, and heart defects.

PHYSICAL EXAMINATION

Every woman should have a complete physical exam early in pregnancy, unless she has had one within the last year. This is to make sure there isn't anything on a physical level of which the woman is unaware that might negatively impact her pregnancy or her baby's health. I will not attempt to teach this here, because competency requires considerable hands-on training. Complete physical examination can be performed by a backup physician or other health provider, whereas routine assessments and pelvic examination as described below are essentials of midwifery practice. Learn more about physical examination from a comprehensive midwifery text, e.g., Holistic Midwifery: Vol. I, *by Anne Frye, or* Nurse-Midwifery, *by Helen Varney. The most definitive reference remains Barbara Bates'* Guide to Physical Assessment.

The first checkup provides an opportunity to ascertain the expectant mother's general state of health. Beyond that, a core purpose of this visit is to establish some degree of physical intimacy and trust. Keep this in heart and hands as you work with her. And record your findings as you go (see Prenatal Care Record, Appendix D).

Begin by **establishing her estimated date of delivery** (EDD). Take the first day of her last menstrual period (LMP), count back three months from this date, and add one week (this is known as Naegele's rule). Also record her previous menstrual period (PMP), note the interval between that and the LMP, and compare with her average cycle length. This way, you make certain that the LMP was a true period and not just implantation spotting. The baby's gestational age (GA) is simply the number of weeks pregnancy has progressed since the LMP.

Before doing any physical assessments on the expectant mother, always ask her permission and obtain her consent. This may seem a formality to you after a while, but it is crucial in upholding her role as director of her care, with yours as assistant.

Proceed by **checking her weight**, noting her pre-pregnant norm and total gain thus far. Assuming her starting weight was normal for her height and frame, an average gain is about a pound per week. Some women are very sensitive about changing body image, and need to be reassured that an ample weight gain is both desirable and essential for the baby's health and their own endurance, particularly during labor and the immediate postpartum. It is noteworthy that most European midwives do not routinely check their prenatal clients' weight, relying instead on maternal hemoglobin levels, general vitality, and the baby's rate of growth as better determinants of a healthy pregnancy. Considering the degree to which women in the U.S. tend to be anxious about their weight, easing up on this routine evaluation might benefit both mother and baby.

Then **check the mother's urine** with a testing strip, looking for protein or glucose. If using a broad-spectrum strip, check for the presence of blood, ketones, and nitrates. Many midwives encourage clients to test their own urine, and have cups and testing strips available in the rest room. Findings of blood or protein require a second, clean catch sample, to rule out contamination from vaginal discharge. Anything over a trace of protein may indicate preeclampsia, blood is suggestive of UTI, and ketones signal inadequate food intake and/or dehydration (more details in Chapter Three). Always explain any unusual findings to the expectant mother immediately.

Next **check her blood pressure**, which may be somewhat elevated due to tension and excitement. There are two assessments made when taking blood pressure: the systolic reading (high number), which indicates the pressure in the arteries when the heart is actively pumping, and the diastolic reading (low number), which indicates pressure when the heart is at rest. Normal blood pressure levels during pregnancy range from 90/50 to 140/90, although readings above 130/80 are cause for concern.

In essence, diastolic pressure assesses baseline intravascular tension, whereas systolic pressure indicates cardiovascular tolerance for exertion. Medical texts claim that only the systolic reading is influenced by emotional state, but I've found overall high readings to be fairly common at the initial visit, most likely from general nervousness. If so, I simply reassure the mother and take her blood pressure again before she leaves. If her reading remains high, I schedule a recheck in several days. Women with repeated pressure readings above 130/80 in early pregnancy may have undiagnosed essential hypertension (see Chapter Three).

It pays to treat any rise in blood pressure seriously, and to begin stress-reduction or other therapies in earnest should blood pressure exceed 130/80. If additional symptoms of generalized edema or proteinuria develop, preeclampsia should be suspected and the expectant mother immediately referred to physician backup.

Along with the blood pressure, **check pulse and temperature** to establish the mother's baselines. Since heightened reflexes can be a signal of preeclampsia, it's wise to **establish baseline reflexes** as soon as possible. Use a reflex hammer, and note degree of reflex irritability.

You should also **perform a breast exam**. Your primary goal is to determine the overall structure of breast tissue, and identify any abnormalities. The norm is bilateral symmetry, which nevertheless allows for dramatic variation in breast structure. I have on occasion been alarmed to find something quite unusual in one breast, only to be reassured by discovering the exact same lump or tissue formation in the other. Of the several standard techniques for performing breast exam, I prefer the following:

1. Begin by observing the woman's breasts while she is sitting upright. Look for symmetry, note nipples pointing in an unnatural way, any puckering or pull around the areola, or irregularities in skin texture. Also have her place her hands on her hips and push against her hip bones, and observe as above.

2. Have her lie down and continue your exam by pressing your fingertips across the entire surface of the breast in a circular fashion, working inward toward nipple. Be sure to feel directly beneath the nipple, then squeeze it gently to check for any secretion. **Colostrum**, recognizable as a thick yellow discharge, may be evident after the first few months of pregnancy. Occasionally women have greenish or bloody discharge which proves perfectly normal, but should still be evaluated by an expert.

3. Use the same pressing motion over the upper chest (pectoral muscles), checking for any lumps or masses. Generally, you will feel only muscles and ribs in this area.

4. Focus on the upper, outer quadrant of the

breast, as this is the area that contains the most tissue and is therefore the most likely site for abnormal growth. Feel more deeply into this area by grasping underlying tissue and rolling it to assess structure. Small/moderate sized breasts will have a bar of tissue extending from armpit to nipple; larger breasts will have an extension of this tissue downward from the nipple to the bottom edge of the breast. Repeat this lifting/rolling motion on any other area of the breasts that has thick (or unusual) tissue.

5. Finally, feel along the outer edge of the breast and into the armpit, feeling deeply for any lumps (likely to be enlarged lymph nodes).

6. Repeat the entire procedure on the other breast, and compare one breast to the other to establish symmetry.

Explain to the expectant mother what you are doing step-by-step, then have her repeat the exam in your presence (one breast at a time). Many women give up on self-exam either because they feel the technique is too complicated, or because they become alarmed upon finding their breasts to be lumpy/irregular instead of smooth. Reassure her that every woman's breasts are lumpy, so her best bet is to identify all the lumps on one side, then compare to the other to be sure they match. If her breasts are particularly dense or difficult to feel, consider having her lean forward to palpate them. This new technique is thought to allow better access to deep breast tissue much the way mammogram screening does.

Some midwives postpone the **pelvic assessment** until the second visit. As you and the mother have had little contact thus far, this may be the best approach. If she has experienced sexual abuse, she will probably have a strong reaction to internal examination. (Although questions on the medical history form address this issue, you will not yet have this information if using the take-home format.) Every midwife should be fully aware of signs of both sexual and physical abuse, and how to respond appropriately. More information on this subject can be found in Chapter Three.

In any case, always ask the expectant mother's permission before beginning the pelvic assessment. If she has not already put her shirt back on after breast exam, see if she would like to do so, or would like a blanket/sheet to cover up. If her partner is present, don't assume she wants him/her there for this portion of the checkup; be sure to ask what she prefers. Internal exam is an intimate event, and most women have had enough rough, insensitive exams to feel more than a little nervous. Proceed gently. Put on a glove, apply lubricating jelly to your fingers, and ask permission to touch her. Always be guided by her muscular reaction—never, ever force your way. Maintain eye contact if she's open to it, and continually reassure her with your findings.

Once you and she are comfortable, **check her cervix**. Note its condition (consistency, length, patency) and its position (central, posterior, or anterior). Note any growths at or from the os, which may be respectively cysts or polyps. If the cervix feels irregular, insert a speculum and do a visual inspection. This is routine with Pap smear, which some midwives use as the starting point of their initial pelvic assessment (see Lab Work in this chapter for instructions on taking a Pap smear).

If she is less than 17 weeks, you may confirm the EDD by doing a **bimanual exam** to size the uterus. Press up firmly on the cervix while using your other hand to palpate the fundus (top of the uterus). As you bring your hands together, you will get an idea of how large the uterus has grown. At 10 weeks, the fundus barely clears the pubic bone; at 12 weeks it is generally a few centimeters above the pubis; at 16 weeks it is midway between the pubic bone and the umbilicus.

If uterine size does not seem to conform to the EDD, re-evaluate the menstrual history. If the woman has used oral contraceptives and has not had regular menses prior to conception, her dates may be incorrect. Breastfeeding mothers may conceive with the first postpartum ovulation before ever having a period. Other women are uncertain of their dates because they've continued to bleed after conception, perhaps for several months at the time menstruation would ordinarily occur. If the uterus does not seem to be enlarged, do a pregnancy test before proceeding further. Nothing could be more embarrassing than doing prenatal care on a woman who is not pregnant!

Next **check her pelvic dimensions**. Take a look at the illustration below, but don't be overly concerned with pelvic type. This initial pelvimetry (bony assessment) is for diagnosing any gross abnormalities in the bone structure which might present an obstacle to normal delivery.

Before you begin pelvimetry, you must measure your fingers/hand in certain dimensions. Measure first from from the inside of your thumb joint to the tip of your middle finger. Then make a fist, and measure across your fingers (between the knuckles). Note these measurements in centimeters.

There are five basic steps in performing pelvimetry. The first is **assessing the depth of the sacral curve**. Begin by finding the coccyx—with fingers just inside the vagina, turn pad side toward you and press straight down as far as you can reach. When you feel the hardness of bone, *keep pressure on this point* as you rotate your thumb up (so it faces the mother's chin). Keeping fingers firmly on the bone, trace the sacral curve by sweeping upwards towards the sacral promontory (see illustration, page 20). The sacral curve should be deep and rounded, like a half circle. If the sacrum feels flat or heavy, note the possibility of android pelvis and reduced inlet and/or mid-pelvic dimensions. Typically, the sacral curve is so deep that you can only trace it for several inches; rarely will your fingers continue all the way up the curve to reach the sacral promontory.

As you attempt to reach the sacral promontory by bringing your fingers to a horizontal plane, you perform your second assessment, **estimating the size of the pelvic inlet**. Unless your fingers are

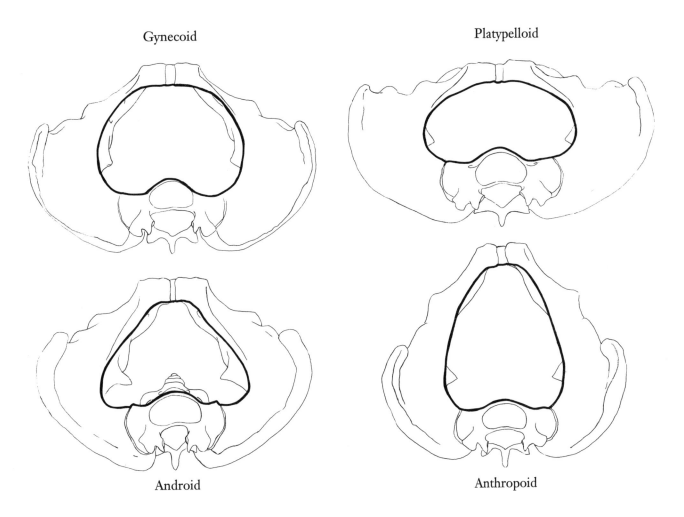

Gynecoid

Platypelloid

Android

Anthropoid

Basic Pelvic Types

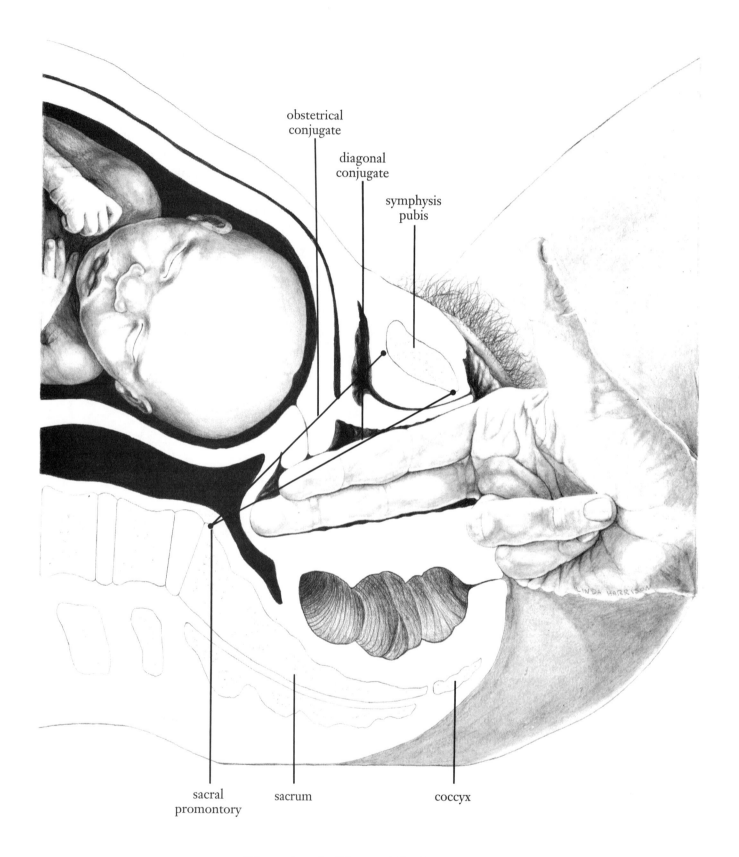

obstetrical
conjugate

diagonal
conjugate

symphysis
pubis

sacral
promontory

sacrum

coccyx

Measuring the Diagonal Conjugate

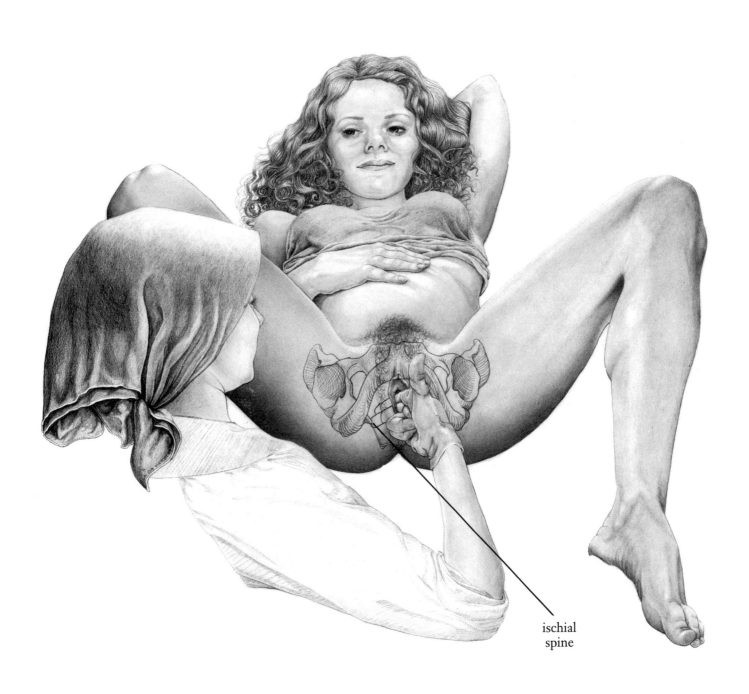

ischial
spine

Finding the Ischial Spines

unusually long or the inlet dimension is foreshortened, you'll feel nothing at all, and can simply note the inlet to be "adequate." If you can reach the promontory, measure the **diagonal conjugate** by making an estimate based on your reach. From this, subtract the 1.5 cm. thickness of the pubic bone to obtain the actual inlet dimension the baby must negotiate, termed the **obstetrical conjugate**. A measurement of 10.5 cms. or greater is considered adequate.

The next step is **assessing the contour of, and distance between, the ischial spines**. First, withdraw your fingers almost to the introitus, then bend them directly sideways—if right handed, to approximately eight o'clock. The ischial spine will initially feel like a bump of ligamentous tissue. A definite indication that you've found the spine is the woman's characteristic flinching response as you touch nerve attachment points in close proximity. At this, disregard the natural inclination to pull your fingers away, and press a bit more deeply to determine whether the prominence is blunt and barely noticeable, or sharply pointed and protruding. If you have difficulty, press your fingers more firmly to the side wall and pull the tips towards you. Note the contour of one spine, then repeat the procedure for the other at the four o'clock position. Complete your assessment by opening your fingers to measure the distance between spines, or **interspinous diameter**, which should be at least 10.5 cms.

Next, as you slowly and gently withdraw your fingers, lift them, pad side up, to **assess the angle, or width of the pubic arch**. You should be able to fit two fingers beneath the arch, and spread them slightly apart.

Once your fingers are out, **assess the outlet dimension or intertuberous diameter** by making a fist and gently pressing it between the ischial tuberosities. Find the tuberosities first by following the pubic arch to its lowest point, somewhat below the introitus. If your fist is of average measurement—around 8.5 cms.—it should fit comfortably, with some play side-to-side.

This completes the pelvic exam. Make detailed notation throughout of your findings; these may have a bearing on your management of labor. And be sure to tell the expectant mother (and her partner, if present) what you're doing and checking for as the exam takes place. Perhaps your assistant can show points on a model pelvis while you're explaining procedures. Women occasionally ask if the shape or size of their hips has any bearing on labor. Explain that there is a difference between the true pelvis, which includes all dimensions from the inlet downward, and the false pelvis, which includes the illiac crests/hip bones, above. This disconcerting terminology nonetheless serves to illustrate that hip size is unrelated to pelvic capacity.

It should be noted that there is far from universal agreement among midwives regarding the best time to perform pelvimetry. Some midwives prefer to wait until the last trimester, when hormonally-induced softening of the four pelvic joints—**the symphysis pubis joint, the sacrococcygeal joint, and the two sacroiliac joints**—may dramatically increase any borderline aspect of the pelvis, particularly the transverse or outlet dimensions. I personally think performing pelvimetry early helps assuage women's nearly universal fear of being "too small" to give birth vaginally. *And because adequate pelvic size is ultimately determined by that of the baby, you can truthfully reassure any woman at this point that there is plenty of room.* Don't worry if pelvic tissues feel tight in early pregnancy, as changes during the third trimester are really quite remarkable.

Beginning midwives often find the **three Ps** context of passage, passenger, and powers helpful for appreciating the relative significance of pelvimetry. The **passage** is defined as the bony pelvis and musculature, the **passenger** is obviously the baby, and the **powers** refer to uterine activity during labor. A woman might have a relatively small passage and medium-sized baby, yet if her powers are strong, she may give birth easily. On the other hand, a woman with generous passage and average-sized baby might have difficulty in labor if her powers are weak due to poor health or lack of support.

In recent years, pelvimetry has been replaced in conventional medical practice by cesarean section, forceps delivery, and vacuum extraction, i.e., "If the baby doesn't birth spontaneously, we'll just cut

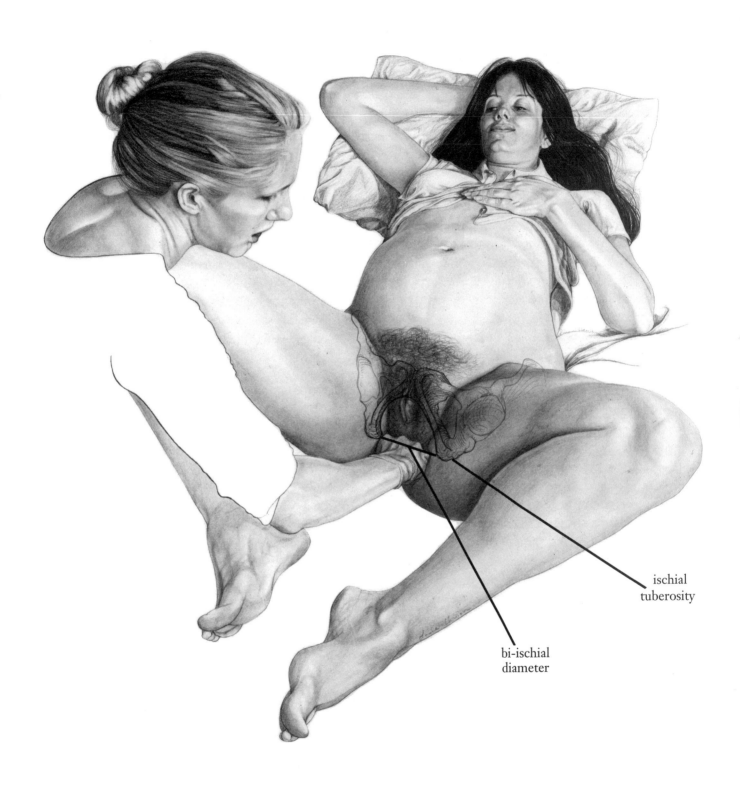

ischial
tuberosity

bi-ischial
diameter

Checking the Outlet Dimension

or pull it out." And due to the relative nature of pelvimetry's significance, some midwives have chosen to discard it altogether. Yet certain traditions in midwifery practice, such as the skill of manually repositioning a malpresenting baby, or safely delivering a breech at home, depend largely on the mastery of pelvimetry. As our practice is based on limiting the use of technology and artfully facilitating vaginal birth, we must uphold our competencies in this regard. Pelvimetry is rapidly becoming a lost art—midwives must seek to preserve it.

If the expectant mother is at least 18 weeks pregnant, **assess the fundal height**. Using a soft tape measure, place one end at the upper edge of the pubic bone, then stretch the tape to the top of the uterus. Record your measurement in centimeters. Make sure to dip in deeply at the very highest point of the fundus (which may be slightly off-center, depending on the baby's lie).

If the mother is at least 24 weeks pregnant, you can **perform uterine/fetal palpation**. This is generally a pleasurable and relaxing part of the visit for everyone involved. Your evaluations of the uterus and baby include determinations of fetal lie, attitude, presentation, and position; estimation of fetal growth; assessment of amniotic fluid volume; and evaluation of fetal responsiveness. Maneuvers used to evaluate the baby are commonly known as Leopold's maneuvers.

Fetal lie will be either longitudinal, oblique, or transverse. Begin by feeling in the fundus to see if any obvious part can be identified—the head feels very hard and very round, the butt is softer and more irregular in contour. If nothing is immediately apparent in the fundus, feel along the sides of the uterus. If the poles of the baby's body (head or butt) are at the sides, the baby is either in transverse or oblique lie. Although common at 24 weeks, the baby finds these dimensions increasingly confining as it grows, and will generally seek the roomier, longitudinal aspect of the uterus by 28 weeks.

If you've found either head or butt in the fundus, feel along the sides of the uterus for the back and small parts, and then above the pubic bone to determine the **presentation**. If the lie is longitudinal, it will be either breech (the butt) or cephalic (the head); if the lie is transverse, the shoulder presents. Of this presentation, the part used to determine the position of the baby is called the **denominator**. For example, with a longitudinal lie, cephalic presentation, the denominator is the occiput bone at the back of the baby's head (see illustration, page 91). In breech presentation, the denominator is the sacrum, and with shoulder presentation, the acromion process.

We determine **fetal position** based on the relationship of the denominator to the mother's pelvis. For example, if the baby is head down, with its back and occiput to the mother's right side, we call this position right occiput transverse (ROT). If the baby is head down, with back/occiput to the mother's left but turned slightly toward her spine, we call this left occiput posterior (LOP). If the baby is breech, with sacrum to the mother's left but turned slightly towards her pubic bone, we call this position left sacrum anterior (LSA). See illustration, page 36 for more examples.

Less commonly used is the term **presenting part**, which refers to the part of the presentation lying directly above the cervix. This is determined not by palpation, but by internal exam.

Attitude is a more subtle assessment of the degree of fetal head flexion. A well-flexed cephalic presentation will manifest a continuous curve of back and head from fundus to pubic bone. This is obviously more difficult to determine if the baby is posterior. Deflexion of the head can be corrected most effectively around 35 weeks gestation (see diagram, page 46).

Palpation is obviously an art learned by experience. Among women of the Yucatan peninsula, the word for prenatal visit is the same as that for massage. I've noticed that midwives spend much more time on palpation than physicians do; this is yet another of our endangered arts for which technology (sonography) has become a substitute. In combination with continuity of care, careful palpation renders evaluations of adequate fetal growth/responsiveness and normal amniotic fluid volume easy to track week-to-week. These assessments are especially critical if factors predispose to fetal growth retardation, if the uterus is large for dates, or if pregnancy is prolonged (see Chapter Three).

If the expectant mother's partner is present, encourage him/her to feel the baby too, and teach the mother how to palpate herself.

Next, **take fetal heart tones** (FHT). The fetal heart should be audible by 20 weeks with standard fetascope; if you cannot hear it within the following week, use a doppler or refer for a sonogram. Normal FHT range is 120 to 160 beats per minute, but younger babies are considered normal up to 170 BPM. The heart rate is generally higher at the beginning of pregnancy, slowing ten to fifteen points as the baby grows. In addition to the BPM rate, **check for variability** by listening for several fifteen second increments, determining BPM for each and noting the overall range, e.g. 132 to 148 BPM. Variability may not be noted until 28 weeks. It occurs in response to manual stimulation, uterine contractions, or the baby's own movements, and is considered a sign of neurological health, as it portends an ability to handle the stress of labor. Don't forget to invite the expectant mother's partner, friends, or other children to listen to the baby—it's a nice way to end the first visit.

*   *   *

To consolidate our discussion of lost midwifery arts, it is noteworthy that since the first edition of *Heart & Hands* was published just eighteen years ago, skills of pelvic assessment, fetal and uterine palpation, fetal heart auscultation, and fundal height assessment have been almost entirely replaced by ultrasound scanning. Yet research has demonstrated repeatedly that neither maternal nor fetal outcomes are improved by this technology. Moreover, routine ultrasound scanning has recently been shown to pose significant risks of fetal growth retardation (see *Pursuing the Birth Machine*, Marsden Wagner, M.D.). Benefits of scanning occasionally outweigh the risks, but generally, ultrasound technology is grossly overused for reasons that have nothing to do with good care, e.g. to have hard-copy records in the event of lawsuit, or to generate office revenues. New studies have demonstrated what midwives have suspected all along—that fundal height assessment and fetal heart auscultation as described in this chapter are just as efficacious in determining fetal well-being

as the use of ultrasound. Once aga[i] must take the lead in reanimating an[d] these traditional skills and competencies.

NUTRITION AND EXERCISE

Base your **nutritional advice** on the expectant mother's three-day record of her food and fluid intake, including all supplements. Don't forget to ask for this when you're scheduling the initial visit, so she can bring it with her. Nutrition is the trunk of the tree of health as regards pregnancy and postpartum—there is hardly a perinatal complication that cannot be forestalled or mediated to some degree by good nutrition.

There are innumerable theories concerning optimal nutrition, but it is not my purpose here to survey them. My own method of determining whether the expectant mother's diet is adequate does not involve adding up micrograms of this mineral or that, but I do have a good working knowledge of the nutritional content of most foods and herbs and so can appraise a diet at a glance. It is helpful to have on hand a comprehensive reference such as the U.S. Government's Agricultural Handbook, *Composition of Foods*. This will aid you in settling disputes about how much zinc is in mushrooms, calcium in tofu, etc.

Above and beyond a good quality, well-balanced diet, I recommend the following daily supplements to compensate for devitalized soil, stress, air pollution, etc.: 1) vitamin E—400 units; 2) vitamin C—500 mg.; 3) folic acid—800 mcg; and 4) iron—75 mg. of a chelated, organic brand. Whenever a woman has symptoms that indicate possible deficiencies, begin by helping her improve the quality of her diet. Devitalized soil aside, food comes first. Assimilation of supplements is unpredictable, and as normal doses for the mother are very high indeed for the fetus, many must be taken with caution. The only safe quantities of vitamins A and D are the minimum daily requirements. Supplemental iron is routinely labeled with toxicity warnings, so doses should remain below 100 mg. daily. Although non-toxic, high quantities of vitamin C taken near the time of delivery can cause newborn withdrawal symptoms, including scurvy.

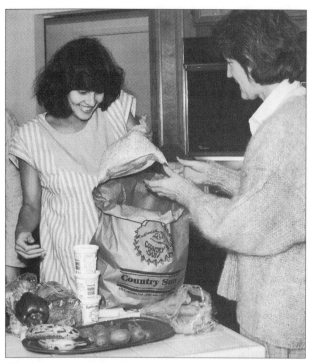

The midwife supports her client in purchasing and preparing the best quality foods possible.

Similarly, a neonatologist in my childbirth class suggested that neonatal hypocalcemia might result if a mother ingested large amounts of calcium near term to raise her pain threshold in labor. Supplements should be supplemental!

Other key minimums for the prenatal diet are 80 grams of protein, and at least two quarts of fluid daily. Calcium is important, but the best sources are not necessarily dairy products; sesame butter/tahini is excellent, as is orange juice "plus calcium" (the acidity of citrus facilitates absorption). Iron can be readily obtained from organ meats, but pumpkin seeds, dried fruits, and almonds are also good sources. Adequate intake of calories is also crucial for accelerated metabolic functions; pregnant women need at least 3,000 calories daily, and nursing mothers, 4,000 per day.

Expectant mothers who eat organically-grown foods, raw or lightly steamed vegetables, freshly squeezed juices, and high-quality protein will feel and look better than those who eat commercially-grown produce or "fast food." One with a conventional "good" diet may nevertheless appear tired and dragged-out, while another, choosing from top-grade food sources without thought or plan, looks absolutely radiant. Quality counts, but

beyond that, how food is selected and when it is eaten also makes a difference. Every expectant mother has a natural, inner voice of hunger telling her what to eat, how much, and when. This may lead a woman to devour six oranges at one sitting, or to crave a particular protein source to the exclusion of all others. Women who have had several children often recall that certain foods seemed central to their well-being with each of their pregnancies, and not necessarily the same ones every time. But keep in mind that this natural voice of hunger only operates in women free of addictions to sugar, caffeine, alcohol, or marijuana.

When confronted with a diet lacking essential nutrients, remember the cardinal rule of nutritional counseling: always begin with praise for whatever is outstanding. In terms of making improvements, base your suggestions on the mother's likes and dislikes. For example, if breakfasts are missing on her report, survey which breakfast foods she enjoys, then point out those with the most nutritional value.

Consider a diet greatly lacking in variety a warning of inadequate resources or poverty. Any woman who has been pregnant will tell you she would never limit herself to just a handful of foods, unless she was sick or had no choice. Although nausea may be a factor from 6 to 12 weeks, nutritional analysis generally occurs after this time. If obtaining food is a problem, refer the mother to public assistance. Sometimes a letter from the midwife verifying pregnancy and stating that the mother is at risk due to inadequate weight gain/food intake is necessary to help her qualify. Every midwife should be knowledgeable regarding social services available in her community. Once funding is obtained, have the expectant mother dictate a list of everything she likes to eat, then help her formulate meals based on her best choices.

An important tip when dealing with ethnic dietary preferences: do not attempt to replace core ethnic foods with other, albeit healthier, selections. For example, it would be foolish to suggest that an Asian woman substitute brown rice for white rice—if you are concerned about her need for whole grains/B vitamins, find an altogether different source. The same goes for sweets or treats; asking a woman fond of chocolate to substitute carob is a waste of time. In short, work around the less than perfect, emotionally-based aspects of the expectant mother's diet. If your expectations are unrealistic she will become evasive, and should some complication or concern necessitate another diet report later in pregnancy, it's unlikely her report will be completely truthful.

Exercise helps pregnant women keep in touch with their ever-changing physical and emotional needs, as well as promoting circulation, elimination, and overall good health. But every expectant mother must be cautioned to immediately desist any activity that causes her pain or discomfort. Regardless of pre-pregnant fitness, her body is different now. Any woman in the habit of exercising compulsively is particularly at risk for ignoring her body's subtle calls of distress. The goal of prenatal exercise is to achieve a sense of balance and harmony, not to reach new heights of performance. Vigorous activity must be blended with adequate rest and rejuvenation.

A mother under stress, with baby concurrently experiencing a growth spurt, may find her stamina reduced and her appetite increased—symptoms that may alarm her unless she tunes in to her situation and trusts her body. Rather than increasing her activity, this woman needs deep relaxation, extra food for energy, vitamins for stress reduction, time to reflect on both her own and the baby's needs, and plenty of sleep.

On the other hand, the woman accustomed to high levels of physical activity who is also able to listen to her body should continue her routine as long as she is comfortable, and then taper off gradually. Any sudden, abrupt drop in activity can cause constipation, circulatory problems, or nervous irritability for the active/athletic woman.

Yoga is my preference for prenatal exercise as it integrates mind and body, movement and rest. At the end of a long day, yoga can dissolve fatigue, and boost energy levels in the evening hours. Yoga helps the body recuperate by stimulating master glands, which in turn keep hormone levels in balance. This creates harmony throughout the entire

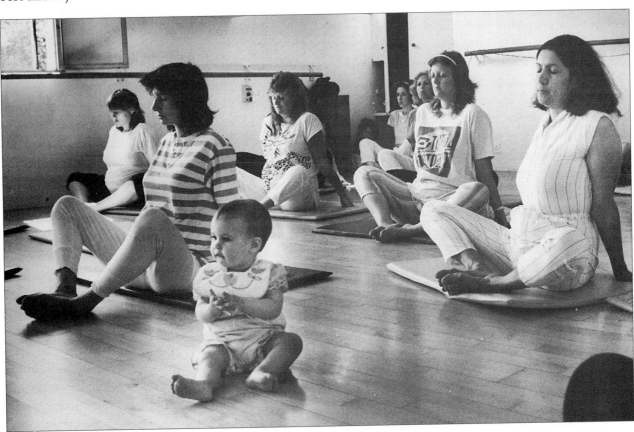

Exercising with others is fun, and helps you relax with your pregnant body.

system. Many women also feel that it fosters their intuition and creativity.

Mothers who work full-time during pregnancy need special consideration. It's hard for them to be spontaneous, to eat when and what they want, rest when they should, and be active when they feel like it. Bending the sharp edges of routine on the job can help, but cutting back work hours is better. Pregnancy is a precious time of preparation for birth and motherhood, requiring a somewhat flexible schedule.

Encourage every expectant mother to join a prenatal exercise or support group. These venues are great for helping women discover universal hopes, fears and anxieties in pregnancy, at the same time diminishing anxiety and self-consciousness about changing body image.

SCREENING OUT

This may seem like harsh terminology, but it's part of a process that involves parents' as much as midwives' decisions. On what basis do you decide that home birth is not appropriate for a woman or couple?

Beyond preexisting medical problems revealed by initial phone screening, certain physical contraindications such as contracted/abnormal pelvis, extreme obesity, or hypertension may have become evident at the initial visit. Psychological contraindications are more complex. An irresponsible attitude, hostility in response to basic suggestions, or an otherwise rigid belief system should give the midwife pause. Poor diet, particularly if the expectant mother is averse to changing it, may indicate deep-seated indifference. Excessive use of drugs, alcohol, or cigarettes has similar implications. If you sense at the end of the first visit that you won't be comfortable working with the woman and/or her partner, suggest they consider other alternatives. This is also appropriate if you feel that she/they were not quite comfortable with you. But if you like the expectant mother and she responds positively to your approach, make room for change. I've worked with women who began pregnancy smoking, drinking, or using recreational drugs, and in a matter of weeks had cleaned themselves up quite nicely. Women who are open to

new information and who have the desire to make the health and welfare of the baby a priority deserve an opportunity to try. Make recommendations, provide handouts/suggested reading, and see what happens at the next visit.

As a beginner, the hardest thing to grasp regarding screening is the relative significance of risk factors. To this end, Oregon and Michigan state midwifery associations have developed point systems, assigning five points to absolute contraindications such as bleeding disorders, heart disease, etc., and four or less points to less serious concerns like borderline anemia, lack of exercise, marginally supportive partner, or less than optimal nutrition. In both states, midwives agree to consult with their peers regarding any situation where women have either a single risk factor of five, or *a combination of factors* totaling five points or more. Although the two states agree regarding conditions meriting five points, they vary considerably on how other points are assigned. Ultimately, risk-screening is somewhat subjective, and as such, requires a sophisticated ability to make judgement calls best learned from training with an experienced midwife.

LAB WORK

If the expectant mother has had any prenatal care from a doctor or clinic, she has probably had initial lab work performed. Have her make a written request for release of her records, mailed directly to you.

The **complete blood count** (CBC) or prenatal panel helps you determine whether the mother is anemic. Both her **hemoglobin** (HGB) and **hematocrit** (HCT) are critical indicators. HGB is the amount of hemoglobin per red blood cell, and HCT is the percentage of red blood cells per total blood volume. HGB should be 11 or above, and HCT should be 33 or more. Because red blood cells are the oxygen carriers, low HGB/HCT readings mean that both baby and mother will suffer some degree of oxygen deprivation. The mother will be easily fatigued and more prone to infection, while her baby may suffer from intrauterine growth retardation. If the mother is anemic at the onset of labor, there is risk of fetal distress, incoordinate or prolonged labor, postpartum hemorrhage (from tired uterus), and infection. Even a moderate blood loss may be serious for an anemic woman because her blood is poorly oxygenated to begin with, thus she is predisposed to shock. (See Anemia, Chapter Three, for more information.)

As you scan the CBC, check to see that the **platelet count** is within normal range. If low, clotting abnormalities may result.

Lab work also includes **gonorrhea culture (GC)** and **syphilis screening** (VDRL/RPR). A positive GC indicates gonorrhea at the cervix or in the vagina, which can cause a potentially blinding eye infection to the baby unless eyedrops are administered within the first two hours postpartum. Gonorrhea is usually asymptomatic, so every woman should be screened. Syphilis can cause miscarriage, malformations, prematurity, fetal death, or neonatal infection. Therefore, the desired result on the VDRL/RPR is NR, or non-reactive.

Both the GC and **Pap smear** are usually done in conjunction with the initial pelvic exam. The Pap smear tests for irregular cells at the cervix; this is crucial because hormonal changes in pregnancy may precipitate abnormal cell growth. It is not difficult to perform a Pap smear, and as it should be repeated again at six weeks postpartum, it's wise to learn this simple procedure. The lab will supply microscope slides, cardboard slide holders and fixative; you will need long-handled sterile cotton swabs, wooden spatulas or cytology brushes, a flashlight, and a speculum (some labs supply all but the latter two). You may prefer to use disposable plastic speculums so you won't have to bother with resterilizing. The mother may wish to take her speculum home to check her cervix some time in the future.

If linked to initial pelvic assessment, begin with the Pap and GC to prevent lubricating gel from contaminating test results. (Plastic speculums are pre-lubricated, so you won't need gel until you do the internal exam.) Once the cervix is in view, identify the squamo-columnar junction—the most common site for abnormality—where red endocervical cells lining the cervical canal meet the pinker mucosal cells covering the cervix and vagina. Take a cotton swab or wooden spatula, and

gently rotate at this juncture (sometimes located just inside the cervical os) to obtain your sample. It is not necessary to scrape, use force or draw blood, as cells come away freely in cervical secretion. Gently roll the swab in two straight lines along the slide. (Do not press hard or rub back and forth, as this may destroy the cells.) Immediately spray the slide with fixative, air dry, and mark with client's name and date. The lab will also provide the necessary identification slips, and will usually pick up weekly (or you may ship instead). The average lab charge for a Pap smear is $10 to $20.

While screening the Pap for abnormal cells, the lab may discover other conditions such as monilia/vaginal yeast, herpes virus, or **human papilloma virus/HPV**. HPV can manifest as **condyloma accuminata**, i.e., visible genital warts, or as flat lesions difficult to see. This viral infection has become today's leading sexually transmitted disease. Like herpes, HPV resides in nerve ganglia in the genital area. There is no cure for this virus, only topical treatment for the warts. HPV is dangerous in that it is considered the chief precursor to abnormal cervical cell growth—the missing link in the mystery of cervical cancer. Any woman with HPV is advised to have Pap smears more frequently, about every six months. Venereal warts or lesions are generally painless and may go unnoticed unless fully visible, thus a woman can have HPV at the cervix and not know it.

While you are doing the Pap smear, use a flashlight to look for signs of HPV or condyloma accuminata as you simultaneously check the cervix for unusual discharge or inflammation. If the latter are evident, the mother may have gonorrhea, **chlamydia**, or other vaginal infection. Chlamydia is the second most common sexually transmitted disease in the United States. It is four times more common than gonorrhea, although the two often occur together. Frequently the woman will notice no symptoms, but her partner may have discharge or pain and burning with urination. Perform routine cultures at this time.

Chlamydia poses dangers to both mother and baby. Untreated, it can lead to urinary tract or uterine infection during pregnancy, or to sepsis in the event of prolonged rupture of the membranes

(PROM). The baby has a 70 percent chance of contracting the organism during delivery, which can cause severe conjunctivitis or even pneumonia. The prevalence of chlamydia, combined with its generally asymptomatic presentation, argues for routine use of eye prophylaxis for every newborn.

The usual treatment for the mother is tetracycline, contraindicated during pregnancy because it causes discoloration of fetal tooth enamel. Erythromycin is nearly as effective, and is safe for pregnancy. The woman's partner must also be treated, and they must use condoms/latex barriers for sex until additional screens for both confirm the infection to be fully resolved.

Another possible cause of cervical/vaginal inflammation is **group B streptococcus** or GBS. This common bacterium lurks harmlessly in up to 40 percent of women, but may have serious consequences for the baby. The rate of fetal infection is low—only two babies per 1000. However, 10 percent of these babies die, and up to half suffer long-term damage ranging from seizures to mental retardation. The first symptom may be apnea (cessation of breathing); spinal meningitis is another common manifestation.

Unfortunately, treating strep in pregnancy is almost pointless. Even after a full course of antibiotics in the last trimester, women often have positive cultures again at term. Nevertheless, it's wise to screen for group B streptococcus at 35 to 37 weeks so you know where you stand in the event of prolonged rupture of the membranes, as this condition more readily predisposes the baby to infection (more on this in Chapter Five). A vaccine for strep B has recently been developed by a Harvard physician, and is currently being tested by The National Institutes of Health. A recent FDA safety alert warns that GBS antigen screening has proven to be highly unreliable, and should not be substituted for the usual culture technique.

Yet another infection that may be sexually transmitted is **hepatitis B**. Screen for this by blood test to determine the presence and quantity of surface antigens (HBsAg). Hepatitis B virus is transmitted through blood or blood by-products, saliva, vaginal secretions, or semen. This disease is highly contagious—women who are HBsAg pos-

itive have high risk of transmitting the disease to their newborns who, if female, may become carriers and transmit the disease to their own offspring. Infected newborns are generally asymptomatic, but a small percent become jaundiced at three or four months postpartum. As HB has been isolated in breast milk and has generally reached epidemic proportions, many pediatricians think it wise to immunize all babies as soon as possible after birth.

Although transmission to the fetus occurs rarely in pregnancy, expectant mothers with active infection should be hospitalized, and all family members screened. Active infection from hepatitis B can lead to life-threatening conditions such as cirrhosis of the liver and hepatocellular carcinoma. On the other hand, carriers are often asymptomatic. But their blood work will show the presence of HBsAb, with long-term core antibodies indicating infection contracted at birth. A midwife colleague of mine recently found a client of hers to be a carrier. This woman already had several children, but neither they nor her husband tested positive, and no special care was required in her case.

Hepatitis C accounts for 20 percent to 40 percent of viral hepatitis in the United States. Although method of transmission is similar to that of HB, hepatitis C is unique in that it can be transmitted to the fetus during pregnancy. Newborn vaccination is recommended.

HIV screening is advisable for all women, particularly those who have engaged in high-risk behaviors of unprotected sex, sharing of needles, etc. In California, state law requires informing all women of the availability of, and recommendations for, HIV screening. Testing can and should be done anonymously, either on-site (available in every state and almost every county) or through the mail. The ELISA test is highly sensitive, but has a false positive rate of up to 10 percent. Only if a repeat ELISA proves positive will the more specific Western Blot for HIV Antibodies test be run.

If the expectant mother is found to be seropositive, her baby has a 25 percent to 50 percent chance of contracting the virus. Depending on weeks gestation, she may wish to terminate the pregnancy. In any case, she will need a tremendous amount of support. She must be advised of all HIV-related symptoms, and you may wish to consult with backup regarding the advisability of continuing primary care.

It bears mentioning that research shows that a significant number of HIV-positive newborns spontaneously seroconvert to negative within the first year of life. And research regarding transmission through breast milk is far from conclusive, although it is generally not recommended that HIV-positive mothers breastfeed since some babies unaffected in pregnancy have contracted the virus through breastmilk.

As a health worker, you must define your protocol for assisting anyone who has a highly infectious and life-threatening disease. Immunization is available for hepatitis B, and may soon be available for HIV. In the meantime, even universal precautions (described fully in Chapter Four) offer some, but not absolute protection—there is always a marginal risk of needle-stick or other inadvertent exposure to infectious body fluids. Identify the standard of care within your midwifery community, know your limits, and communicate promptly with your clients should the need arise.

Rubella antibody titre indicates whether or not the mother has immunity to German measles. The test is done by a diluting process that detects the presence of antibodies. For example, a rubella titre of 1:48 means that antibodies can be detected even though the sample has been diluted a number of times. It is proof that the mother has had rubella or has been immunized, even if she can't remember when. An unusually high reading (greater than 1:64) may indicate recent or current infection. Repeat the titre in this case, and consult with backup. If the mother's titre is low (less than 1:10), it means she is susceptible to infection and should be immunized after the current pregnancy and at least three months before the next, to minimize her chances of contracting the disease while pregnant. Were that to occur, her baby would have a 20 percent chance of heart, vision, or hearing defects.

The mother needs to know her blood type too, in case need arises for emergency transfusion. This information is an absolute must for the midwife's records. The four blood types are O, A, AB, and B,

with an accompanying **Rh factor**, either positive (+) or negative (-).

The Rh factor is an antigen present in the red blood cells; 83 percent of women have this factor and are Rh (+), 17 percent don't and are Rh (-). If a woman is Rh (-) and her baby is Rh (+), there is a 2 percent risk of **isoimmunization.** This occurs if fetal blood enters maternal circulation due to intrauterine trauma, premature separation of the placenta, or placenta praevia, causing the mother to produce antibodies against her baby's positive cells and rendering it severely anemic. Isoimmunization is rare with a first baby (as rare as the traumas that can cause it to occur) unless the Rh (-) mother has had abortions or miscarriages without receiving RhoGAM, the anti-antigen which blocks the development of antibodies. Since even a first-time mother may have had an undetected miscarriage at some point, every Rh (-) woman is screened for antibodies early in pregnancy, and again at 24, 28, 32, and 36 weeks. If antibodies are detected, the baby will be tracked closely and may need a transfusion while still in utero.

It is now standard of care to administer RhoGAM prophylactically during pregnancy at 28 to 30 weeks. RhoGAM injection during pregnancy conveys passive immunity; it will not protect subsequent pregnancies. As RhoGAM is commonly formulated with chemicals such as mercury that may be harmful to the fetus, its use prenatally is somewhat controversial. The expectant mother must make her own decision.

Immediately after the birth, you must take a sample of cord blood from the baby and draw blood from the mother to determine whether there is a need for RhoGAM, and if so, appropriate dosage. RhoGAM must be administered within 72 hours to be effective.

Urinalysis is also a part of standard prenatal screening. Besides protein and glucose, a complete urinalysis detects the presence of bacteria, with values of + 4 or more indicating urinary tract infection (UTI) necessitating a urine culture. This will determine exactly what kind of bacteria are involved. Urine cultures are often accompanied by antibiotic sensitivities, which show which antibiotics are most effective in eliminating the infection. This information is helpful to have on file if the need to consult arises. Whenever values are +2 or +3, begin by repeating the urinalysis. Even the slightest symptoms of UTI are cause for immediate screening, and all women with previous history should be screened periodically to rule out insidious infection.

The **PPD** is used routinely to screen for tuberculosis, an increasingly common infection in crowded urban areas and among Native American, Asian, Middle Eastern, and military populations. Initial infection is often self-healing, so a woman may remain infected and appear asymptomatic. Although congenital infection is rare, postpartum infection of the newborn commonly occurs due to contact with the mother or other infected family members. A mother with an initial infection during pregnancy should be treated at once, whereas treatment will generally be postponed if infection is asymptomatic.

Certain women should also have **genetic screening**. If both parents are of Mediterranean descent, the fetus is at risk for B thalassemia. TaySachs disease can affect fetuses of Jewish couples. Or if the parents are African-American, they may be carriers of the sickle-cell gene. Parents who have previously given birth to children with defects will undoubtedly be concerned about the likelihood of recurrence. Refer all parents at risk to genetic counseling. This can be an area of tremendous anxiety and it would be irresponsible for a midwife to reassure a couple without being on good technical ground.

Every woman age 35 and over should also be advised of her options for genetic screening. **Amniocentesis** can be used to rule out Down's Syndrome or other chromosomal defects associated with advanced maternal age. The incidence of Down's for a woman of 35 is one in 365, equal to the risk of miscarriage or infection caused by the procedure; by the age of 40, the incidence increases to one in 100. Amniocentesis is performed by inserting a needle through the abdomen and into the amniotic sac, then withdrawing a sample of fluid. Ultrasound is used simultaneously to visualize the baby. The procedure cannot be performed before 14 weeks because there is not sufficient fluid, 14 to 16 weeks is optimal. It may take several weeks to get results.

Chorionic villus sampling is done at 10 to 12 weeks: an obvious advantage over amniocentesis in case some abnormality is found and the woman decides to terminate the pregnancy. However, the procedure carries greater risks of miscarriage and infection, as the requisite sample of placental tissue must be obtained through the cervix. And because chromosomal construction of placental tissue does not always reflect that of the fetus itself, there are a significant number of false positive and false negative findings. More disturbing are results from a study recently performed at Oxford University, showing a possible link between the procedure and subsequent fetal anomalies. Chorionic villus sampling is contraindicated for women with a history of cervical incompetence, miscarriage, or premature labor.

Alpha-fetoprotein screening is a blood test detecting neural tube defects only. These include anencephaly, microcephaly, hydrocephaly, and spina bifida. Unfortunately, the test has a 20 percent false positive rate, so that ultrasound may be necessary for a final diagnosis. Numerous states require informing parents of the benefits and risks of alpha-fetoprotein screening.

Decisions regarding genetic screening are very personal and often agonizingly difficult. Should a woman decide against it, she will undoubtedly be reminded of her decision over and over, as total strangers ask if she has had "the test" and whether her baby is a boy or a girl. Amniocentesis has becoming increasingly routine; in response to the threat of malpractice, some physicians recommend it for any woman over 30. There is no easy answer, but a session with a genetics counselor can help a woman assess her risks realistically. The midwife should be prepared with up-to-date handouts and referrals.

Glucose testing to rule out gestational diabetes is routine from 26 to 28 weeks, although it may be performed earlier if there are predisposing factors in the health history. Most common is the **glucose screen**, which requires the mother's blood be drawn one hour after she ingests 50 mg. glucose (a thick, syrupy drink). If values exceed 140 mg./dl.,

FETAL DEVELOPMENT

The **embryonic period** of fetal development includes the first through seventh weeks of life post-fertilization (or, from the LMP, the third through the ninth week). The **fetal period** includes all fetal development after the embryonic period and before the time of birth.

Growth and development begin at the moment of fertilization. The **pronucleus** of the sperm and that of the ovum fuse to form a **zygote**. Each pronucleus contains only 23 chromosomes (the **haploid** number); when they fuse, the normal 46 chromosomes (**diploid** number) are restored.

Also determined at the moment of fertilization is the sex of the individual. The pronuclei are carried in the sex cells, or **gametes**, of both sexes. The male gamete carries either and X or a Y chromosome. The female gamete carries only an X. An XX combination is female, an XY, male.

Immediately after fertilization, the zygote undergoes **cleavage** and becomes a morula. As the morula develops and fluid enters the mass, it becomes a blastocyst. When the **blastocyst** implants in the uterine lining (on the tenth or eleventh day after fertilization) the embryonic period begins.

Development during the embryonic period, dating from the LMP:
- The **heart** starts to beat around the beginning of the sixth week.
- The **ears, arms, legs, facial,** and **neck structures** begin to form at the end of the sixth week.
- The **brain** and **eyes** begin to develop during the seventh week.
- The **nose, mouth,** and **palate** begin to form in the eighth week.

- The **neck is established, urogenital development begins,** and all other essential structures are present by the end of the ninth week.
- The fetus can **swallow, make respiratory movements, urinate, and open and shut his/her mouth** by the end of the twelfth week.

The embryonic period is a critical one in terms of exposure to teratogens, which may cause congenital malformations or death.

Development during the fetal period, dating from the LMP and taken by lunar months:
- **Fourth lunar month** (13 to 16 weeks): eyelids are fused, body growth accelerates, fingernails develop, reflexes manifest, sex is distinguishable, fetus reaches a weight of about .25 lb.
- **Fifth lunar month** (17 to 20 weeks): toenails develop, fetus hiccups, vernix covers the body, fetus reaches average weight of .75 lb.
- **Sixth lunar month** (21 to 24 weeks): hair growth prominent, fetus covered with fine, downy hair (lanugo), buds of permanent teeth form, fetus makes crying/sucking motions, brown fat (source of heat and energy for the newborn) forms, weight 1.25 lbs.
- **Seventh lunar month** (25 to 28 weeks): eyes begin to open and shut, the fetus grows longer, gains significant weight: average 2.25 lbs.
- **Eighth lunar month** (29 to 32 weeks): fat deposits smooth body contours, thick vernix, rhythmic breathing motions, average 3.75 lbs.
- **Ninth lunar month** (33 to 36 weeks): skin smooth, baby looks chubbier, weight 5.5 lbs.
- **Tenth lunar month** (37 to 40 weeks): fetus well proportioned, lanugo disappears, vernix decreases, weight reaches an average of 7.5 lbs.

further testing is recommended. Many midwives find glucose screening unreliable for their clients, most of whom eat very little sugar and are thus less tolerant to the dosage used in testing. Beyond this, controversy rages as to whether or not gestational diabetes poses a significant risk for women with neither historical nor clinical signs (see Chapter Three for more details).

If a woman comes to her initial visit with no previous lab work and you are unable to do it yourself, send her to a public health facility or women's health center with a full list of requisite tests, including vaginal cultures. But make every effort to acquire these lab skills as soon as possible—your clients will greatly appreciate the continuity of care, and you will enjoy the autonomy of practice.

ROUTINE CHECKUPS

The scheduling of prenatal visits is fairly standard: up to 28 weeks gestation, every four weeks; from 28 to 34 weeks, every two weeks; from 35 weeks onward, once weekly. The main reason for the increasing frequency of visits is that complications for mother and baby are more likely to arise at the end of pregnancy. It is also important that the midwife have additional personal contact with the expectant mother as pregnancy progresses, in order to foster trust and intimacy.

Routine at every visit are urine dipstick for protein and glucose, blood pressure evaluation, fundal height measurement, fetal auscultation, and uterine/fetal palpation. Weight may be checked less frequently, but nutrition and exercise should be checked each time.

At 28 weeks, certain assessments from early pregnancy should be repeated. Call for another three-day diet report, as needs for protein, calcium, and iron intensify during the last trimester. Check the HCT/HGB again, for if the mother is anemic, you may need time to find an effective solution. This is also the cutoff point for routine glucose screening. Otherwise, caregiving during the last trimester should focus on more personal aspects of helping the mother prepare for labor and impending parenthood.

Throughout the pregnancy, there are many appropriate topics for discussion: books and articles read, experiences in childbirth class, partner/family preparation, postpartum support, sexuality, aspects of newborn care, rest and relaxation, work and play. Take your cues from the mother, but avoid the rut of discussing the same subjects over and over. Your task is to expose expectant parents to issues and concerns they may not have considered, in preparation for the many-faceted experiences of birth and child rearing.

Don't forget to inquire about the mother's general well-being at every visit, as there are a number of physical complaints that may arise from time to time (see next section).

And always take good notes! For guidelines, refer to the section on Charting in Chapter Eight.

COMMON COMPLAINTS

Ligament pains are experienced as pelvic sensitivity and vague pain when walking, and are caused by stretching of the ligaments which support the uterus as they adjust to its increasing size and weight. Many women don't realize that the uterus is suspended by ligaments, which run from its base to the pelvic bones. The uterus is very movable, more or less a floating organ (see illustration, page 35).

Morning sickness is due primarily to elevated levels of estrogen and human chorionic gonadotropin (HCG). This low-grade, persistent nausea is called morning sickness because it is much more likely to occur when the stomach is empty, although it may also occur in response to evening cooking odors. Women widely acknowledge that mental conflict or emotional turmoil contribute to their experience of morning sickness. Therefore, emotional support and stress reduction are crucial. Encourage the expectant mother to ask her partner for some pampering or special attention, or help her with this if need be. Also have her try B-complex—specifically, 50 mg. B-6 at bedtime and again at mid-day. Other remedies include crackers or plain yogurt upon arising, and ginger or raspberry leaf tea. Many women report that small meals and nearly continuous eating, particularly high protein foods, seem to help. This makes sense, as another possible explanation for morning sickness is low blood sugar levels, primarily from fasting during sleep but potentially reoccurring throughout the day (metabolic changes of pregnancy make it harder for the body to regulate blood sugar levels).

Should nausea progress to vomiting, recommend ground ginger capsules with meals and maintain daily contact, at least by phone. As mentioned earlier, if vomiting progresses to hyperemesis gravidarium, the mother is at risk for severe dehydration and should be seen by a physician immediately.

Indigestion and heartburn are often related to fetal growth spurts and the resulting displacement of stomach and intestines. The best remedy

round
ligaments

utero-sacral
ligaments

Supporting Ligaments of the Uterus

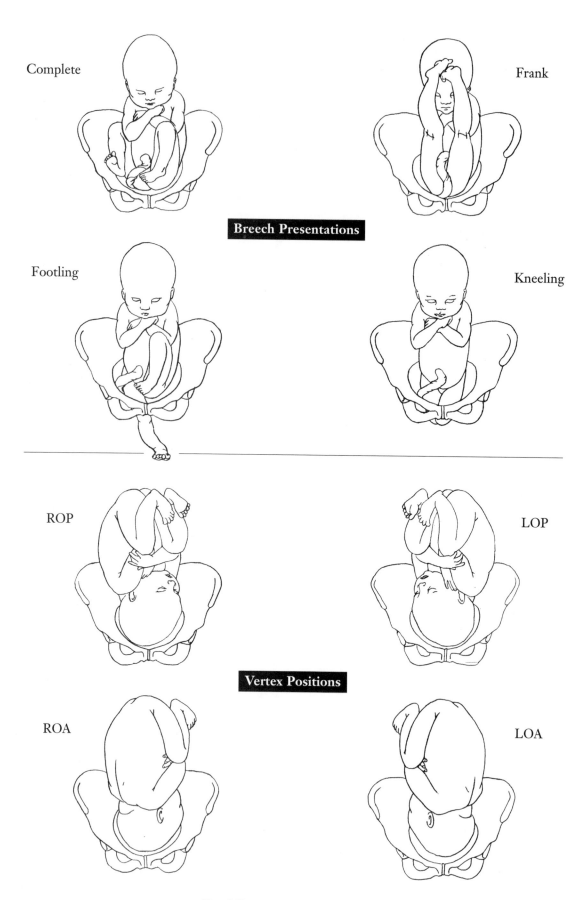

Complete

Frank

Breech Presentations

Footling

Kneeling

ROP

LOP

Vertex Positions

ROA

LOA

Fetal Presentation and Position

seems to be frequent, smaller meals, with digestive enzymes like papaya and bromelain taken as needed. Advise women not to eat too much before lying down, and to eat leisurely. Digestion slows naturally in pregnancy to increase absorption of essential nutrients, thus food must be chewed more thoroughly. And since the gall bladder functions less efficiently, reducing fat intake can help.

Fatigue has a relationship to nutrition and general state of health. But in early pregnancy, fatigue is directly related to hormonal changes and major physiological adjustments, and can actually serve the positive function of helping the mother tune in to her body's changing needs. If problematic after the first trimester, review the diet. Sometimes women get into ruts regarding food and exercise, and need to break away from familiar patterns. A wide variety of foods, especially fruit and vegetables, provide diverse vitamins and minerals needed for increased vitality. Daily exercise and social interaction serve to stimulate body and mind. Encourage every expectant mother to experiment and find what works best for her, and make her aware that her needs will change as pregnancy progresses. (This is good preparation for flexible, resourceful parenting.) If fatigue is extreme or persistent, rule out anemia with a repeat HCT or prenatal panel.

Headaches and other minor pains often respond to relaxing teas such as hops, skullcap, and chamomile. Yoga is another remedy, as it is emotional clearing wrought by talking through problems and concerns. Headaches may also result from dehydration, so stress adequate fluid intake.

If the mother complains of **backache**, see that she is getting sufficient but not overstrenuous exercise, and suggest pelvic rocks to keep the lower spine flexible. These can be performed on hands and knees, alternately arching the back like a cat and bringing it back to normal position. She can do the same motion standing, sitting, driving in the car, anytime. She should also use her stomach muscles to maintain good posture; suggest she hold her stomach taut periodically throughout the day.

If she indicates that backache is near waist-level, rule out the possibility of kidney infection (pyelonephritis) by **checking for CVA tenderness.**

Do this with the mother in a sitting position, her back fully exposed. Prepare her first, then make a fist and gently strike the area nearest her waist and adjacent her spine, on either side. In order to pound firmly enough to secure your diagnosis, you may wish to place your other hand across the area to cushion your blow. If the woman jumps or otherwise indicates pain, note whether her sensitivity was to the left or right, and refer her immediately to a backup physician. (If there is no CVA tenderness, chart this "No CVAT.")

Varicose veins of the legs and vulva are caused by high levels of progesterone relaxing smooth muscle and hindering venous return throughout the body, particularly in the extremities. Hereditary factors may also play a part. Standing or sitting with crossed legs for long periods makes things worse, but exercise helps by stimulating circulation, as does elevating the legs and buttocks periodically. Six hundred to 800 units of vitamin E daily may also be beneficial, but have the mother taper down to 400 units by the seventh month, as excessive quantities may cause retained placenta. For best absorption, this fat-soluble vitamin should be taken separately from other supplements and with milk, cheese, or other fatty food sources.

In the absence of hypertension or proteinuria, **swollen ankles** are a normal result of impaired circulation in pregnancy, or excessive periods of standing. The diet should be improved with more protein, fresh vegetables, and plenty of fluids, and moderate exercise should be taken regularly. Elevating the feet and legs helps too.

Constipation can be caused by hormones or diet, but plenty of fluids and fibrous foods should take care of the problem. Sometimes women eat well but mistake thirst for hunger, and must learn to distinguish the two impulses. Regular physical activity is critical.

Vaginal infection, particularly yeast/monilia, is common during pregnancy. Characterized by a white, curd-like discharge, yeast is a naturally occurring vaginal organism which tends to overgrow in pregnancy due to increased vaginal alkalinity caused by elevated progesterone levels. It can be controlled by inserting vaginal sponges (be sure to boil first to remove mineral deposits) or cotton tampons soaked in acidophilus culture. Saturate either of these with solution, squeeze out lightly, insert and change every three hours. Cotton underwear is essential. Yeast infection at term increases the risk of newborn thrush.

Bacterial vaginosus (also known as garnerella or hemophilus) is another common vaginal infection. Although ordinarily benign and transient, this infection can complicate pregnancy by causing premature rupture of the membranes, preterm labor, and chorioamnionitis.

Commonly detected by the woman because of fishy odor (noted particularly after lovemaking), bacterial vaginosus may produce a thin, grey or white discharge which tends to adhere to vaginal walls. Seldom is there vaginal irritation or itching. The best way to test for BV without a microscope is by symptoms/odor in combination with the whiff test. Touch a cotton swab with discharge sample to a bit of KOH solution, and if it lets off a potent fishy odor (amine), you have bacterial vaginosus.

One natural remedy is to insert a peeled, unnicked clove of garlic into the vagina, changed three times daily. Follow with five days acidophilus treatment, as described above for monilia. If this does not work, medical treatment is indicated. (It is also important that the woman abstain from intercourse during treatment, and that her partner be checked if symptoms persist.)

Trichomonas infection is characterized by a thin, malodorous, highly irritating yellow-green frothy discharge. The usual treatment, Flagyl, is contraindicated in the first half of pregnancy. The following herbal douche formula is effective for both trich and yeast, and although a bit of trouble to prepare, it's worth it. Unlike harsh medicinal formulas that strip mucous membranes, this blend is gentle and nourishing. Douching is generally not recommended during pregnancy, but is safe as long as the pressure is kept to a minimum—a hand-held squeeze unit is best—with warm water, not hot. Never insert the nozzle into the vagina more than a few inches.

Garlic suppositories may also work for trichomonas or severe monilia, used in combination with the douche.

Keep in mind that trich is sexually transmitted, thus the expectant mother's partner must also be treated. Men may have relatively minor symptoms (such as twinges of pain with urination or slight discharge), but because the organism can be harbored in the urethra, men must take oral medication. Condoms must be used for sexual activity until both partners are cured.

All vaginal infections respond positively to certain dietary factors: plenty of dark green vegetables, good-quality protein, whole grains, and ample fluids. Unsweetened cranberry juice or concentrate in capsules can help increase vaginal acidity (also useful in treating UTI). Yeast thrives on sugar, so eliminate sugars completely, including any excessive intake of fruit, whether fresh, dried, or juiced. Eating plenty of yogurt with acidophilus can help, as does brewer's yeast.

Douche for Vaginal Infections:

One part each of:

Comfrey root	Yarrow
Mugwort	Rosemary
Peppermint	Alum

Steep in a non-metal container using boiled spring water. Allow to cool. Douche with one pint strained solution twice daily for two days. On the third and fourth day, douche as usual in the morning, but for yeast infections add one part acidophilus in the evening, and for trichomoniasis, one part myrrh in the evening.

Herpesvirus hominus #2 is at epidemic proportions and has thus become a common complaint. Small, painful blisters are the prime symptom of this sexually transmitted viral infection. The initial outbreak is usually severe, much like a bad flu. Once the accompanying sores disappear, the virus remains in nerve ganglia affecting the genital area, and infection may recur repeatedly. Susceptibility to outbreak is increased during times of severe stress or exhaustion. Some women have outbreaks every few months, while others go into full remission or have no symptons for many years. If a woman reports recurring episodes, inquire as to the number, severity, and usual location of lesions, and note in the chart.

Herpesvirus can have a devastating effect on the baby's central nervous system. If initial outbreak occurs during the first trimester, consult with backup. If there are active lesions when labor commences, vaginal delivery is generally prohibited unless sores have closed and can be kept from contact with the baby. Do cultures on both the sores and cervix in the event of any outbreak during pregnancy. Weekly cultures are no longer deemed necessary in the last trimester—a visual inspection of the cervix at the onset of labor is considered sufficient to rule out current infection. But if membranes rupture prior to the onset of labor, screen the cervix within two hours, as the baby may be rapidly affected by herpesvirus without the barrier of intact membranes.

Treatments for herpes during pregnancy are basically comfort measures. Most important is to keep the affected area dry and cool—no nylon underwear, panty hose, or tights. Hot baths tend to aggravate the infection. Local applications of lysine ointment, cold milk, zinc oxide, A&D ointment, ice, and calendula cream (marigold extract) are all reputed to be healing and soothing. Certain dietary changes may help; one mother reported cutting her usual five-day cycle in half by beginning stress supplements (B-complex) and protein drinks at the first sign of infection. Increased lysine intake may also help, in supplemental doses of 500 mg. daily. Elimination of coffee/black tea, chocolate, alcohol, and sugar makes a difference, as does getting plenty of rest. Intercourse is prohibited until all sores are completely healed.

COMMON FEARS AND COUNSELING TECHNIQUES

Certain fears regarding pregnancy and birth are universal. These cross-cultural concerns of expectant mothers are rooted in survival instincts; they function to alert a woman to the needs of her developing baby and prepare her for motherhood. Almost every expectant mother wonders if her baby will be normal and healthy. Most women have certain fears of labor, and wonder if they will be able to tolerate it. These worries are often alleviated simply by realizing how commonly they occur.

Besides these fears, there are special concerns unique to our times and culture. The expectant mother of today often has anxiety regarding her forthcoming role; she may fear losing her career-related identity and being buried in domesticity. She may also find herself uncertain about her relationship with her partner—the more sensitive and emotional she becomes, the more nervous and erratic his/her behavior may be.

As she brings these concerns into the open, you may need to do a bit of counseling. Your primary goal should be to focus the mother on her own problem-solving capabilities. At the same time, it is crucial to sympathize with her distress. Validating the hormonally-enhanced sensitivities of a pregnant woman can be one of the heavier demands placed on the midwife. Or it can be a lot of fun, if spiced with humor and a bit of personal disclosure. In midwifery practice, the counseling relationship works best as one friendship, unless there are more serious problems necessitating referral.

What are some basic techniques for counseling? As the midwife receives impressions and reflects them back without judgment or distortion, she **mirrors** her client. She may also try **pacing** the mother's breathing rhythm, or **matching** her speed and style of self-expression as a means of establishing trust. **Active listening** requires that she use all parts of herself—not just her ears, but her heart and soul—to fully receive what her client is trying to communicate. Sensing moments of truth or reckoning, she then gives **positive reinforcement**.

Contrary to the medical model's premium on detached objectivity, personal involvement is essential in the midwife/client relationship. Why so? By being personally committed to help a woman work through her problems, the midwife inspires commitment in return. And by letting her own character shine through, she helps her client feel confident and courageous enough to accept newly revealed truths about herself and her life. All this serves to **elicit responsibility**, for when the mother embraces her realizations and begins to make them manifest, the ultimate aim of counseling is achieved.

Truth be told, midwives need to be needed. We are healers in a traditional sense, with strong

HERBS AND HOMEOPATHY IN PREGNANCY

by Shannon Anton

The following is a list of herbs contraindicated during pregnancy: Goldenseal, Ephedra, Cotton Root Bark, Blue Cohosh, Pennyroyal, and Birthroot. For more information, refer to *Wise Woman Herbal for the Childbearing Year*, by Susun Weed.

Goldenseal: As Goldenseal has become popular, it has also been overused and over harvested. Once abundant and easily wild crafted, it is now endangered in certain areas. To harvest Goldenseal you must take the root, thereby eliminating a significant portion of, or the entire, plant. Goldenseal is also extremely strong medicine; overuse taxes the liver and kidneys. There are only a few conditions for which it is a traditional remedy; other potent and more appropriate remedies abound. Do not use it for cold and flu, as you would echinacea tincture. There are a few appropriate uses for it postpartum, but do not use it at all during pregnancy. If you must use Goldenseal, preserve its potency and stretch its volume by tincturing it.

Buying Herbs

Dried herbs should hold a deep color and smell strongly of their substance. Faintly colored herbs with little scent have been stored incorrectly or for too long a time, and their potency is questionable.

Herbal tinctures are comprised of either fresh or dried herbs preserved in a liquid form. Herb qualities are extracted using alcohol or glycerin, then the mixture is strained and stored. Tinctures are taken in drops from an eye dropper, or by dropperful. When buying tinctures, try to find out how they have been prepared. Tincture from fresh, wild or organically grown plants is the best. The company Herb Pharm consistently provides quality tinctures prepared with care and respect for the plants.

Working with dried plant material for tinctures is fine. But consider taking a class from an herbalist to have opportunity to observe herbs as they grow, and to learn directly from the herbs about their properties and uses.

Using Homeopathy

While homeopathy is a rich and exact healing tradition, there are beginners' rules, that make it easier to work with these marvelous allies. Homeopathic remedies must be properly stored or they are antidoted (negated). Store homeopathics out of sunlight, protect from heat and extreme cold, and never keep near strong aromatic substances like herbs, camphor, peppermint, toothpaste, perfumed products, etc. Avoid storing them in your medicine cabinet, or in your birth bag near your herbal tinctures.

If possible, one must avoid eating or drinking for 15 minutes prior to taking a remedy (in labor, this cannot always be achieved).

The strong potencies listed here are not for everyday use; birth is exceptional in its requirements. Potencies of 6x or 30C are applied in most other situations. Unless you are sure of your expertise, never treat issues outside of birth with these stronger potencies.

In critical situations, as when resuscitating an infant or dealing with maternal hemorrhage, dosing and then dosing quickly again is appropriate. Once relief is experienced or a shift is noted, discontinue the remedy. If symptoms return, apply the remedy again.

I urge you to read *Homeopathic Medicines for Pregnancy and Childbirth* (Moskowitz) to better understand the nature of homeopathic medicines, and to further research the following remedies.

Pregnancy Support

The most basic and well known nutritional herbs are also beneficial for pregnancy. Herbal infusions are a simple and delicious way to take herbal nourishment. To make an herbal infusion, use one ounce of fresh or dried herb (a good handful) per one quart boiling water (removed from heat). Steep at least four hours in a covered, non-metal container. You can mix two herbs per quart water, or double the batch and mix three or four. You may also want to add honey and/or lemon. If you like, brew peppermint tea separately and add it to your infusion for taste.

Nettle leaf provides excellent support for kidneys, is rich in vitamins A, C, D, and K, calcium, potassium, phosphorous, iron, and sulfur. It prevents leg cramps and postpartum hemorrhage, eases postpartum pains, nourishes the circulatory system to reduce hemorrhoids, and encourages abundant breast milk.

Dandelion leaf is nature's special gift to nourish and revitalize the liver, and also provides great kidney support. Rich in calcium and potassium, vitamins A, B complex, C and D, iron. Essential in the prevention and treatment of preeclampsia, also a reliable digestive aid.

Red Raspberry leaf is the classic uterine toner and pregnancy tonic. Prepares the uterus to function at her best. Can ease morning sickness and gently aid digestion.

Red Clover leaves and blossoms greatly nourish the whole reproductive system, and nourish and balance the endocrine system. Rich in calcium, magnesium, and trace minerals.

Lemon juice and water safely detoxify the liver during pregnancy (or at any time of stress).

Remedies in Pregnancy

Nausea

Nausea can be greatly relieved with **Ginger** tea. Pour one cup boiling water over three to five slices of fresh ginger root. Let steep five minutes and sip slowly.

Homeopathic remedies can be extremely effective for easing morning sickness. The remedies are specific to symptoms. Research **Pulsitilla, Sepia, Nux Vomica,** and **Ipecacuanha**. Additional remedies to consider include **Antimonium Tartrate, Argentum Nitricum, Petroleum, Sulfur,** and **Tabacum**. Good references are *Homeopathic Medicine for Women* by Trevor Smith, MD, and *Homeopathic Medicines for Pregnancy and Childbirth* by Richard Moskowitz, MD.

Anemia

Anemia is often diagnosed in pregnancy. Herbal/green sources of iron include **Dandelion, Nettles, Kelp,** and **Parsley. Yellow Dock Root** improves absorption. **Floradix Herbs + Iron**, a concentrated herbal and food compound, is an excellent tonic.

Heartburn

Slippery Elm lozenges greatly relieve the worst heartburn. Also try chewing raw **almonds**, raw **papaya**, or papaya enzyme tablets.

Sleep Difficulties

Apart from deep relaxation and exercise during the day, a silky eye pillow filled with flax seed and lavender has proven to be my own best remedy for sleeplessness. Stronger remedies include: 1/2 dropperful of **Motherwort** tincture, **Skullcap** tincture, **Catnip** tincture, or **Valerian** tincture. Or, during the last trimester: 1/2 dropperful of **Hops** tincture.

Some women are awakened by anxiety or worry that keeps them from getting back to sleep. Homeopathic **Aconite** 30C is very effective to calm and quiet nervous tension and fears. Use this remedy only during anxious episodes.

Back Pain, Sciatica, or Carpal Tunnel Syndrome

Chiropractic care can be crucial: joints softened by pregnancy may become misaligned, and if readjusted, other remedies can be more helpful. Even if you are unfamiliar with chiropractic care, don't hesitate to try it in pregnancy

St. John's Wort (hypericum) oil is the best remedy I've found for nerve or muscle pain. Apply it directly over the sore area, as well as a bit above and below. Especially if used before sleeping, St. John's Wort brings amazing relief. Depending on the severity of pain, use it straight from the bottle or dilute one ounce in six ounces of almond or olive oil. Arnica oil can also be beneficial, though it is St. John's Wort oil that earned the reputation of "miracle cure" during the middle ages. For nerve pain, **St. John's Wort** tincture may be taken orally, 1/2 dropperful tincture every few hours.

Homeopathic remedies include **Hypericum** 30C, taken every two hours during painful episodes, and topical application of a gel compound, **Arni-flora** (made by B&T).

Hemorrhoids

Red Clover and **Nettle** infusion nourishes the circulatory system and prevents or improves hemorrhoids, especially if taken routinely.

Grated raw **potato** may be used as a compress directly on hemorrhoids, or a thin slice of raw potato may be inserted into the rectum to shrink and relieve painful swelling.

The classic standby, **Witch Hazel Extract**, is very effective. Apply directly on hemorrhoids or use compresses. It may also be taken orally as homeopathic **Hamamelis** 30C when hemorrhoids flare up.

Constipation

Hydration is of utmost importance when dealing with constipation. Plenty of vegetables and whole foods offer sufficient bulk to avoid constipation. For additional bulk, **Psyllium seed** (the main ingredient in Metamucil) can be added to oatmeal or taken in capsules; take lots of water with it. **Prune** juice is the faithful elixir our grandparents knew and loved; it works great.

Diarrhea

Even pregnant women get the stomach flu. The biggest concern is keeping enough fluid down to prevent dehydration. Often, plain water is abrasive to the system. Add **honey** or **maple syrup** to warm or room temperature water, and sip slowly. To stop diarrhea, here are two proven remedies:

Rice water: Cook white rice with 4:1 ratio of water to rice. Cook only until rice is tender, then pour off excess water and drink it.

Tea x 3: using black tea and boiling water, brew one cup of tea. Save the tea bag, and dump the tea. Use the same tea bag and brew a second cup. Repeat a third time, and drink.

Both of these remedies are complemented by **polarity** therapy. To practice this, the woman and her partner face each other and fully relax. The partner places one hand on the woman's right shoulder and one hand on her left hip. Waiting until both hands feel "even" or seem to pulse together, the partner then gives the woman warning that a change is coming, and shifts hand positions to hold the woman's left shoulder and right hip. When the energy in both hands feels even again, the partner slowly removes both hands.

Rescue Remedy, a Bach Flower Remedy, is helpful in any case of physical/ physiological upset.

Breech Babies

Besides the usual postural exercises for turning a breech baby, two additional remedies have proven effective. Homeopathic **Pulsitilla** 30C taken several times a day can also encourage the breech to rotate.

Even more reliable is **moxa** treatment. Moxa is a roll of tightly compacted **Mugwort**, used in traditional Chinese medicine. When lit, moxa looks rather like a cigar. The ash of burning moxa is extremely hot, so care must be taken in handling. Place the burning end near the outer, lower corner of the pinky toenail; heat at this "point" facilitates rotation of the breech. Treat the toes on both feet two or three times daily until a change occurs—and don't worry, women know how hot is hot enough! Moxa treatment is most effective when done on a slant board.

Preterm Labor

The sooner preterm labor symptoms are addressed, the better your chance of getting them to stop. In times of threatened preterm labor, good hydration is critical.

In addition, **Magnesium** supplements have proven invaluable in preventing preterm labor in any woman with predisposing factors, or forestalling it if it occurs. Too much magnesium causes diarrhea; reduce intake as necessary, and space doses throughout the day. Follow this routine until 37 weeks. If preterm labor begins, extra doses of magnesium and plenty of fluids should be taken at once, along with a deep, warm soak in the tub.

Homeopathic **Mag Phos** 30C is also useful. Using a non-metal cup, put seven pellets in a half cup of hot (not boiling) water, and stir with a non-metal stick 100 times. Slowly and continuously sip little sips of this remedy until it is gone. Contractions should slow or stop within an hour. Continue to monitor for preterm labor symptoms: if labor is not slowing or is accelerating, or if cervical change is occurring, consult a physician.

Postdates

In addition to the famed **Evening Primrose Oil** remedy, the cervix may be softened with homeopathic **Cimicifuga** 30C, taken once an hour for eight hours. Follow with homeopathic **Caulophyllum** 30C, taken as above. If the cervix is already soft, go right to Caulophyllum. Often, one dose of Caulophyllum 200C before bed will result in labor during the night.

maternal instincts nourished by giving. On the other hand, our natural desire for closeness must at all times be tempered by respect for our clients' privacy and pace. We must avoid becoming co-dependent by projecting our own needs and concerns into our caregiving relationships. Working in partnership with other midwives can keep us from going overboard in this respect, and help us maintain the necessary balance between personal involvement and objectivity.

Men with questions and concerns about parenting may have difficulty communicating these directly. Regardless of encouragement, it remains difficult for many men to identify and express deep feelings. Pride may be a factor, along with general embarrassment over matters considered too personal to discuss. Impart information discreetly; supply reading materials, handouts, or make referrals to childbirth classes/expectant parents groups.

PARTNER PARTICIPATION

Frequently, the partner of a woman planning to birth at home desires his/her own vital role in the experience. Some want to assist with delivery. This requires healthy intimacy between partners, and a good understanding of the mechanics of labor and delivery. There is no reason why her partner shouldn't catch the baby, barring an unforeseen complication or the expectant mother's last-minute desire to have him/her by her side. For many women, the act of easing the baby into their partner's loving hands brings total release and ecstasy.

Whenever an expectant partner professes interest, provide reading material with clear, reasonably detailed information on assisting delivery. At the same time, describe the sensual aspects of birth—how the baby's head will look and feel as it descends and emerges. Then schedule a delivery practice a few weeks before the birth, perhaps at the home visit, using a model pelvis and baby doll to demonstrate. If you do a vaginal check on

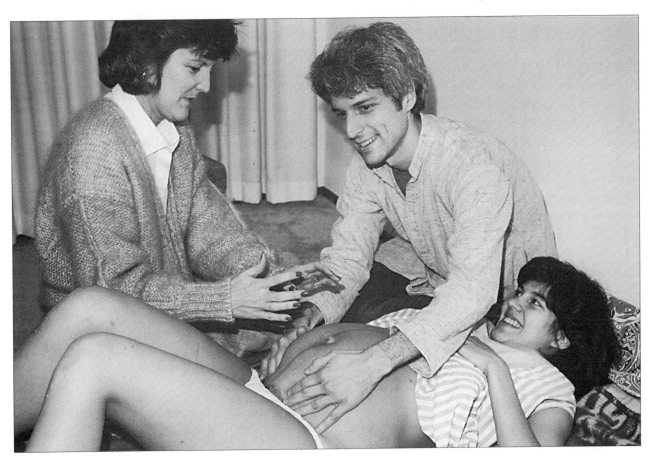

This father is discovering how to feel his baby's position.

the mother and she is willing, you can show her partner how to combine vaginal massage with perineal support during delivery. You can also demonstrate techniques of perineal massage/support using your hand to simulate the birth outlet, with stretched skin between thumb and forefinger serving as perineum.

Some fathers see "making the catch" as a kind of virility test, a chance to conquer the mystery of birth. Be sure to emphasize the need for sensitivity and awareness of what is happening to the mother; he must at all times follow her lead. I remember one father who paid minimal attention to prenatal instruction and had a pretty rough time during the delivery. He massaged so vigorously that he actually pushed the baby's head back in as it began to crown! I put my hand over his to slow him down, gave him more instruction, and fortunately, calmed him enough to make his work effective.

Ideally, the partner's preparation is mostly personal, an extension of the couple's intimacy. Here is Frank's story:

I wanted to share the birth process with my mate and felt that my involvement was necessary and my right as a father. Practicing exercises and massaging Bridget almost every night put me in tune with her body and spirit. By participating in this way I believed that my mind and body would appreciate the mystical aspects of birth when the time came.

My participation was not limited to prenatal classes, exercises, and reading material. This was our second pregnancy and once again my goal was to catch the baby and cut the cord. I had performed this mighty ritual during our first birth. That labor was only three hours; Bridget went immediately into hard labor-transition. Even though it was hard to absorb this rapid labor I still made the catch. Lydia was small, yet perfect to the touch. I caught her and held her close to my joyful, tired body.

I did not catch our second child. His shoulders were stuck and thus we needed assistance. His birth was twelve hours long, which let Bridget and me absorb ourselves at every stage. We touched, massaged, showered, and supported each other in every way. This made up for not catching Paul.

During this second birth I felt fully in touch with Bridget sexually and spiritually. I noticed that my sensitivity was greater than before, and my love for Bridget and my family grew with every phase of the encounter. Patience, listening, and empathy were at their peak. I felt then that I truly understood both birth and Bridget.

Here's the joint perspective, with comments from both father, Eugene and mother, Pamela.
Eugene:

Every man should catch his own baby. I didn't realize that, when my daughter was born eight years ago. We had her at home, I cut the cord, and it was the high point of my life. Yet it would have been even better if I had caught her.

I didn't because I was ignorant. I didn't know how easy it was, and nobody told me that I could or should. But when my son was born, I found out that catching your baby is the next best thing to having it. I urge all fathers to do it, to insist on it.

I enjoyed being down there between Pamela's legs. At my daughter's birth I was at her mother's side and didn't have the intimate perspective. This time I could see what was going on.
Pamela:

I was not sure where I wanted Eugene to be—at my side or at my feet. But as our cycle was near completion I realized that this was the only time we, the three of us, would be connected in that intense moment of birth. Watching Eugene's concentration, his hands and the message of love that they carried, and seeing my baby's head in the mirror helped me to stay focused. Soon I was feeling those irresistible urges to push and feeling my baby's body moving through the passage. First the head, then swoosh the body into the hands of the man I love. A beautiful baby boy was born so right. The connection is made and is never lost.
Eugene:

When Lenny slithered into my hands I immediately felt bonded to him. I was the first one able to see that he was a boy. That was a special thrill. Though Pamela carried Lenny and gave him up like ripe fruit, I was his first contact with the world as a whole person. In this first, total contact I knew he could feel my protective, loving feelings. And when I gave him to Pamela, completing the cycle, I felt truly satisfied.

Sibling Participation

Children who will be at the birth need preparation too. Have picture books available to lend for this purpose. Many parents worry needlessly that their children will be frightened by the sights and sounds of birth. To mediate these fears, send the family to a birth video or film showing. Mothers can make "birth noises" with small children for fun, helping them to be better prepared.

It is, however, a good idea to include an adult-companion for siblings (other than the mother's partner) who can take them out if they become upset during the birth and decide they want to leave.

The atmosphere at clinic is most important. Here's one mother's story of her experience in preparing her three-year-old daughter:

From the beginning of our second pregnancy we wanted to include Lydia in the birth. We felt that this would ease the transition from being an only child and lessen any jealousy that might arise. A home birth would enable her to comfortably share this joyous family occasion. Although some friends and relatives thought she was too young to participate, our midwife and other friends invited to the birth supported the idea.

Our preparation started with prenatal exams in the home of our midwife, Elizabeth. Lydia accompanied us on all of these visits, and with each one became more interested in the proceedings. We tried to explain each step to her and encouraged her to take part by imitating Elizabeth. The relaxed atmosphere and obvious enthusiasm of everyone in the room made her more comfortable.

In preparation for the actual birth we asked a friend who is close to Liddy to look after her during labor and to try to gauge whether she wanted to be in the room while the baby was born. We were happy that she slept through most of my labor because this reduced the chance that she would become bored, plus Frank and I were better able to concentrate on each other and the birth.

Liddy entered the room in the arms of a friend just as I was pushing the baby out. She was very calm, putting to rest our fears that the intensity of pushing might upset her. Even after the birth, much of my attention went out to Lydia, who seemed a bit shy at first. But a few hours later when the four of us were alone, she warmed up considerably and has continued to show a deep affection for her little brother. We feel that bringing her to clinic and letting her attend the birth has a lot to do with her present warmth and tolerance.

The Last Six Weeks

The emphasis of caregiving shifts dramatically during this final phase of pregnancy. The birth is imminent, and that is the focus. Parents have last-minute preparations to consider and more questions than before, while the midwife attends more assiduously to assessing readiness of both mother and baby. She carefully palpates the baby for position, size, and growth, and also checks for descent, flexion, and engagement. These additional assessments can be done abdominally or by internal exam.

Lack of flexion can be corrected if the head is not too far down in the pelvis; in fact, the deflexed head can and should be prevented from engaging. The maneuver is simple—facing the mother's feet, press the occiput down into the pelvis while pulling up on the sinciput, tucking the baby's chin to its chest.

Internal exams are not mandatory, but may help satisfy the mother's curiosity regarding her readiness for labor. When examining near term you should: 1) check the cervix for dilation and effacement, 2) note the station (level of descent) of the baby's head, and 3) note any increase in vaginal lubrication or softening of the vaginal musculature common when birth is imminent. If a first pregnancy, the cervix will often be somewhat closed until labor begins, with perhaps a centimeter of dilation, whereas a woman who has had children before may be two or three centimeters dilated at term. **Effacement**, or softening/shortening of the cervix, depends largely on how far the baby has descended and how much pressure it is exerting on lower uterine tissues. If the baby's head is still high and the cervix posterior, it is rare to find much effacement.

The degree of effacement is recorded in terms of a percentage. An uneffaced cervix feels thick, firm, and about an inch long. A cervix 50 percent effaced feels softer, "mushier" with a less

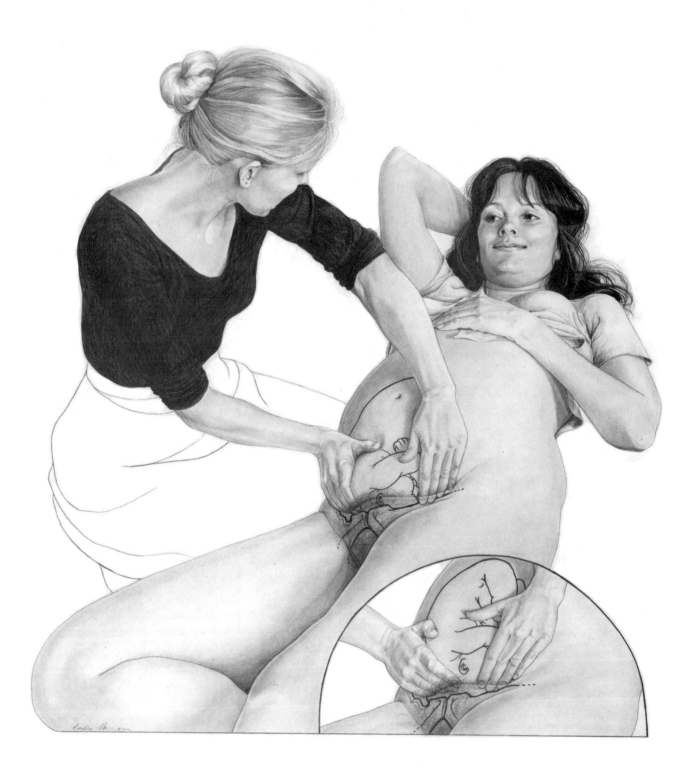

Checking for Flexion and Engagement

distinguishable neck, just half an inch or so in length. Sometimes the cervix is almost fully effaced but the os feels ring-like, with a clearly defined and somewhat rigid edge. Other times, the cervix effaces unevenly because the baby's head comes down at an angle (asynclitism) and puts pressure on either the anterior or posterior aspect. Sixty to 80 percent effacement is fairly common in the final weeks before labor commences. Rarely, women are 100 percent effaced (cervix paper-thin and smooth against the baby's head) with little or no dilation at term, but with great propensity for precipitous labor. Other women dilate to five or six centimeters weeks before labor begins; these labors are also apt to be quick.

If you find the cervical opening to be rigid/ taut, or you know the expectant mother to have scar tissue there from previous infection or surgery, have her do self-massage with evening primrose oil (available at the health food store). This will soften the tissue and break up adhesions, preparing the cervix for dilation. This can also be done in early labor, in case it is prolonged. Help the mother find her cervix in case she has never felt it before, and direct her to massage twice daily for several minutes. (This is contraindicated for any woman with a history of premature labor until at least 37 weeks.)

The phenomenon of **false labor** commonly occurring in the final weeks of pregnancy is characterized by irregular contractions. Instead of increasing in duration and frequency, they eventually just taper off and stop. Little or no dilation takes place because uterine action is incoordinate.

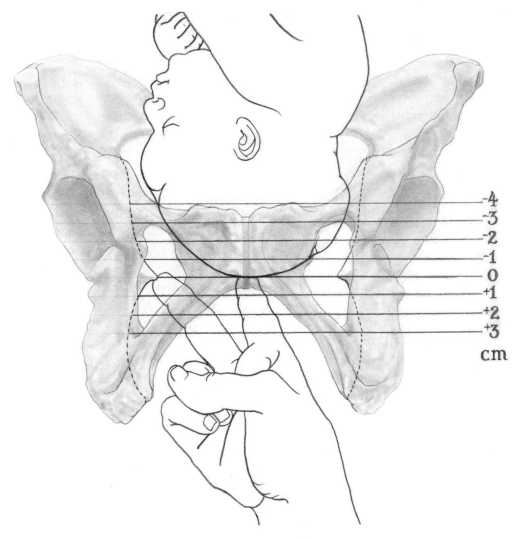

Estimating Station

Uterine muscle is comprised of three layers—the external, longitudinal layer, the internal, circular layer, and a middle, connective layer. In incoordinate labor, only certain long muscle segments contract, and all must work together harmoniously in order to pull open circular muscles at the cervix. Still, the term "false" is both discouraging and somewhat misleading, as these contractions usually accomplish some cervical softening or effacement, or may facilitate the baby's descent/engagement.

Descent is measured according to the relationship between the level of the presenting part and that of the ischial spines (which mark the midpoint of the pelvis). If the head is one centimeter above spine level, the station is termed - 1. The head can be as high as - 2, - 3, or - 4 and still be felt internally. If the top of the head is exactly level with the spines, it is at O station and considered to be **engaged**. If the head is a centimeter or two below spine level, it is at + 1 or + 2 station. Rarely will the presenting part be lower than + 2 before labor begins.

Checking for station is difficult for beginners. It's essential to have some clinical experience with pelvimetry to be certain you can find the spines. Insert two fingers, bend the middle one and place it on the spine, then extend the index finger to find the presenting part. Your reading will only be accurate if you keep both fingers on the same horizontal plane. Note how many centimeters up or down you must move your index finger to touch the presenting part, then take your reading. After a while, assessment of station is based primarily on a qualitative sense of how well the head (or butt) fills the pelvis, and ceases to be such a mysterious and painstaking procedure.

Vaginal muscle awareness and control are essential for avoiding vaginal/perineal tears. If the expectant mother can learn the difference between contracted and relaxed states of her vagina and perineum, she will be able to create either at will. Encourage her to do some exploring; have her place her fingers inside and contract her muscles around them, in order to learn which motions work for her. Being able to stop the flow of urine—a common way to learn vaginal muscle

awareness—does not necessarily indicate a full range of control.

My favorite exercise is the classic "elevator." In this exercise, the pelvic floor muscles are pulled up like an elevator ascending to the first floor, second floor, third floor, fourth floor, fifth floor, then are held for 30 seconds, and let down slowly to the fourth floor, third floor, second floor, first floor and finally, to the basement—the place from which we give birth. Yet another exercise that imparts control of the internal muscle most likely to tear at birth (the bulbocavernosus) is a quick, snapping movement lower down in the vagina, near the introitus. These exercises are also useful postpartum to help restore vaginal tone and speed tissue healing.

The advantage of vaginal/perineal massage is that it increases circulation and makes tissues supple, healthier, and more liable to stretch easily. Some women feel awkward about massaging themselves, but this anxiety can often be alleviated with some instruction and gentle encouragement.

Sometimes women prefer their partner's help with this. Massage often flows into lovemaking and that's fine; fingers and/or penis make for great vaginal massage. But sexual interaction is not essential preparation for birth, especially if unpleasant emotions inhibit letting go. An expectant mother's relationship with her baby is unique and distinct from that with her partner. She can feel more or less open to him/her sexually, and still respond completely to the eroticism of giving birth.

Sometime in the last few weeks of pregnancy, it's a good idea to **carefully examine the mother's external genitals** so if tearing occurs, you have some idea of how she looked previously and can more easily approximate tissues. Many women have caruncles—hymenal skin tags irregular in shape—which can confuse your suturing efforts. And check for any scar tissue from previous repair that might require extra attention/support during perineal distension.

HOME VISITS

Home visits are obviously an essential part of home birth preparation. It is good to do at least two; one early in pregnancy to see the mother and her supporters in their own element, and another around 35 weeks to be sure that supplies are in and last-minute concerns are fully addressed. An extra home visit may be wise if a woman complains of problems at home, or reports feeling unsettled in her environment. It's also a good idea when her partner hasn't come to prenatals for a while, whatever the reason.

The last home visit should probably include a review of prepared childbirth techniques; this is especially critical if the expectant mother and her partner have not had classes. School-aged children can be included in dinner discussions, then afterwards can feel mom's belly and listen to the baby's heartbeat. Every member of the birth team should be present at this gathering, so that roles can be clearly delineated in advance.

Use this visit to appraise the home for order and cleanliness, and see that a table top or some other protected area will be available for laying out supplies. One of your most crucial assessments is for *adequate heat in the birthing room*— newborns quickly lose body heat, and are almost impossible to resuscitate if cold. And appraise sleeping arrangements for baby; beware of the crib or cradle in a separate part of the house. Emphasize the importance of skin-to-skin contact in the early weeks, and debunk fears about bringing the baby to bed. You might come prepared with handouts or other reading material, should your discussion progress to baby care or other postpartum concerns.

If the mother has felt shy or awkward with vaginal exams at your office, perhaps her own bed will be better. If she agrees, her children might be allowed to watch so they will be less likely to be alarmed at intimate procedures during the birth.

This is a perfect time to discuss any unresolved concerns the expectant mother or her partner may be harboring with regard to the birth. Because this is a leisurely visit and the mother is in her own environment, she may become more vulnerable than ever before and reveal her deepest fears. Consider this visit time well spent, as the birth may be shorter and smoother because of it. The main purpose of this visit is to affirm the mother's home as the birth place, and to inspire confidence and intimacy among the entire support team.

LAST-MINUTE CLIENTS

What about mothers calling for help just weeks before their due date? In general, the last-minute scramble to obtain all necessary information and develop intimacy in short order will challenge even the most competent midwife. If the expectant mother has had previous care and her records are available, your task is less daunting. Without prenatal records, you have no established maternal or fetal baselines from which to extrapolate norms during labor. And if her dates are at all uncertain, you have no point of reference regarding the baby's maturity except its current size. You also have very little time to assess the mother's needs and expectations of you, or to assert your own. All this increases your liability, and you must decide if the additional effort and risk can be justified.

Your decision to assist must be based on a strong sense of rapport, and the conviction that the mother and her supporters are utterly committed to home birth. If they are coming to you from another midwife's care, explore their reasons carefully to make sure they're not just chasing rainbows. Get right down to it: what do they want from you? Make a home visit as soon as possible, and schedule longer clinic appointments. You must still cover all essential information on emergency care, the mechanics of labor, and birthing techniques. Some last-minute clients expect a major

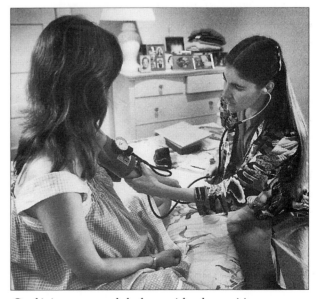
Combining a prenatal check-up with a home visit.

discount; explain that providing care in these short-order circumstances requires a challenging condensation of your services.

Tina, a midwife practicing in rural Hawaii, shared this tale of assisting a true last-minute client. Her account also serves to exemplify how the midwife's work can overflow into her personal, home and family life:

This lady-in-waiting called me two days after her due date—I'd met her before, and I said sure, I'd find time to see her. But I made no promises, as I'm wary of "last-minute goodies." She had no support, no man, not even a place to call home. She'd seen a doctor three times, but didn't feel comfortable or prepared for the hospital situation.

There she was on my doorstep; I had just returned from one of my huge food shopping expeditions. So I put the groceries away, made some tea, sat down with the woman and felt out the situation. She looked pretty tense, had been having contractions all night but didn't want to go to the hospital. She didn't even know if she wanted to keep the child. Very much alone, she felt she had other things to do with her life besides mothering. But she did have enough incentive to give the baby a good beginning with a natural birth and breast milk. She also was willing to give herself some time to feel out motherhood.

It was early afternoon, and I got the feeling that she was definitely in labor and would have her baby that night. But I didn't even know this woman, didn't even know if I liked her! All I knew was that she was confused and I wanted to help her. She couldn't have her baby at my place—too much traffic with five children. So I told her I'd go to the hospital to ease the doctor confrontation and serve as her support person and coach. She seemed relieved with my decision. She took a walk outside in the banana patch for about an hour and came back a different woman: resigned, courageous, strong. She began squatting for most of her now regular contractions. I suggested that she lie down and rest in the loft where it was quiet and where Adrian (my

one-year-old) was sleeping. The older children came in from playing and we gathered around the table for dinner.

No sooner were the dishes cleared than we heard some serious "Oh-oh-ohs" from the loft. I dropped everything and got ready to examine her, but she was already on her way down the ladder saying she had to go to the bathroom. She came back out to kneel on the living room floor and her water bag broke. "Can I check you?" said I. "No, no, no, oh, oh, oh," said she, "I've got to go to the bathroom again." Then she really began complaining, she said she wasn't comfortable at all, couldn't see any point in all this discomfort, wanted to go to the hospital and get drugged out. She got off the toilet and leaned on the sink, but was still pushing.

Uh, oh . . . what's this? Oh god, quick, wash those hands, catch that baby, plop, flop, she's out, gorgeous! Her mother was stunned but finally uttered something, and the baby gave a cry back. Relief, release. I wrapped the babe in a towel, set another towel on the floor so they could lie down, and waited for the placenta. I opened the bathroom door and there were some little faces eager to greet the baby; the children all heard that first cry. Haydon (nine and a half years old) announced that it happened at two minutes to eight. Chana (eight years old) got a blanket for the baby. Nara (six years old) got my birth kit so I could clamp the cord, and also a bowl for the placenta. Then I announced bed-time but of course I wasn't heeded; the excitement was too much.

I assisted the mother with baby holding and bonding and the placenta came out fine. "Now," I thought, "if I can just get them up off this floor and onto a bed in the living room to check for tears . . . hmm, well, she was standing and there was no support." So after a good nursing session I suggested she go to the hospital to be sutured and stay for a few days. She would rest better there and wouldn't have to think about her personal care for a while.

They came to stay with us for several weeks before finally leaving the island. We really fell in love with the baby—it was quite an experience for all of us.

SELF-CARE IN PREGNANCY

Prenatal care is more than just the checkups you receive from your practitioner every few weeks—it is the care you *give yourself* each and every day! Here are some of the main components of self-care in pregnancy, with a rating system to help you see how well you are doing. Enter one of the following with each category:

4: Do this automatically, naturally
3: Do this consistently but with definite effort
2: Do this occasionally, with some resistance
1: Just can't seem to do this, or haven't thus far

Nutrition

_____ Eat from the four basic food groups daily
_____ Take supplements that I know I need
_____ Drink at least two quarts of water, juice, etc. per day
_____ Pay attention to my inner voice of hunger and respond accordingly
_____ Treat myself to something I know is especially good for me and the baby
_____ Indulge myself in favorite foods (that are also healthful) for pure pleasure

Exercise and Relaxation

_____ Take fresh air and (if available) sunshine daily
_____ Do something to work up a sweat each day
_____ Stretch out my back, legs, shoulders, and neck daily
_____ Do exercises specific to pregnancy several times a week
_____ Dance, move rhythmically and freely with music
_____ Do vaginal exercises daily
_____ Completely let go at least once every day
_____ Practice progressive relaxation at least twice a week
_____ Have my partner (or someone else) massage me at least once weekly
_____ Dress in clothing that allows freedom of movement and is comfortable
_____ Deliberately release areas where I know I hold tension, several times daily
_____ Allow myself the necessary comforts to curl up and take it easy before bed

Emotional Wellbeing

_____ Let myself cry whenever I feel like it
_____ Ask for support, acknowledgment, touch, sex from my partner whenever I need it (if applicable)
_____ Vent my frustrations before they become explosive
_____ Feel free to be loving and tender with my partner (if applicable) day-by-day
_____ Feel loving and tender with myself at least once each day
_____ Give myself time alone, and find new ways to enjoy it

Intellectual Preparation

_____ Read something on pregnancy at least once a week

_____ Formulate and ask questions of my care provider

_____ Take stock of my status in pregnancy by reviewing my daily or weekly activities and looking for areas that need improvement

_____ Discuss technical aspects of pregnancy, birth, and parenting with my partner and/or supporters on a regular basis

_____ Work on developing my birth plan by noting ideas and preferences as that arise

_____ Attend information sessions or film series on birth whenever possible

Social Preparation

_____ Meet with other pregnant women at least once a week

_____ Talk to mothers of infants or pregnant women in public places

_____ Observe infant behavior and family interaction whenever possible

_____ Ask for concrete support from friends and relatives for needs in pregnancy and postpartum

_____ Think about the changes having a baby will bring and formulate ways to adapt

_____ Support my partner (if applicable) in talking to other new parents, reading about parenting, or discussing the baby with me.

There are several different ways to score this exercise. First add up your total score in each section; this will give you a general idea of areas where you are strong and those where you could use improvement. Your overall score can be viewed as follows:

110-144: yes, you are enjoying being pregnant and are taking good care of yourself.

80-109: you are doing well enough, but could stand to focus a bit more on the pregnancy. Look carefully at your areas of resistance, and see what you can do to discipline or motivate yourself more.

36-79: well, perhaps you are very busy with other things, but you definitely need to give your pregnancy some attention. Try combining an activity where you scored low with one where you scored high; for example, if you get outside every day but can't seem to take your vitamins, make it a prerequisite before leaving the house (like locking the door, turning off the lights, etc.)

You'll feel much better if you care for yourself regularly!

CHAPTER 3

Problems in Pregnancy

The challenge in caring for problem pregnancies is to differentiate psychological and physical factors, for they often overlap. One must be wary of oversimplifying physiologic complications with a psychosomatic view; on the other hand, emotional disequilibrium for an extended period of time can definitely cause physical illness or jeopardy. The hallmark of a competent midwife is her ability to enlist the expectant mother in unraveling the personal aspects of her condition, while promptly securing medical consultation or assistance as needed.

Physical problems still in incipient stages call upon the midwife to utilize her insight and expertise to formulate, with the mother's assistance, a remedy as holistic as possible, i.e., one combining health-giving physical treatments with self-awareness practices. Safe leeway for finding the most effective remedy always depends on close and continued surveillance of the mother's condition. Whenever pregnancy becomes complicated, prenatal checkups should be scheduled more frequently—perhaps as often as every few days, with phone contact in the interim. Don't hesitate to consult with another experienced midwife or another expert within your network of health care providers.

The following section on physical complications will not address every pathological condition of pregnancy, but will focus on those pertinent to low-risk women already established as good candidates for home birth.

For more information, consult a medical textbook or your backup physician.

PHYSICAL COMPLICATIONS

ANEMIA

Nutritional anemia is common in pregnancy, due partly to dietary quirks and partly to the normal physiology of pregnancy. Iron-deficiency anemia, which accounts for 95 percent of nutritional anemias, is caused by a diet specifically low in iron. However, supplemental iron is seldom enough to remedy the problem. Adequate protein is necessary to build new red blood cells, and adequate folic acid must be available to maintain the integrity of cell membranes. Vitamin C is crucial for iron absorption, whereas dairy products interfere and must be taken separately. If stress is a factor, vitamin C, the B-complex vitamins, and trace minerals may also be depleted, and increased intake is advisable. The best approach is to dramatically revamp and improve the entire diet by adding more fresh fruit and vegetables, high-quality protein, whole grains, mineral-rich seeds and nuts, and nourishing herbal teas.

Take care with iron supplements, as this mineral is toxic in large quantities. I recommend ferrous peptonate or gluconate, in low doses (25 to 50 mg.) spread throughout the day, and no more than 100 mg. total. Supplemental iron is difficult to assimilate; often, no more than a third is absorbed. The unused portion can irritate the kidneys and intestines and cause indigestion, constipation, and black stools. This is particularly true of ferrous sulfate. If the mother is vegan, she can try one of several brands of iron which contain no animal products.

If a woman is anemic in early pregnancy (HCT <33 or HGB <11), suggest 100 mg. iron taken with 500 mg. vitamin C each day. Repeat blood work in three to four weeks. An extremely anemic woman may benefit from higher doses of vitamin C and iron, but emphasize dietary changes too. Good food sources for iron include prunes and prune juice, molasses, almonds, raisins, dark greens, and liver (organic is best). Around 28 weeks, HCT/HGB readings may dip temporarily due to hemodilution, i.e., increased blood volume causing a relative decrease in the percentage of red cells. For this reason, all women should be checked for **physiologic anemia** at the beginning of the last trimester, and advised as indicated to bring the HCT/HGB to optimal levels by the time of the birth. Remember that it takes several weeks to build red cells, and effective therapy for one woman may do nothing for the next.

Anemia creates numerous problems for the mother. Fatigue and diminished vitality affect her appetite, her resistance to infection, and her general enjoyment of pregnancy. She is more susceptible to premature labor. And labor itself may be prolonged, complicated by incoordinate uterine action and maternal exhaustion. Once her uterus is tired, it is less likely to contract efficiently after delivery and she is at risk for postpartum hemorrhage. And with less oxygen-carrying red blood cells in her system, she may go into shock more rapidly than normal. To top it off, anemia can be particularly devastating in the postpartum period, as it renders the new mother more susceptible to infection, poor healing, difficulties with establishing a milk supply, and postpartum depression.

The baby of an anemic mother may be growth-retarded or lack sufficient body fat, important for its insulation and stress-resistance during the early weeks. Normally, it will store enough iron in the last six weeks of pregnancy for its first six months of life, but if the mother's intake is inadequate, she may have to begin feeding solids before either she or the baby are ready. During labor, fetal distress and/or need for immediate resuscitation may occur due to decreased oxygen levels in the maternal bloodstream. For all of these reasons, a woman wanting home birth should strive to keep her HCT/HGB levels up throughout most of her pregnancy.

Before treating the mother for iron-deficiency anemia, double check the blood work to rule out a 5 percent chance of megaloblastic anemia, caused by a deficiency of either folic acid or vitamin B-12. How do you identify this problem? Take a look at her prenatal panel, and notice the figures given in the MCV, MCH, and MCHC categories. **MCV/Mean Corpuscular Volume** indicates the average size of her red blood cells. **MCH/Mean Corpuscular Hemoglobin** indicates the average amount of hemoglobin per cell. **MCHC/Mean Corpuscular Hemoglobin Concentration** indicates amount of hemoglobin per cell relative to cell size. In iron-deficiency anemia, the MCV is normal but MCH and MCHC are lower than usual; this type of anemia is a microcytic (small cell) anemia. In B-12 and folic acid anemias, the MCV is elevated but the MCH and MCHC are normal; these anemias are macrocytic (large cell) anemias.

If it appears the expectant mother suffers from a macrocytic/megaloblastic anemia, further testing will be necessary to determine whether a deficiency of folic acid or B-12 is at fault. In the meantime, carefully reassess the mother's diet. Sources of folic acid include egg yolks, orange juice, and all dark greens like spinach, chard, kale, collard greens—the darker the green, the better. Four large servings of the above per day would barely be enough to remedy a minor deficiency during pregnancy. So advise the mother to combine food sources with supplemental folic acid, about 2400 mcg. daily. Folic acid is vital to cell production, and deficiency can lead to neural tube defects, like spina bifida (see Chapter Five).

B-12 is found almost exclusively in dairy foods and animal products and will therefore be lacking in the diet of complete vegetarians unless a supplement is taken. This vitamin is important in the formation of all body systems, and correct replication of the genetic code within each cell. B-12 deficiency is associated with central nervous system damage in the newborn, and should the deficiency persist into childhood, there will be slow, insidious and irreversible brain damage by the fifth year. Thus it is absolutely essential for all vegetarian mothers to be certain of adequate intake. This is often a touchy point because most vegans dislike supplements in general, and believe their diets to be perfect. Regardless, B-12 supplements are absolutely necessary, and will be virtually useless unless specifically designed to be taken sublingually. Absorption of supplemental B-12 is negligible via the digestive tract, and in severe cases of deficiency, intramuscular injections are the only remedy.

There are certain types of hereditary, microcytic anemias such as thalassemia or sickle cell anemia that may render MCV values unusually low. If the MCV is below 80, and the woman is of African, Mediterranean, or Asian descent, consider ordering a hemoglobin electophoresis, a test which determines normal hemoglobin.

PROBLEMS WITH WEIGHT GAIN

Determining whether weight gain during pregnancy is either inadequate or excessive depends partly on pre-pregnant weight. The average weight gain in pregnancy is about a pound per week; underweight women may gain more, and overweight women may gain less. In either case, intensive nutritional counseling may be necessary to assure that adequate nutrients and calories are taken during pregnancy. As a rule of thumb, the expectant mother should gain at least ten pounds by 20 weeks.

What causes weight gain in pregnancy? There is increased water retention due to hormones, increased fatty insulation deposited over belly and backside, increased weight in the breasts, increased blood volume, plus the obvious weight of the enlarged uterus including amniotic fluid, placenta, and fetus. Most women lose an average of fifteen pounds at delivery or a few days thereafter; the remainder is used for sustenance during the first few months postpartum. Making breast milk, getting up several times a night to nurse, and dealing with the stress of a new baby definitely burn up the fat reserves!

If a woman seems to be gaining weight more rapidly than usual, check for a fetal growth spurt. It's not unusual to see a gain of five pounds in two weeks linked to a corresponding increase of three or four centimeters in fundal height. Occasionally, the mother gains weight *just before* a growth spurt, so wait a week or two before jumping to conclusions. Double check her diet to see if she's made any deleterious changes (perhaps due to something she has read or heard). If so, reiterate nutritional basics, and remind her to heed her instinctive sense of hunger. Excess sugar intake may signal a need for more protein. Suggest she have vegetable snacks instead of highly caloric fruits and juices; see what fruit she likes, and find a vegetable with equivalent vitamin and mineral content. Also recommend low-fat protein sources like cottage cheese, fish, or chicken breast in place of high-fat sources like ice cream or hard cheese. Be sensitive to the expectant mother's response to your ideas, and try to work positively around her attachment to certain foods.

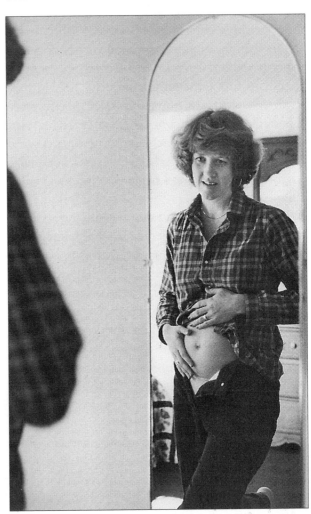

Your pregnant body takes some getting used to, but once you feel the baby move it all makes sense.

A woman with a history of eating disorders may require additional care from an expert. Anorexic women often have great difficulty conceiving, and may also have problems maintaining the pregnancy. Women with recent history of bulimia face similar challenges. Even when pregnancy seems to be well established, increased appetite combined with changing body image may re-activate prior eating disorders. Women who have suffered from bulimia are particularly at risk for hyperemesis gravidarium, and women who have been anorexic, for malnutrition. Schedule prenatal visits more frequently, and plan to see the expectant mother in her home (where you can share meals together) as often as possible.

Any woman who claims she must "watch her weight" should be taken seriously. If she defines eating as an out-of-control, emotionally-based activity, she may never learn to trust her instincts for nourishing herself and her child. She may have strong feelings of guilt associated with eating, and may have suffered years of criticism from family or friends regarding her appearance. Do take history in this regard, but don't dwell on the negative aspects. Encourage her to bring variety to her diet, honor cravings for treats from time to time, and find some type of physical activity she can embrace. Brisk walking is a good beginning; prenatal exercise classes are ideal.

How about the underweight woman who doesn't seem able to gain much during pregnancy? She may be somewhat hyperactive, used to running around constantly, more or less "living on air." Help her slow down enough to tune into her pregnant body, particularly if she shows any nervous symptoms such as insomnia, dizziness, or fainting. Your slender client may love fresh squeezed juices, raw vegetables and vegetable proteins like tofu and nuts, but unless she gets enough calories each day, she will not look and feel her best. Thin women often complain of feeling bloated, heavy, or "clogged-up" with more food, especially carbohydrates. Suggest smaller meals, with an extra one at bedtime. Encourage continuous snacking throughout the day, with baggies full of goodies in her purse or car at all times. Explain that her body makes nourishing the baby a priority, and if she is underweight, she has little to spare for herself. Thus she is at risk for anemia, preeclampsia, premature labor, prolonged labor, postpartum hemorrhage, poor recovery, and postpartum depression. With her cooperation, set a goal of around 25 pounds weight gain.

The expectant mother's partner must also understand her liability with inadequate food intake; see that he/she understands the nutritional demands of pregnancy and is fully supportive. Make sure the mother is not dieting or trying to control her weight in order to please her partner! Discuss the physical transformation of pregnancy with both of them, emphasizing positive aspects of rosier complexion, fuller, more sensitive breasts, warm pregnant glow, and increased sexual appetites.

Miscarriage (Abortion)

The proper technical term for miscarriage occurring before 20 weeks is **spontaneous abortion**—beyond this point, it is termed **fetal demise**. In the vast majority of cases, the cause of spontaneous abortion is abnormal development of the fetus or placenta due to chromosomal abnormalities. Less commonly, a mother may miscarry due to viral infection, severe malnutrition, substance abuse, or an antibody effect towards the father's sperm.

Threatened abortion is presumed whenever the mother has vaginal bleeding in the first half of pregnancy, particularly if combined with cramping or persistent backache. But keep in mind that one in four women experience bleeding in the first trimester, while only one in ten actually abort. With threatened miscarriage, blood loss may be either dramatic, or slight but continuous for days/weeks. **Inevitable abortion** ensues if the membranes rupture or if the cervix dilates.

Is there any intervention that can keep a threatened miscarriage from becoming inevitable? Probably not, but certain measures may be worth a try. If symptoms are acute, recommend bedrest and complete cessation of all sexual activity. If there is cramping without bleeding, a glass of wine may halt uterine activity and forestall miscarriage. But if it does become inevitable, console the mother as best you can, and focus on helping her through the physical aspects of the process.

If she wishes to go through her miscarriage at home, be certain she is not anemic and keep close watch for possible hemorrhage. *Two cups of blood is the maximum safe blood loss.* If miscarriage extends for more than a day or two, the mother is at risk for infection and must check her temperature several times daily. Persistent bleeding or pain are signs she must see a physician to determine whether the abortion is complete, i.e., everything has been shed. She may also wish to save remnants of her miscarriage (commonly referred to as "the products of conception") and have them tested for possible causative factors.

Occasionally, women have light bleeding for many weeks with no distinct episode of resolution. This may be due to **missed abortion**, i.e., the fetus has died but is retained in utero. The mother may notice that her breasts have returned to their normal size, or that she has lost several pounds. Upon examination, her uterus may seem scarcely normal sized, or may be small for dates. The most conclusive sign of missed abortion is lack of fetal activity and/or heart tones.

In case of suspected missed abortion, it is important to make a determination via sonogram as soon as possible. Although rare before 20 weeks, coagulation disorders such as **disseminated intravascular coagulation** (DIC) may result from retained products of conception, seriously complicating the termination of pregnancy with risks of catastrophic internal bleeding. The incidence of DIC increases exponentially the longer the mother has been pregnant, and the longer the fetus is retained after it has died. If a client with signs of missed abortion notes excessive bleeding from the gums, nose, or minor injury sites, she is extremely high risk. Have her seen by a backup physician immediately.

I've had one case of missed abortion in my practice. The mother came for her first visit at eighteen weeks, reporting brown spotting for the last week or so. She did have a history of previous miscarriage, although she also delivered a baby at term (whose birth I assisted several years earlier).

Her uterus felt normal sized for dates. I couldn't hear the baby with the fetascope but was not concerned, as this is often the case until 20 weeks. At 20 weeks, she came in again and reported what she thought was fetal movement, but the brown discharge had been almost continuous since her last visit. This time I was alarmed at not finding the fetal heart, and although the uterus felt slightly larger than the last visit, I sent her for a sonogram. She called from the hospital to report a missed abortion; it was unclear exactly when the fetus had died, but development appeared to have arrested at 12 weeks. She was screened for DIC and was negative, but immediately scheduled a therapeutic abortion because she couldn't stand the agony of waiting.

For any type of miscarriage, emotional support and counseling are crucial in follow up. Women often express guilt over some behavior or attitude they think may have caused the miscarriage, and many are anxious about their future prospects of carrying to term. Occasionally, miscarriage is **habitual**, i.e., occurs more than three times, in which case genetic or other factors may be at fault. Refer a woman or couple with this problem for consultation with a specialist.

Studies show that women grieve as deeply with miscarriage as they do with fetal demise, stillbirth, and neonatal death. Feelings of shame, guilt, and embarrassment are common, and need to be validated and worked through. *Ended Beginnings* (Panuthos and Romeo) is an excellent reference in this regard. Support groups for women who have miscarried may also be available through your local birth resource center.

ECTOPIC PREGNANCY

Ectopic pregnancy refers to implantation occurring outside the uterine cavity. Ninety-five percent of the time, the blastocyst implants in one of the fallopian tubes. Depending on the portion of the tube in which implantation occurs, the fetus may either be expelled into the abdominal cavity as it grows too large or may cause the tube to rupture, usually between 10 and 13 weeks. This is a serious, life-threatening complication. With tubal rupture, the mother will lose the baby and is at risk for severe internal hemorrhage, which may lead to shock or even death. Ectopic pregnancy and/or rupture may be misdiagnosed as pelvic inflammatory disease, severe gastro-intestinal upset, or appendicitis, particularly if the woman does not yet know she is pregnant.

The primary cause of tubal pregnancy is pelvic inflammatory disease, which leaves behind scar tissue that may partially occlude the tube, cause reduced ciliation and/or the formation of blind pockets. Ectopic pregnancies have more than doubled in recent years due to the prevalence of sexually transmitted diseases, trauma from intrauterine devices, and infection following abortion. Prior ectopic rupture and reconstructive surgery (tuboplasty) also predispose a woman to ectopic pregnancy.

Symptoms of tubal pregnancy include pelvic pain (more than cramping) and often, spot bleeding. (One of my colleagues, whose practice has had more than its share of ectopic pregnancies, now routinely does a bimanual exam on any woman with first trimester bleeding to look for uterine enlargement and rule out any luteal/pelvic masses.) Pain becomes quite severe with actual rupture, and may be referred to the shoulder area. A definite sign that the mother is suffering from tubal rupture (as opposed to miscarriage) is that the degree of shock far exceeds what would normally be expected for the amount of blood loss.

If an expectant mother calls to report symptoms that lead you to suspect tubal pregnancy and/or rupture, contact your backup physician immediately and have her call an ambulance for transport. Even if per initial phone consultation, avoid sending her to the emergency room as the wait may be life-threatening.

Emotional recovery from tubal pregnancy is complex. The woman is faced with the fact that she has nearly lost her life, along with what may have been a long awaited child. Her future fertility will likely be affected. And her partner may struggle with multiple shocks of finding her pregnant, nearly losing her, then losing the baby. See to it that the women and her partner are offered counseling and support.

HYDATIDIFORM MOLE

This extremely rare complication occurs in one per 1500 pregnancies in the United States. The hydatidiform (high-duh-tit´-uh-form) mole is an abnormal development of the chorionic villi, which ordinarily form the membranes and placenta, but in this case become a mass of clear, grape-like vesicles filling the uterus. In 95 percent of cases, hydatidiform mole appears to be caused by an abnormal sperm inactivating the chromosomes of the ovum. This is called a **complete mole**, and there is no fetus. In the remaining 5 percent of cases, there is fetal tissue present, though chromosomes from sperm and ovum are abnormal in number. This is called a **partial mole**. Molar pregnancy is more common in women over 40.

Light brown bleeding is the most outstanding symptom, persisting for weeks or even months (though rarely past the first trimester). What distinguishes hydatidiform mole from other complications correlated to light brown bleeding (such as missed abortion or ectopic pregnancy) is that the uterus is generally large for dates, and feels woody hard or doughy to the touch. Blood work shows abnormally high HCG levels (which are typically subnormal with missed abortion and ectopic pregnancy).

Hyperemesis occurs in 25 to 30 percent of all cases, but tends to develop later than usual in pregnancy, generally at the onset of the second trimester. The mole almost always aborts spontaneously, but occasionally must be surgically removed. Approximately 10 to 20 percent of molar pregnancies progress to invasive cancer, thus follow-up examination and testing are necessary for at least a year. (A former student of mine related that during her training as a nurse-midwife, she took care of a woman who had metastasis to her brain from cancer originating in molar pregnancy!) If you suspect hydatidiform mole, refer to a physician promptly.

As with ectopic pregnancy, attend also to the mother's emotional recovery, or need for psychological support.

BLEEDING LATE IN PREGNANCY

Occasionally, vaginal bleeding a bit heavier than spotting occurs after intercourse in the second or third trimester. The cervix has increased vascularity during pregnancy and is often quite friable, i.e., easily abraded with friction. If the mother also has a vaginal infection, the mucosa will be irritable and additionally prone to bleeding during and after sex.

Another possible source of bleeding is a **ruptured cervical polyp.** Polyps are small, tongue-like protrusions at the cervical os, visible by speculum exam. Bleeding from a ruptured polyp is sudden and somewhat dramatic, but tends to resolve quickly and completely. However, if blood loss is significant and persistent in the second or third trimesters, it is probably due to either placental abruption or placenta praevia.

Placental abruption refers to a premature separation of the placenta. It may be caused by cord entanglement, multiparity, smoking, or physical trauma. Forty percent of cases are linked to hypertension or preeclampsia. There are several types of abruption. **Marginal abruption** refers to separation at the edge of the placenta only, causing blood to flow from the vagina. **Concealed abruption** refers to separation of the center portion of the placenta while margins remain attached, so that bleeding is concealed. **Complete abruption** refers to total separation of the placenta. These are all rare, particularly the last. Fortunately so, because abruption may prove fatal for the baby, and sometimes for the mother. If abruption occurs during labor and delivery is imminent, the fetus will probably survive and the mother will be fine. But if it occurs late in pregnancy or early in labor, even emergency cesarean delivery may not be quick enough to save the baby, and depending on the degree of abruption, the mother's life may also be in jeopardy.

Symptoms of abruption vary depending on degree. In cases of concealed abruption, bleeding is not evident but there is acute abdominal pain, distinct from that of uterine contractions in its persistence and location. The uterus is woody hard and exceedingly tender to the touch. With marginal abruption, bright red bleeding is apparent but abdominal pain may be less noticeable, partic-ularly in hard labor. In either case, the mother should be rushed to the hospital, unless she is about to deliver. Administer oxygen and treat her for shock with feet elevated, head down and body warmed with blankets.

Repeated episodes of light bleeding or heavy spotting with no report of abdominal pain may indicate **placenta praevia,** i.e., placenta implanted low in the uterus. Why does blood loss occur in this case? In late pregnancy, the lower uterine segment begins to thin and distend as the presenting part of the baby enters the pelvis; if the placenta is imbedded in this area, small portions will detach whenever underlying uterine tissues stretch. There are varying degrees of placenta praevia: **total praevia,** in which the placenta completely covers the cervical os; **partial praevia,** in which the os is partially covered; **marginal praevia,** in which the edge of the placenta is at the edge of the os, and **low-lying placenta,** in which the placenta is close to the os but does not actually reach it.

Prospects for vaginal birth depend on the location of the placenta at the onset of labor. Total and partial praevia necessitate cesarean delivery. A marginal praevia will inevitably separate as the cervix dilates, and depending on degree of maternal blood loss, may also require cesarean section. Vaginal delivery is more likely with a low-lying placenta, but maternal blood loss must be carefully monitored. Placenta praevia is also associated with an increased risk of postpartum hemorrhage, due to poor contractability of the lower uterine segment.

Placenta praevia may manifest as early as 24 weeks. If so, the placenta will appear to migrate upwards as the lower uterine segment develops with advancing pregnancy. I had one case like this in my practice; I couldn't believe this client's bleeding was due to praevia because it occurred so early. The mother was put at bedrest for a number of weeks until a sonogram showed that the placenta was out of the way, and she had a perfectly normal vaginal delivery.

Diagnosis of placenta praevia must always be done by sonogram. As *Williams Obstetrics* admonishes, "Examination of the cervix is never permissible unless the woman is in the operating room with all the preparations for immediate cesarean section, since even the gentlest examination of this sort can cause torrential hemorrhage." *Never, never do a vaginal exam when there is bleeding in late pregnancy!* Have the mother suspend all sexual activity until a diagnosis is made.

GESTATIONAL DIABETES

As *Williams Obstetrics* clearly states, "Gestational diabetes is a diagnosis still looking for a disease." This term for decreased glucose tolerance during pregnancy was coined in 1979, when blood glucose levels for pregnant women (as distinct from the general population) were first established. The validity of these levels remains controversial, as the samplings on which they were based included pregnant women at high risk and in poor health, as well as pre-diagnosed diabetics. No screening was done with regard to diet—even the abnormally low fasting glucose levels of women suffering from malnutrition were used to establish baselines. The data do show a correlation between elevated blood glucose levels in pregnancy and a tendency to develop diabetes later in life, but no correlation to increased risk for the fetus or other prenatal/intrapartal complications. The midwife's greatest concern is that if a client in her care has an abnormally high glucose screen, conservative medical protocol may determine this woman to be high risk and no longer suitable for home birth, or may funnel her into an excessive regimen of risk screening which may negatively affect her experience of pregnancy and ability to labor with confidence.

Gestational diabetes is said to complicate from 2 to 5 percent of all pregnancies. Predisposing factors are thought to be family history of diabetes, unexplained fetal death or stillbirth, obesity, recurrent candida (yeast infection), polyhydramnios, preeclampsia, recurrent glucosuria, age over 35 years, large baby in utero, or previous delivery of large baby (over nine lbs.). Significantly, the supposed correlation between gestational diabetes and stillbirth has recently been disproven. Common sense dictates that a combination of the above factors plus others—such as poor nutrition, smoking, substance abuse, or high stress levels—might indicate a need for testing. This is a moot point, though, as far as the medical standard of care is concerned; glucose screening is routine at 28 weeks. Many midwives consider this to be just another profit-generating, malpractice-averting diagnostic trend (similar to the bilirubin testing craze of the early 1980s).

There are several tests typically used to screen for gestational diabetes. The most common is the **glucose screen**: the mother ingests 50 mg. liquid glucose and her blood is drawn an hour later. This test renders an exceptionally high number of false positives. Nevertheless, if the mother's blood glucose exceeds 140 mg./dl., she is usually referred for an **oral glucose tolerance test** (OGTT). After fasting the night before and up until test time, her blood is drawn to establish baseline glucose levels, and she then ingests 100 mg. glucose syrup. In the commonly used three-hour OGTT, blood is drawn at one, two, and three hours. During this time, the mother must not eat or smoke. If two of the following levels (using whole blood, not plasma) are met or exceeded, a diagnosis is made:
1) fasting, above 90 mg./dl.;
2) one hour, above 165 mg./dl.;
3) two hours, above 145 mg./dl.;
4) three hours, above 125 mg./dl.

Many women report nausea, vomiting, headache, bloating, or profuse sweating with liquid glucose. An alternative, published in *The American Journal of Obstetrics and Gynecology*, is the **jelly bean test**, with 18 jelly beans substituted for 50 mg. glucola.

The most reliable test is probably **the two hour post prandial**. If a fasting blood sample is desired as baseline, the mother must eat nothing for twelve hours. Then, after eating a full meal high in calories and complex carbohydrates, she has blood drawn two hours later. Readings will be more accurate if she exercises lightly after eating. Normal levels are 120 to 140 mg./dl.

If diabetes is present in pregnancy, the most obvious effect is **macrosomia**, or baby large for gestational age. Because glucose readily crosses the placental barrier, even mild degrees of elevated maternal blood sugar can cause a significant rise in the baby. The fetal pancreas reacts by greatly increasing production of insulin, which leads to an increase in growth. The baby of a diabetic mother is therefore at risk for size-related complications during delivery (such as shoulder dystocia), and may also develop respiratory distress (increased fetal insulin interrupts the production of surfactant in the lungs). It may also have severe problems with **hypoglycemia** (low blood sugar) or **hypocalcemia** (low calcium levels) after the birth.

Negative effects of maternal diabetes include a four times greater chance of developing preeclampsia, ten times greater incidence of polyhydramnios, and a high risk of postpartum hemorrhage.

Treatment for diabetes in pregnancy depends on degree; in severe cases, insulin therapy is recommended. Nutritional therapy is central; a diet very high in protein and complex carbohydrates, with ample calories and limited sugars, is usually recommended. Chromium picolinate supplements are reported to helpful. Regular, aerobic exercise is also encouraged. Blood sugar levels are tested daily to ensure the diet is working. Monitoring of the fetus via non-stress testing and/or biophysical profile begins around 36 weeks (see section on Postmaturity, this chapter, for more information).

HYPERTENSION

Hypertension/high blood pressure may manifest in several ways during pregnancy. Essential hypertension is a preexisting condition indicated by initial and subsequent readings of 140/90. Gestational hypertension is high blood pressure which develops during pregnancy, usually after 28 weeks. These two types can be confused if a woman begins care in her last trimester, and hypertension is detected. In this case, you must obtain records of previous care, either during the pregnancy or before. Home birth is contraindicated for the woman with essential hypertension, and may be contraindicated by gestational hypertension, depending on degree. *Note: I have deliberately avoided the use of more common terminology for gestational hypertension, pregnancy-induced hypertension or PIH, because most texts use this term as synonymous with preeclampsia. It has been my experience that hypertension can exist independently of other clinical signs of preeclampsia.*

Keep in mind that blood pressure fluctuates dramatically with emotional upheaval and tension.

In *Holistic Midwifery*, Frye mentions a study done by K. Dalton at Cambridge University, showing fluctuations as great as 40 points systolic and 22 points diastolic in ten minute intervals! Therefore, no conclusions should be drawn unless readings are high on at least two occasions a full six hours apart. It helps to do repeat readings with the woman on her left side, as this position serves to induce relaxation and is thought to render the greatest accuracy.

To some degree, hypertension is relative to a woman's baseline readings. A rise of 30 points systolic pressure is considered definitive, as is a rise of 15 points in the diastolic reading. Thus a woman with baseline pressure of 90/60 might be diagnosed hypertensive by an otherwise normal finding of 120/76. But be sure to use first trimester baselines when applying this rule, as second trimester readings may be considerably lower than usual due to vascular relaxation/vasodilation.

Severe and prolonged hypertension may cause intrauterine growth retardation, as attendant vasoconstriction can affect the flow of oxygen (and nutrients) to the baby. For the same reason, elevated blood pressure during labor can cause fetal distress. If readings rise to 160/100, medical intervention will be necessary to prevent severe vascular damage from occurring. Therefore, any woman showing a consistent rise in blood pressure during pregnancy, no matter how slight, should be treated to prevent the problem from progressing. Here are some suggestions:

1. **Exercise is critical** whenever the pressure is just starting to rise, and as long as it is no more than moderately elevated. Exercise increases circulation and forces blood vessels to stretch and dilate, which reduces the pressure inside them. Most effective are aerobic activities, such as brisk walking, hiking, or swimming. Have the mother start out slowly, depending on what she is used to. One of my midwife colleagues advises all of her clients to work up a sweat every day, as a preventative measure.

If blood pressure goes above 140/90, rest takes precedence over physical conditioning. The mother should lie on her left side for extended periods, to allow optimal uptake of oxygen.

2. **Deep relaxation** goes hand in hand with exercise. Women who live in a state of chronic tension may have little experience of complete release for days at a time, even while sleeping. Relaxation practice can help relieve tension in the voluntary muscles, which in turn reduces tension in the involuntary system. A calm state of being also contributes to emotional stability, which helps prevent extreme reactions to challenging situations.

3. **No stimulants whatsoever.** These include coffee, black tea, certain carbonated beverages, chocolate, nicotine, and cocaine. The last two in particular have been proven to cause vasoconstriction and low birth weight. Strong spices like mustard, black pepper, ginger, and nutmeg should also be avoided.

4. **Good diet and healing herbs** help immensely when used in combination with the above measures. Improper eating and abnormal weight gain place stress on the system; encourage the expectant mother to eat plenty of high-protein, low-fat foods, whole grains/complex carbohydrates, and lots of mineral-rich fresh fruits and vegetables. Watermelon, cucumber, parsley, and onion specifically reduce blood pressure, and garlic is a must. Contrary to popular opinion, salt is a necessary nutrient and should be used according to taste. (See Gail and Tom Brewer's excellent book, *What Every Pregnant Woman Should Know*.)

   Herbs like hops, skullcap, passionflower, hawthorne, and chamomile (listed in order of potency) can be used to induce relaxation; these are perfect for the mother with elevated systolic pressure who mostly needs to calm down. Increased fluids are crucial, as is increased intake of calcium, potassium, and magnesium. In an analysis of nearly 2,500 women, those who took 1,500 to 2,000 milligrams of calcium a day were 70 percent less likely to have hypertension in pregnancy than those who did not take the supplements. Cayenne pepper replicates the effects of aerobic exercise by causing vasodilation and increased circulation. Chinese herbs and acupuncture are also helpful.

5. **Counseling** may be the first step if you're

working with a woman so tense and distracted she can hardly take responsibility for herself. Assist her in getting to the roots of her anxiety—this can release a lot of tension and help her find new enjoyment in the pregnancy. If she is enabled to work through whatever is troubling her and can feel good about herself and her situation, attending to messages from her body won't seem so difficult or overwhelming.

I've had two experiences with gestational hypertension that bear repeating. The first mother made immediate changes in her diet and began exercising every day. Relaxation was difficult for her as she had a very active work schedule that couldn't be altered. But she tried to moderate her activities with a more relaxed attitude and periodic meditation. In a matter of weeks, her blood pressure was down from a high of 150/86 to 120/70. Pride in this accomplishment motivated her to consolidate her new routine. Toward the end of pregnancy, her blood pressure rose again to 136/80; she was experiencing much emotional tension on the job. She began to use relaxant herbs daily, and by her next visit, her blood pressure was back to baseline. Throughout labor, it was steady at 120/70.

The other mother showed a rise in her blood pressure to 130/86 at about 30 weeks. We gave her suggestions concerning diet, relaxation, and exercise to help her nip this problem in the bud, but she was decidedly indifferent. Her diet was not the best—she ate a lot of red meat and refined foods, and was already 35 pounds overweight when pregnancy began. Her blood pressure was 140/90 at her next visit, and she became angry and defiant in response to suggestions of what she might do for it. When we saw her a few days later, readings of 140/100 prompted us to suggest physician consultation. At this, she burst into tears and expressed a flood of anger towards her mate about working too much and neglecting her needs. They asked for more time, and went home seriously resolved to work on their situation. Two days later, her blood pressure was still 140/90 and continued to rise for the next few exams, so we referred her for hospital birth. She was given intravenous magnesium sulfate (standard treatment for hypertension) during labor, and delivered without further complications.

Occasionally you will have a client who manifests a sudden rise in blood pressure just two or three weeks before term, with no other clinical problems. If she is well hydrated and not unduly stressed, don't worry. Recent research suggest this may actually be a healthy compensatory mechanism to increased circulatory volume and other metabolic demands of late pregnancy.

On the other hand, a slow and steady rise to maximum safe levels suggests the mother should give birth promptly at term. If her cervix is ripe/partly effaced, suggest induction via castor-oil, acupuncture, or other non-pharmaceutical means. As soon as contractions begin, check frequently to be sure that her blood pressure is stable. It is also important to listen to the baby to be certain that any elevation in blood pressure is not causing hypoxia.

Often, women troubled with borderline hypertension prenatally show a drop in their readings during labor, a sign that the problem was not really pathological. And it is not uncommon for previously normal pressure to jump as high as 140/90 with the most rigorous transition contractions. But a steady rise during labor may herald preeclampsia or lead to vascular damage, and should not be allowed to continue at home (see Chapter Four for more details).

PREECLAMPSIA

One of the primary purposes of routine prenatal care is to screen for preeclampsia. The exact cause of preeclampsia is unknown, but this dangerous disease poses a threat to the lives of both mother and baby. Early signs include generalized edema, sudden and excessive weight gain, hypertension, and protein in the urine, generally occurring after 26 weeks. **Hemoconcentration** (as revealed by an abnormally high hematocrit) may be the earliest sign, due to reduced blood volume. This is in dramatic contrast to the usual dip in hematocrit readings from hemodilution typical at this stage of pregnancy.

It is currently believed that preeclampsia may be the direct result of protein deficiency/malnutrition. Inadequate albumin in the bloodstream causes fluid to leak from the cells, resulting in decreased blood volume and generalized edema. Reduced blood flow to the kidneys triggers a compensatory rise in blood pressure, and reduced blood flow to the uterus accounts for fetal growth retardation in pregnancy and fetal distress in labor. If hypertension becomes severe, vasospasm and irritation of cell walls cause microthrombi (tiny clots) to form. These micro-thrombi stretch the filtering slits in the kidneys so that large protein molecules begin to slip through, leading to proteinuria. Microthrombi can do significant harm to other parts of the body; they can cause impaired circulation to the liver leading to epigastric pain/liver damage, or in severe cases, can lead to DIC as the body exhausts its clotting factors.

Nutritional guidelines for preventing preeclampsia include a minimum of 80 grams protein daily, combined with ample calories, plenty of complex carbohydrates, and fresh fruits and vegetables. Adequate fluid intake is also crucial. Preeclampsia is suspected when hemoconcentration is noted, and diagnosed when hypertension and an additional sign from the aforementioned list are present on two occasions at least six hours apart. The preeclamptic mother should immediately rest in bed on her left side, while the backup physician is contacted.

Check for edema by observing the mother's hands and face. If present, edema causes facial features to look coarse; the hands and fingers will feel puffy/inflexible, and all rings will usually have been removed. Ankle edema is physiologic and therefore not significant, but edema of the upper shins, breastbone, or sacrum is definitive. Check for the degree of edema by checking for pitting, i.e., press a fingertip into the skin and see whether or not a depression remains. The rating system is as follows: 2mm. depression equals + 1; 4mm. equals + 2; 6mm. equals + 3; 8mm. equals + 4. Pitting of + 2 or greater is a sign of preeclampsia.

When checking for **proteinuria**, the mother should take a clean catch to prevent vaginal discharge from affecting results. This is done by washing the labia/vaginal opening with a towelette, then allowing a bit of urine to flow before collecting the sample. Anything over a trace is significant.

Hyperreflexia is a transitional sign, indicating that preeclampsia has progressed to a more serious stage. Check for hyperreflexia by checking for **clonus**. Have the mother in a sitting position with knees bent. Support her calf with one hand, and dorsiflex her foot (bending toes upward towards her knee). Maintain this hold for a moment, then release. Ordinarily the foot will fall back to its natural position with no extraneous movement; if you notice jerking while it is dorsiflexed or oscillation as it falls, the test is positive. (It is wise to check all reflexes at some point in early pregnancy to establish baselines.)

Once a mother is diagnosed to have preeclampsia, you may be able to co-manage care with her backup physician. She should be seen twice weekly, and should be advised to report any of the following signs that might indicate that her condition has worsened: 1) severe headache; 2) epigastric pain (pain in upper abdomen); 3) visual disturbances; 4) decreased output of urine; 5) extreme nervous irritability; or 6) decrease in fetal movement.

One of my clients became preeclamptic at 37 weeks. I knew it as soon as she walked into my office; her face had that coarse look I'd so often heard about. We had made a home visit in early pregnancy, at which time her diet was clearly excellent. However, just a week ago we'd gone to her house again, and had been served a vegetable dinner with no protein whatsoever. I was concerned and intended to bring it up at this visit, but was obviously too late.

The remarkable thing in this case was the mother's blood pressure; it never went higher than 120/76, but as her baseline was only 98/56, she was clearly hypertensive. We referred her immediately to backup, and alternated visits twice weekly with her physician. Her condition remained borderline—periodic facial edema with blood pressure high but stationary, proteinuria from a trace to + 2. She took bedrest as much as possible, and we transported as soon as labor was established.

What are the dangers of preeclampsia? As mentioned earlier, reduced uterine blood flow may lead to fetal growth retardation and hypoxia/fetal distress in labor. There is also higher incidence of placental abruption (about 8 percent) which can lead to fetal death, or jeopardize the mother's life with severe hemorrhage. If preeclampsia progresses to eclampsia, convulsions in labor may threaten the lives of both mother and baby. A grim picture indeed, but not without hope if dietary changes are made immediately, and the woman is kept under close surveillance by her midwife and backup.

POLYHYDRAMNIOS/HYDRAMNIOS

This is a term referring to excess amniotic fluid. It occurs in approximately 1 percent of all pregnancies, often in conjunction with multiple pregnancy, toxemia, or diabetes. It is also associated with fetal anomalies, particularly with atresia of the esophagus, hydrocephaly, anencephaly, or spina bifida.

Polyhydramnios may occur suddenly and acutely at around 24 weeks, but this is rare. It is more common to notice a slight elevation in fundal height at the onset of the last trimester, with a steady increase in the weeks that follow. Difficulty palpating the baby at a time when it should be snugly filling the uterus may also be noted. Sometimes it is possible to confuse a thick uterine wall with excess fluid; in both cases, heart tones will be difficult to hear and the baby confusing to feel. But polyhydramnios is distinguished by a gelatinous, vibrational quality when palpating, known as **fluid thrill**. This is in direct contrast to the more solid feeling of thick uterine muscle.

A woman with noticeable hydramnios should be seen again in several days regardless of gestation. If you find an additional increase in fluid, send her for a sonogram to determine the cause. She may have twins, or other underlying complications. Once polyhydramnios develops, hospital birth will be necessary unless it is borderline. Polyhydramnios predisposes the woman to serious complications in labor—placental abruption, uterine dysfunction, and postpartum hemorrhage—all due to overdistension of the uterus. Fetal malpresentations and cord prolapse are also common.

I recall my frustration with diagnostic ultrasound as regards one mother I assessed to have a considerable degree of excess fluid, whose sonogram reportedly showed no such thing. Her fundal height was elevated nonetheless from 28 weeks, reaching 42 centimeters at term (with head in the pelvis). Early labor was characterized by spastic, painful incoordinate contractions. We transported, and imagine my feigned surprise when membranes ruptured at the hospital in a quantity sufficient to bring the entire staff running! At this point, the uterus began to work more efficiently, and labor progressed normally. However, the mother sustained a fairly severe postpartum hemorrhage.

Another woman I assisted developed polyhydramnios before I had any idea she might be carrying twins. The extra fluid really alarmed me; her fundal height at 25 weeks was 29 centimeters, a rise of six centimeters in just three weeks, with an accompanying weight gain of nearly eight pounds. Less than a week later, her fundal height had increased three more centimeters, and she had gained three more pounds and was almost impossible to palpate. I made no mention of twins, but she brought up the possibility. Sure enough, her ultrasound showed two babies plus extra fluid within normal range for multiple pregnancy. Two weeks later she went into premature labor, and no wonder, with a fundal height of 39 centimeters at only 28 weeks!

However, not all women carrying twins have excess fluid. Good nutrition and adequate rest can minimize polyhydramnios, along with other side effects of multiple pregnancy such as anemia, varicosities of the legs and vulva, and premature labor. If you are co-managing the care of a woman with polyhydramnios, check her cervix weekly to look for changes that might portend premature labor.

OLIGOHYDRAMNIOS

Oligohydramnios is an abnormally small amount of amniotic fluid. It is often associated with a marked increase in fetal mortality, due to underlying conditions such as intrauterine growth retardation, post-maturity syndrome, and congenital anomalies. Reduced amniotic fluid also renders the fetus more susceptible to cord compression and fetal distress/hypoxia during labor. Amniotic fluid volume varies considerably from woman to woman, but oligohydramnios is readily detectable when the fetus is tightly compacted in the uterus and fundal height is lagging. Continuity of care enables the midwife to notice small fluctuations in amniotic fluid volume without having to resort to serial sonography.

Studies have shown that amniotic fluid can be increased by adequate hydration—in other words, the more fluid the mother drinks, the more amniotic fluid she will produce. It is nevertheless true that well women with healthy pregnancies do not usually have oligohydramnios. Consider it a sign of something amiss that must be quickly identified. (Please refer to sections on Intrauterine Growth Retardation and Postdatism later in this chapter, and Fetal Anomalies in Chapter 5.)

DIAGNOSING TWINS

A fundal measurement above gestational age in weeks should immediately lead you to consider twins. But first, rule out other possible causes of a uterus large for dates (see section on LGA later in this chapter). Next, consider your clinical findings. Have you noticed an abundance of small parts when palpating? Does the head presenting at the inlet feel somewhat small relative to fundal height? Twins are sometimes missed if one is tucked behind the other's body.

Unless a woman is subjected to serial sonography, twins are usually discovered by 30 weeks, with clinical confirmation through the auscultation of two heart beats. But take care—what appears to be two heartbeats may be just one, audible over a wide range. If you note a 10 to 15 point difference in rhythms with distinct patterns of variability, you most likely have identified twins. When in doubt, order a sonogram.

Twins occur about once in every 90 births. There are two types: identical/ monozygotic (one egg, one sperm) and fraternal/dizygotic (two eggs, two sperm). Identical twins share a placenta but have separate amniotic sacs, whereas fraternal twins also have separate placentas. It is important to identify twins as soon as possible because twin pregnancies carry extra risks and potential problems for mother and babies. Maternal anemia is much more common, as is the incidence of premature delivery. Women with twins need expert nutritional counseling, as well as recommendations for moderating activity and getting adequate rest. Guidelines for recognizing and reporting signs of premature labor should be provided immediately. Occasionally, **twin to twin transfusion syndrome (TTTS)** may cause blood to be shunted from one identical twin to the other, putting the "donor" baby at risk for growth retardation and other complications.

In the area where I practice, delivery of twins at home is out of the question. However, I have diagnosed twins a number of times and have continued to give prenatal care, later attending the births in hospital. A midwife can provide special assistance to a woman carrying twins by focusing on the emotional and practical aspects of caring for two babies. And if she can enable the mother to maintain her pregnancy to at least 37 weeks, hospital management will be fairly relaxed, with early discharge.

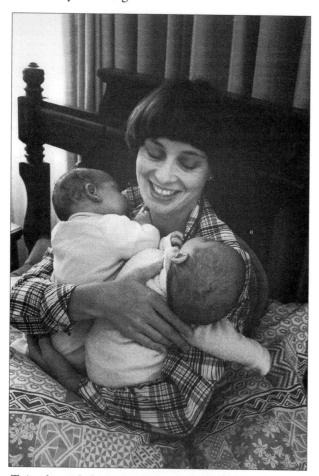

Twice the work, but twice the joy and fulfillment.

The reasons for hospital birth are numerous. One potential problem is cord prolapse. This is more likely to occur with the first baby if it is breech. In fact, most physicians will do an automatic cesarean if the breech is footling or kneeling. The second baby is at even greater risk for cord prolapse, especially if it remains high in the uterus after the first has been born. It may also become hypoxic, as reduced uterine volume may cause constriction of vessels leading into the placenta. For the same reason, there is risk of placental abruption. Finally, there is considerable risk of postpartum hemorrhage from an overdistended and tired uterus.

Only once did I seriously consider doing twin birth at home. The expectant mother was in excellent health, sensitive and cooperative, and both her babies were presenting vertex (head down). We jointly discussed and carefully considered her situation. My hesitation was mostly political; if transport became necessary I knew I could lose my backup. And because the mother had some fears regarding her safety, we decided on hospital birth. Had this couple been really insistent, though, I might have assisted them at home.

You must be certain parents are well aware of what to expect from the hospital experience. If the birth is to be vaginal, ultrasound is standard to assess fetal position, as are double fetal monitoring and intravenous fluids for the mother. There may be many attendants besides the obstetrician: residents, interns, student nurses, and the neonatal team. Based on the options available at your backup hospital or through your backup physician, help the mother and her supporters devise a realistic birth plan. Emphasize the emotional aspects of the experience, and the support you will provide.

BREECH PRESENTATION AND TRANSVERSE LIE

Because of my backup situation and the political climate in my area, I do not deliver breeches at home. If I had a choice, I might do so very selectively. The biggest risk with breech birth is cephalopelvic disproportion (CPD). If the body is born and the head proves too large for the pelvis and is stuck behind the brim, fetal hypoxia and death may result. Certain breech presentations are particularly problematic. For example, if the breech presents footling or kneeling, there is nothing to prevent the cord from slipping past the body and prolapsing.

What are wise criteria for breech birth at home? The expectant mother should have an ample gynecoid pelvis, and an average-sized baby. If she's already had a baby without problem, the risks diminish. However, the baby should either be frank breech (legs extended up over the chest) or complete breech (legs up and crossed), in either anterior or transverse position with head well flexed so it can negotiate the pelvis readily. In order to make certain of these factors, a combination of ultrasound and/or X-ray technology must be used.

Even so, complications may arise that require special expertise. An arm impacted behind the head must be deftly and quickly manipulated, and a deflexed head must be repositioned without delay. These maneuvers are beyond the scope of this section. Suffice it to say, it is not advisable to attend breech birth without the assistance of someone experienced in both basic and advanced techniques (including neonatal resuscitation).

Before presenting breech, the baby may assume a transverse lie. This is common up to 26 weeks, at which point the baby generally finds greater comfort in lying longitudinally. If the baby remains transverse after 27 weeks and is high in the uterus, it's wise to listen carefully around the lower portion of the abdomen for placental sounds (these are swishing, wooshing sounds of blood coursing through placental circulation at the same rate as the mother's pulse). Do this to rule out placental praevia, an implantation over or near the cervical os which would prevent the baby from engaging either breech or vertex. If the baby remains transverse past 30 weeks, a sonogram is in order to locate the placenta precisely.

Rarely, the breech rotates to vertex at the last minute, either in the last weeks of pregnancy or right before labor. Rather than wait and see, have the expectant mother try to rotate her baby with postural tilting if it remains breech beyond 30 weeks. All she must do is lie down comfortably, with her hips elevated on pillows 12 inches or so,

three times daily for 20 minutes. Suggest she do deep relaxation while in this position, and visualize the baby turning. If she feels major movement, have her come in right away to be checked.

If the baby has not rotated after several weeks and is beginning to feel rather snugly encased, external version is another option. This is a tricky maneuver for all but the most experienced midwife, as it requires great expertise in fetal palpation and a highly refined sense of touch. There is also some risk of cord entanglement and/or compression, so the fetal heart must be monitored continuously by another experienced practitioner.

Have the mother drink a beer or glass of wine to promote uterine relaxation, and make sure her bladder is empty before you begin. Position her in a tilt, then gently attempt to massage the baby into position. Be sure to keep the head flexed, and to rotate the baby in the direction it is facing. If any resistance is felt or changes in the fetal heart are noted, the version should be stopped and the baby returned to its original position. Because of the risks involved in this procedure, informed written consent of the parents is essential. Some prefer to be in hospital, so an emergency c-section can be performed quickly in case fetal distress occurs.

Some mothers report massaging their babies into vertex position themselves; others claim that talking with the baby or meditating has served to facilitate rotation. But if, despite all efforts, the baby has not rotated by 36 weeks, you might ask your backup physician to give version a try. Most physicians hesitate to perform external version until 37 weeks, for fear of causing premature labor. However, they generally employ a more forceful technique than that of the midwife, due to the use of terbutaline or other uterine tocolytic in conjunction with the procedure.

If all attempts at version fail, prepare the mother for hospital birth, or possible cesarean if the breech is footling or kneeling. (Also refer to the section on Surprise Breech in Chapter Five.)

PREMATURITY

The medical standard of care defines a baby premature if born prior to 37 weeks gestation, although this limit is somewhat arbitrary. The chief concern with premature delivery is that the newborn's lungs may not yet be mature, leading to the development of **respiratory distress syndrome** (RDS). Signs of RDS in the newborn include **tachypnea** (rapid respirations), **cyanosis** (blue color), **nasal flaring, grunting** (with expiration), and **retractions** (sucking in of the skin between the ribs with every inspiration).

In reality, the lungs are almost always mature by 34 weeks; the 37-week limit permits a margin of error in calculating the EDD. Therefore, if an expectant mother is certain of her dates and her baby's growth pattern is consistent with them, the midwife may consider the baby term and permit home birth as early as 36 ¹/₂ weeks.

Causes of preterm labor include spontaneous rupture of the membranes, vaginal or urinary tract infection, cervical incompetency, polyhydramnios, multiple pregnancy, baby large for gestational age, uterine anomalies, faulty implantation of the placenta, substance abuse, malnutrition, fetal death, and extreme or chronic stress. The latter has yet to be fully acknowledged as a causative factor in U.S. literature, but according to French studies, the proportion of preterm births is higher for women with longer work weeks, women in stressful occupational categories, and women whose work involves prolonged standing or is physically tiring.

Any mother with a history of miscarriage or previous premature delivery is automatically at risk. Monitor her carefully from 24 weeks onward; schedule visits every two weeks, and perform gentle cervical examination each time. Recommend a reduction in her work load. Screen her at the first sign of vaginal infection. If the cervix begins to soften or efface, have her curtail sexual activity, make sure she knows how to distinguish contractions from fetal movement, and see her weekly thereafter. If regular contractions occur or the cervix begins to dilate, immediately refer her to a physician.

Medications commonly used for stopping labor include magnesium sulfate, ritodrine, and terbutaline; these generally do the job but cause the mother nervous irritability and nausea. They are also quite toxic, and should be used no more

than several days. If the cervix is not drastically changed, contractions are mild, and the mother has no history of alcoholism, you might suggest she take a couple of stiff drinks. Alcohol inhibits the action of oxytocin, and thus relaxes the uterus. Before the aforementioned tocolytics were developed, alcohol was given intravenously to stop premature labor.

One of my clients began premature labor at 35 weeks. Her cervix was quite effaced and about two cms. dilated (this was her second baby). She took two shots of vodka in grapefruit juice, stayed in bed, and was fine until the following morning. Her contractions resumed upon arising, so she repeated her previous routine. This went on for almost a week, during which I checked her daily and in spite of regular uterine activity, found her cervix to be unchanged. Contractions then stopped completely. She carried her baby to 41 weeks and delivered at home, but not without difficulties. Severe shoulder dystocia, partial separation of the placenta necessitating manual removal,

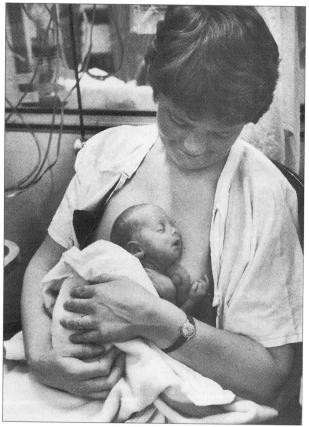

When a baby needs intensive care, the family must be creative, as well as assertive in finding ways to stay close to the baby.

and postpartum hemorrhage made for an interesting trade-off of complications!

Another of my clients carrying twins had a fundal height of 38 centimeters at 30 weeks, with slight polyhydramnios. She began premature labor and was given ritodrine, which did little to stop her contractions. However, as a student of yoga, she discovered that postural tilting several times daily definitely stopped uterine activity, probably by taking pressure off her cervix. Her backup obstetrician at the hospital called in the staff to observe her innovation. Ritodrine was discontinued, and she carried her babies to term.

SMALL FOR GESTATIONAL AGE (SGA) AND INTRAUTERINE GROWTH RETARDATION

With regard to uterine size, causes of SGA include miscalculated dates, fetus transverse or low-lying, hereditary predisposition to small babies, and intrauterine growth retardation (IUGR). The first three are fairly easy to rule out, but the last is a complication requiring special attention.

IUGR is suspected when fundal height has been normal up to 24 weeks gestation, but then begins to fall behind the standard growth curve. Although babies grow more often in spurts than steadily, overall growth should average about one centimeter per week.

The causes of IUGR are numerous; they include malnutrition, anemia, chronic hypertension, substance abuse, fetal infections or malformations, abnormalities of the placenta and cord, and prolonged pregnancy. Chronic stress and overwork are also implicated: a French study by Nayer and Peters reported that neonates born to women who work in the standing position weigh less than those born to unemployed women at comparable gestational age.

Here is an interesting case history. This mother came to us at 27 weeks with a fundal height of 22 centimeters, certain of her dates but carrying a baby very small for gestational age. Her nutrition was poor and she smoked half a pack of cigarettes daily, but she made a commitment to improve her diet and cut back her intake of nicotine. Her baby began to grow in spurts over the next few weeks,

and steadily thereafter. Total maternal weight gain was about 20 pounds. Sonograms at 31 and 35 weeks determined a normal rate of fetal growth, but a baby so small for gestational age that a month was added to the EDD. This seemed arbitrary to say the least, considering a solid menstrual history, and the couple's claim that, as per sexual activity, they couldn't possibly have conceived a month later. Nevertheless, if "sonogram says," we'd best believe it!

Her final checkup revealed her cervix to be slightly dilated and 60 percent effaced. At 38 weeks by original dates, 34 weeks by revised EDD, labor commenced with ruptured membranes. What to do? Was the baby premature, or simply small for gestational age? We palpated a four and a half to five pound baby and so decided on hospital birth. This was a real disappointment to the parents, who had never accepted the revised dates anyway.

After six hours of labor, she delivered a healthy, vigorous baby girl of five pounds, estimated to be about 38 to 39 weeks gestational age. No respiratory distress; lungs were fully mature. Clearly, the ultrasound-based EDD was incorrect. There was some indication of fetal compromise in that the placenta was spongy, shredding, and full of calcifications. But the baby showed no other signs of growth retardation; it was neither wizened nor emaciated, and had excellent Apgar scores of 9/10.

Could this birth have taken place at home? If a baby is SGA, and care begins later in pregnancy when accuracy of dates is more difficult to determine, hospital birth is more or less by default. Premature babies definitely face serious risks at delivery, whereas complications linked to a minor degree of intrauterine growth retardation are more manageable. These include hypoglycemia, i.e., low blood sugar, and hypothermia, i.e., difficulty maintaining body temperature, both due to insufficient body fat. Neither condition is immediately life-threatening, and either can be dealt with initially at home. Still, it is wise to have the baby seen by a pediatrician within the first few hours after delivery.

If, during the last trimester, the fetal growth pattern is persistently slow or irregular, hospital birth may be advisable. Even with minor degrees of IUGR, it is wise to do non-stress testing (see page 72), assess amniotic fluid volume, and have the mother do fetal kick-counts from 34 weeks onward, because there is a correlation between IUGR and stillbirth (for more on these procedures, see section on Postdatism, this chapter).

If you are preparing to assist the birth of a small baby who has grown well in later pregnancy and whom you believe to be term, have oven-warmed flannel blankets and an aluminum outer wrapper (space blanket) ready as insulation. Place the baby skin-to-skin on the mother's body, then wrap in flannels with aluminum blanket over all. It is crucial to keep the head covered at all times—use a stockinette cap so that the mother will not have to fuss with the blankets and can maintain eye contact with the baby. Take the axillary temperature several times an hour until you are certain the baby has stabilized.

Check the baby's blood sugar level by doing a dextrostix (heel stick with test strip). If the level is below 45, contact a pediatrician. Otherwise, encourage the mother to nurse, and afterwards give sterile water and molasses or corn syrup, one teaspoon per cup (never use honey, due to risk of infant botulism). Repeat the dextrostix every two hours, so that you can evaluate whether the oral feeds are raising the blood sugar level. Be sure to chart each time fluid is given, how much, and how well the baby tolerates it. If the baby vomits, intravenous feeding may be necessary; contact the pediatrician without delay.

This baby is also at risk for **polycythemia**, i.e., excess red blood cells predisposing it to severe jaundice. If the baby looks ruddy at birth, do a hematocrit, and if elevated, immediately consult your backup pediatrician. Postpartum visits should occur daily for the first four days, minimum.

LARGE FOR GESTATIONAL AGE (LGA)

Causes of LGA have already been presented in other sections of this chapter; they include miscalculated dates, hydatidiform mole, gestational diabetes, twins, polyhydramnios, maternal obesity, hereditary predisposition for big babies, fetal anomalies, baby high in fundus due to placenta praevia or abdominal muscle tone, fibroids (inter-

nal or external) displacing the baby upwards or positioned atop the fundus, and postmaturity.

Whenever a mother measures large for dates, each of these possibilities must be considered and ruled out. I recall a woman who came to me at 28 weeks with fundal height of 32 centimeters, wide abdominal girth (but not overweight) and + 4 glucose in her urine. On palpating her I felt a good-sized head entering the pelvis, butt in the fundus and small parts everywhere (posterior position, I assumed). I sent her immediately for an OGTT (the only screening for gestational diabetes at that time) and it was negative. Next week, no glucosuria was noted but two heartbeats were audible; a sonogram soon confirmed that she had twins!

A big baby is of concern unless the mother's pelvis is ample. How will the midwife know if a baby is growing too large for the mother, and what can be done about it?

One simple way of determining adequacy of the pelvis relative to the baby's size is by checking for engagement. You must assess not only the station of the head, but also how well if fills up or fits into the pelvis. If the baby is still high, **check for ability to engage** by grasping the head externally and pressing it back towards the sacral promontory, then down into the inlet. If the head feels movable and enters the pelvis readily, things are fine so far. Another way to check is to place your hand above the pubic bone with the mom in a semi-sit position, then have her sit up completely. If the head bulges into your hand instead of slipping into the pelvis, it will have difficulty clearing the inlet.

I've had only one obvious case of cephalopelvic disproportion (CPD) in my practice. This was a first pregnancy, the mother was certain of her menstrual history but the baby had been consistently large for dates. She had a small pelvis with adequate inlet, but android characteristics of close-set ischial spines and slightly flattened sacrum. She was about 5'3" tall; the father, 6' tall. At 37 weeks, I remember feeling alarmed at the size of the baby's head, particularly in the way it overrode the pubic bone and bulged out into my hand. Upon discovering this condition of **fetal overlap**, I encouraged her to give birth anytime she was ready (her cervix was soft, about 60 percent effaced). She finally commenced labor at 40 weeks, dilated completely with the help of pitocin but pushed for two hours without ever engaging the head, and had to be delivered by cesarean section. Her dates proved correct, as the baby showed no evidence of postmaturity. He simply grew too large for her pelvic dimensions.

If a similar situation arose again where we were certain of dates and the mother's cervix was ripe, I might suggest **castor-oil induction** as early as 37 weeks. The diarrhea caused by castor oil releases prostaglandins in the system that stimulate labor. Have the mother take two tablespoons initially with orange juice, followed by another tablespoon in half an hour, with a final tablespoon an hour later. It helps if the mother relaxes with a bath. I've used this formula (minus the bath) for cases of prolonged ruptured membranes where time is of the essence, and have had almost certain success with it. It is definitely worth a try.

Other ways to induce labor include acupuncture techniques, herbal formulas (blue cohosh tincture, a dropperful every few hours), periodic nipple stimulation, and sexual intercourse. If the woman's partner is male, the latter serves dual purposes of stimulating contractions via the release of oxytocin, and ripening the cervix via the high prostaglandin content of seminal fluid. An alternative for ripening the cervix is cervical massage with evening primrose oil.

There are certain risks attendant to LGA deliveries. The uterus is apt to be overdistended and less able to contract efficiently, resulting in prolonged labor, arrested progress, or postpartum hemorrhage. With any degree of maternal exhaustion, the baby is at risk for hypoxia, and may require resuscitation at birth. There may also be some degree of shoulder dystocia. Be prepared!

POSTDATISM

Fetal postdatism becomes a concern if pregnancy progresses beyond 42 weeks, assuming the EDD is correct. Sometimes there is hereditary predisposition for longer term pregnancy, e.g., the expectant mother reports that she herself was born three weeks late, as were all her siblings.

Commonly, there is no obvious physical reason. Perhaps some babies simply need to gestate longer than others—the fruit on our trees doesn't ripen at exactly the same rate, so why should our babies?

Emotional factors may also cause a woman to "hold onto her baby" and go beyond term. Perhaps it's to be her last pregnancy, and she's hesitant to give it up. If this is her first baby, she may be frightened of the responsibilities of parenting and loathe to surrender the special attention she's enjoyed during pregnancy. Sometimes both parents are uncertain about changing roles, and this will prolong the pregnancy. Or if the expectant mother has felt obligated or otherwise compelled to work right up to her due date, she may be taking some extra time to enjoy her pregnancy and wind down in preparation for labor.

When exploring these possibilities, it's important that the mother not feel judged or accused, as this may exacerbate any tension she is already feeling. Encourage her to make her own observations, draw her own conclusions. Such a difficult time, these postdate weeks of waiting!

The risks of postdatism are twofold. If all is well in utero and the fetus continues to grow, cephalopelvic disproportion may become a problem. On the other hand, if the mother ceases to eat and drink in sufficient quantities (perhaps for fear of having a large baby), the fetus may suffer weight loss, fetal distress, or even stillbirth. Once considered to be a "timed organ," the placenta was thought to expire with advanced gestation, but recent research shows this not to be true. It is maternal malnutrition and dehydration that lead to reduced blood volume and oligohydramnios, which in turn can cause cord compression and fetal compromise. *Williams Obstetrics* differentiates the above postdate conditions with the words **post-term** and **dysmature**, the former referring to the baby who is late but otherwise healthy, the latter referring to the baby clearly undernourished as a result of maternal malnutrition/dehydration and resulting cord compression.

Certain assessments can help determine maternal-fetal well-being in the postdates period. Have the mother do **fetal kick-counts** daily, for an hour after her largest meal—she should note about eight to ten movements in this time period. (Although critical for postdate pregnancies, some practitioners recommend that all women begin counting fetal movements at least once daily from 34 weeks onward.)

Another common assessment of fetal well-being is **non-stress testing** (NST), which evaluates fluctuations in the baby's heart rate in response to its own movements. The desired, or positive response is moderate acceleration. The NST can be performed in the hospital by external monitor, or the midwife can simply listen with her fetascope for an extended period and note heart rate changes as the mother reports fetal activity. In recent years, the validity of the NST has been called into question as no correlation has been shown between findings of this test and fetal outcome; nevertheless, it remains standard of care for postdatism.

Amniotic fluid volume is more significant. It can be assessed by serial sonography commencing at 41 weeks, or by careful uterine palpation performed week-to-week by an experienced care provider. Amniotic fluid volume assessment in combination with non-stress testing has less than a 15 percent margin of error—the two taken together dramatically reduce the chance of being either falsely reassured or unreasonably alarmed by the individual results of either procedure.

Depending on your findings from the above, you should either consult with backup, leave well enough alone, or recommend castor oil or other means of induction if the cervix is ripe and the head well down in the pelvis. As previously discussed, this might also be appropriate if you determine that the baby is getting a bit large for the mother's dimensions. As the days and weeks go by, the postdate baby's passage through the pelvis may be made increasingly difficult as skull sutures become less cartilaginous, rendering its head less moldable in labor. Check carefully for fetal overlap, and beware of the previously engaged head rising up in the pelvis.

Current medical protocol for postdatism combines the aforementioned assessments with a few more obtained by ultrasound. In addition to amniotic fluid volume and fetal activity level, fetal breathing movements and muscle tone are evaluated, then combined with NST results to form the **biophysical profile** (BPP). With a scoring system similar to the APGAR assessment, zero, one, or two points are given for each of the five categories cited above, with ten the highest possible score. A total score of less than seven is considered an indication for induction of labor.

Can the midwife's clinical assessments of postdatism provide enough information to substitute for the biophysical profile? In my opinion, the answer is yes. Although fetal breathing movements cannot be assessed directly, these may be presumed adequate on the basis of normal muscle tone, as demonstrated by kick counts. NST is easily accomplished with a standard fetascope. And to reiterate, even the most subtle changes in amniotic fluid volume are readily noted with continuity of care.

The most stressful time in labor for the dysmature fetus is at the onset. Uterine contractions are far more stressful than are Braxton-Hicks, thus any degree of fetal compromise will show up almost immediately. Plan to attend the postdates labor from the very beginning, and take heart tones more frequently than usual.

PSYCHOLOGICAL ISSUES AND DIFFICULTIES

Begin by reviewing basic counseling techniques in Chapter Two. The vast majority of emotional upsets in pregnancy result from hormonal changes: complaints forgotten by the following visit are typically hormone induced. If emotional problems recur, ask for more background. You may uncover problems in the expectant mother's relationships, environment, or health that were unknown to you before.

Occasionally, you'll have a client who becomes increasingly imbalanced or emotionally extreme as pregnancy progresses. Midwives know that pregnancy is a tempestuous time, and generally encourage expectant mothers to use the volatile energy of this transitional phase to take personal inventory and forge new modes of self-expression. After many years of practice, I believe the best way to promote a pregnant woman's well-being is to help her see aspects of herself that are weak or neglected in a positive light, so she will feel motivated to work on herself. Self-reliance and self-love are the cornerstones of connectedness in pregnancy, birth, and parenting.

A woman with an extremely physical nature will often become anxious over changes typical in the first trimester. If highly athletic, e.g., used to competitive sports or marathon running, she will probably find fatigue, nausea, and softening of her muscle tone to be extremely frustrating, even frightening. She is in danger of pushing past physical imperatives for rest and relaxation, and unless she learns to tune into her body, may even be at risk for miscarriage or premature labor.

I had one such client, a black belt in karate and marathon runner who broke down and cried at about 12 weeks, "My body just doesn't work anymore!" I explained that pregnancy is a transformative time of rapid growth, which simply cannot be controlled or forced. I suggested books and articles to help her understand the miraculously complex physiologic changes occurring in her body. I encouraged her to keep hold of her strength, but experiment with pacing herself. During labor, she found surrender for dilation difficult, but really reached her peak with pushing. Afterwards, she viewed her entire experience as positive, and was proud of herself as a mother.

The more emotionally-based woman will usually savor the changes of early pregnancy, particularly the dreamy quality of her heightened sensitivities. She may drive her partner a little crazy with her mood swings, and may forget to eat or get regular physical activity. Help her develop a health plan/schedule, and encourage her to read for factual information. She might also like to keep a diary, which can serve dual purposes of helping her chronicle emotions and observe how they correlate to her day-to-day care of herself. Emotionally-oriented women tend to dilate slowly yet steadily, but may dislike the concentrated effort of pushing. Help expectant mothers who are ethereal in nature prepare for the demands of second stage labor with third-trimester squatting practice, vaginal awareness/perineal massage, or any physical activity requiring endurance (such as aerobic dance, lap swimming, etc.)

The more mentally-oriented woman chooses the particulars of her birth plan methodically. She is extremely well read on pregnancy, birth, postpartum, and related subjects. She will generally practice what she has learned regarding diet and exercise, but may tend to repress her emotions. Ask this expectant mother how she is feeling, and she'll probably answer with a simple "fine," or "I'm OK." This is in marked contrast to the emotionally-based woman, who will talk for twenty minutes on every nuance of her personal situation. It may be difficult to forge a close connection with the self-contained intellectual woman before labor, although massage or other body work can help establish physical intimacy and encourage emotional exchange.

I had one such client whose mother arrived a few days before the EDD. First days, and then weeks went by, and still the expectant mother insisted that everything between them was "just great." The day after her mother left, she went into labor. And she labored beautifully and with perfect control; in fact, she didn't want to be touched or assisted by anyone (including her husband). Caring for the baby was her biggest challenge; she kept trying to get him on a schedule!

Most women are not as extreme as these examples, but many have either the physical, emotional, or mental aspect of personality somewhat underdeveloped. If you can help an expectant mother identify and activate some latent part of herself, she may find new power in synergistic balance, and find new skills for birthing and parenting in her own special way.

And yet, ease or difficulty with dilation, fast pushing or slow pushing, liking one phase of labor and hating another are all in the cards for women, and may vary for the same mother from labor to labor. As midwife Janice Kalman says,

Sometimes birth is energetic, sometimes emotional, sometimes challenging depending on aspects of relationship, or the mother's physical or psychological state that day…it's always Mr. Toad's wild ride as to how these aspects create the warp and weave of the story of labor. The trick during pregnancy is for the midwife to recognize red flags of fear, anger, anxiety, discord at home or about who will be at the birth, and then, facilitate open communication around these issues and help a woman come to her truth, no matter what the outcome.

Certain life situations may particularly expose some women to stress and difficulties in pregnancy. The following sections explore these circumstances in depth.

CHALLENGES FACING SINGLE MOTHERS

It has become increasingly common in our society for women to choose to parent alone. Some women reach an age where "it's now or never," choose the baby's father quite deliberately and then willingly absolve him of any further emotional and/or financial entanglement. Women who become pregnant accidentally by men they barely know, or with whom they cannot hope to establish lasting relationships, have decidedly different adjustments to make during pregnancy. And the expectant mother estranged from but still attached to her baby's father has yet another psychological set.

No matter what their circumstances, most single mothers feel vulnerable because they have no intrinsic support person. Those who choose home birth may fear the impersonal nature of birth in hospital, with no one to protect them. Single mothers definitely need extra nurturing from the midwife. But they also need to meet other expectant mothers, in order to find the companionship necessary to sustain them in their challenging situation.

What is the experience of a single mother during pregnancy? If she is recently separated from the baby's father or other intimate partner, her pregnancy may be a time of unprecedented apprehension and loneliness. All pregnant women have feelings of separateness and uniqueness, but an interested partner lends the comfort of intimacy. For a woman alone, pregnancy may make her feel isolated in a way she can hardly cope with. She feels her baby move, and has no one close to tell. Alone at night, with the baby kicking and disturbing her sleep, she wonders how she will ever handle her impending responsibilities, with everything in her hands, in her keeping. The task all single mothers face is to accept and transmute these anxieties into positive, growth-producing emotions, by actively seeking adequate support.

How can you help the single mother cope with her need for loving companionship? First of all, make sure she has good self-esteem. Encourage her to talk through concerns about her changing identity, while stressing her positive traits, aptitudes, and accomplishments. Be on the lookout for signs of depression—see whether she gets out socially, and how she spends her free time. Just be careful not to assume sole responsibility as confidant. Always remember that after the birth she will have a whole new set of emotional needs, and you will have other expectant mothers counting on you. Don't make the beginner's mistake of engendering the single mother's dependency!

What are the practical concerns of expectant single mothers? Usually, the greatest fear is that the requisite emotional and physical stamina of mothering alone will be just too much to sustain. Occasionally, a single mother will deliberately keep the prospect of parenthood veiled, and will float through pregnancy with little thought to what lies ahead. Your role in this case is to initiate a practical discussion of newborn care. First, ask her how she plans to cope with her own needs in the first few weeks postpartum, and then, how she thinks she might cope with the baby. Does she have an adequate supply of baby clothes and accessories? A diaper service, perhaps? Has she ever diapered or bathed a baby before? How will she feed herself if she cannot find time to prepare food, or get to the store? If there is an emergency (whether physical or emotional), who can she call for help? These are important checkpoints for any expectant mother; for the single mother, the sheer magnitude of what lies ahead makes this line of inquiry especially critical.

What about fears concerning the actual birth? Some of these, such as fear of overwhelming sensation and loss of control, are universal. But the single mother is especially susceptible for lack of an intimate partner. Who will stand by her if she starts to fall apart or become desperate? Besides yourself, she should also have a woman friend or female relative as primary support for the birth.

If the single mother is not currently in an intimate relationship, broach the subject of birth's sexual-sensual intensity by explaining the physiology of the process, i.e., how hormones affect pelvic circulation and how the vagina adapts and expands to suit the baby's contours during delivery. Sometimes it's easiest to talk this over while showing the woman vaginal massage techniques, or discussing the role of vaginal awareness during delivery. Reassure her that masturbation and orgasm are beneficial in pregnancy, and good preparation for giving birth. Your aim is to help her find a comfortable but sexually charged vitality to bring to her labor. Explain the sensations of giving birth as vividly as you can, and encourage her to feel free to to make noise and move uninhibitedly when the time comes.

This brings up a major concern for the single mother: is there love and romance after birth? Are women with babies desirable as sexual partners?

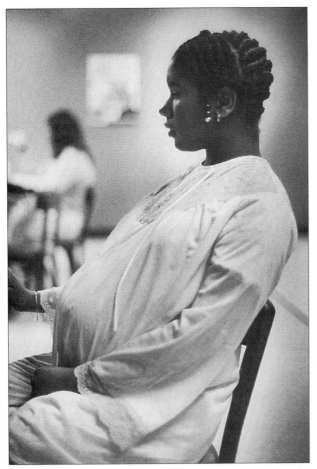

Single mothers must give themselves credit for the courage and strength it takes to go it alone.

Who wants a lover with a child in her arms? In truth, single parenting is now so widespread that a single mother is bound to find company if she so desires. Increasingly, single fathers take physical responsibility for their children. What's more, some single mothers report being pleasantly surprised by a new lover's relief at being spared the pressure to reproduce. Women who combine aspects of nurturer and lover are often uniquely attractive. As one mother put it, "There are oodles of guys who would love a ready-made family." Enable the single mother to feel confident about her current situation and prospects for a loving relationship, and she will approach her birth with enthusiasm.

DIFFICULTIES OF WORKING MOTHERS

"Every Mother Is a Working Mother," the popular bumper sticker reminds us. If expectant, and additionally juggling the demands of a busy career with domestic engineering, a woman may often find herself at wit's end. Much depends on her temperament, how she handles stress and maintains her personal equilibrium. If her life is centered almost entirely on her work, she may need help focusing on pregnancy and her developing baby. Encourage her to stay tuned to her feelings and connected to her body throughout the course of each work day.

Here are some questions for the hard-working mother to help her determine whether her career might be negatively affecting her pregnancy. Does she have problems sleeping? During her free hours, is she generally preoccupied with concerns stemming from her work? How is her sex life? Does she ever make time for deep relaxation/massage/body work? Her answers to these questions will shed light on how well she is supported, whether or not she is able to unwind, and if she makes or finds time for the introspection and surrender so essential in preparing for labor.

The most common problem of working mothers is chronic stress. Stress tends to manifest in aches and pains at night, or insomnia, and may be mediated by increased vitamins B and C, trace minerals, calcium, and protein. Herbal tinctures of hawthorne, passionflower, or hops are sometimes useful at night. Any woman dealing with stress needs an excellent diet, and regular means of emotional and physical release. Relaxation practice and meditation also help, along with a routine of aerobic exercise.

If income from outside work is so essential that an expectant mother must continue even when physical and emotional signals say it's time to quit, suggest that she lie down and relax as soon as she gets home, and keep weekends completely free. Discuss this plan with her partner and significant others so they can lend support. Regardless of their situation, I urge all expectant mothers to quit work at least a week or two before the EDD. Particularly if stressed, women who work to term are frequently overdue (as if making up for lost time).

Often, career women intend to recommence work immediately after giving birth. Emphasize the importance of taking time out to get to know the baby, establish a good milk supply, and develop a workable routine at home. None of this is possible without adequate rest and recuperation. If available in your area, recommend a mother's support group to all your clients. Interesting and intelligent discussions on issues surrounding parenting can reassure career women that mothering is a worthy and engrossing occupation. For your part, explain how a few months of undivided love and attention for the baby establish an intimate foundation that makes parenting more pleasurable and fulfilling in the long run.

An important catalyst for ready adjustment to mothering is the bonding period immediately following birth. If the career woman seems overly concerned with body image, help create a positive one of her as mother by commenting on the beauty of her baby, how great she looked during labor, and how lovely she is with the baby in her arms.

If the new mother must start work soon after birth and intends to breastfeed, make sure she is in touch with other working and nursing mothers. La Leche League International can provide referrals and phone counseling in your area. Better yet, help her find support *before* the birth. Otherwise, she may unconsciously begin withholding nursings during the early weeks, which will invariably lead to a reduced milk supply and early weaning.

An exception to all the above is the woman who chooses her own work hours, who is in tune with her pregnancy, and whose work is so appropriate to her nature that it is health-affirming. For example, one woman I recently assisted had been an artist for many years and was given a grant to do murals around the city. While pregnant, she planned and directed work on her projects, but was free to rest whenever she wanted. Instead of distracting or exhausting her, her work enabled her to stay happy and well.

The working women category also includes student mothers. More so than women working eight-hour shifts, pregnant students can really deplete their resources with late-night studying, and can accumulate tremendous physical tension from sitting still and concentrating over long periods of time. The expectant mother/student needs to assess her best times for effective, relaxed study, then use these and no others. Help her take a realistic view of continuing her studies after the birth—even if she limits in-class hours, she may be so preoccupied with the subject matter that she will find it hard to give her baby adequate attention.

CHALLENGES FOR ADOPTIVE MOTHERS

Begin by looking closely at any biases you have regarding mothers who plan to give their babies up for adoption. The decision to let go of a baby is a painful one—never an easy choice, in the best of circumstances.

The first home birth I ever attended took place in a milk shed in Oregon; I was just five months pregnant. There was no midwife, but the mother had two children already, both born at home, and felt comfortable with the responsibility of birthing on her own. This was in 1971, when humanistic options were virtually nonexistent in hospital.

What was remarkable about this birth was that the mother did not intend to keep her baby, but to give it to a couple who could not have children and were present at the birth to receive it. Besides the astounding energy of the birth process and the mother's remarkable power, what I recall most vividly was her restraint at the time of delivery. For the hands that caught the baby were the adoptive mother's, and it was she who first took the baby to breast. And yes, the women remained friends—the biological mother became an "auntie" mother, and had continued contact with her child throughout the years.

If the notion of giving a baby up for adoption strikes you as an evasion of responsibility or child abandonment, you had better refer the birth mother elsewhere. At the very least, she needs support from her caregiver, and will additionally need the help of agencies and organizations that respond to the emotional and legal needs of birth mothers during the adoption process. And if the biological father is in the picture, he may also need counseling and support. Concerned United Parents, at (800) 822-2777, offers assistance to birth parents, and local social service agencies may have similar contacts in your area.

Every state has its own legal regulations regarding the number of days which must elapse after delivery before consents can be signed, as well as time limits for withdrawal. Even after papers are signed, there is a probationary period lasting an average of six months, depending on locale. In some states, the biological father must also sign his consent. Know the regulations prevailing in your area.

The example presented by my account is that of **open adoption**, which seems preferable in most cases to **closed adoption**, where the identity of the birth parents is concealed from the adoptive parent(s) and the child, although the biological mother may be able to sign a waiver allowing the child to seek her upon reaching legal adulthood. **Agency adoption** is facilitated by licensed social agencies, who meet with prospective adoptive parents and birth parents alike to assess their respective situations. Should your client prefer an agency adoption, advise her to contact the Child Welfare League of America, or the Family Service Association. Private adoptions increasingly result from the efforts of an intermediary, such as a lawyer or independent adoption facilitator. Generally, these intermediaries work for the adoptive parents, and charge a substantial fee. It is crucial that the birth mother hire her own legal counsel to protect her rights, and to make sure the intermediary is above board.

Suzanne Arms, author of *Adoption: A Handful of Hope*, suggests that two midwives may be necessary for the adoption process—one for the biological mother, and one for the adoptive mother. In terms of assisting the biological mother through pregnancy and birth, midwife and author Anne Frye astutely observes that grieving begins during pregnancy, and birth is a major loss, like a death. Thus the biological mother may want to name the baby, take photos of the baby at birth, snip a lock of hair, take hand or footprints, or save a baby shirt or blanket from the time of delivery. And unlike my experience in the milk shed, the birth mother may want and need to nurse the baby, in order to bond sufficiently with it to make peace with her decision. She may also want your assistance in developing a ritual or ceremony to formalize her act of letting go, with the help of family and friends.

Adoptive mothers/parents have their own anxieties during the birth mother's pregnancy and postpartum. Whatever will they do if she changes her mind? How on earth will they cope with the disappointment, especially if the baby has been in their care for some months? Again, if you feel ill-equipped to handle these issues, contact local agencies or other midwives who might share their expertise.

ISSUES OF MOTHERS OVER THIRTY-FIVE

It used to be that any woman over 35 having a first baby was termed an "elderly primigravidia" and considered to be high risk. The main concern was that labor might be inhibited by age-induced rigidity of pelvic bones and muscle tissue, or complicated by deteriorating health. But the standard has changed: as more and more women delay childbearing and maintain their health and fitness throughout the years, age is no longer such an issue.

As for stamina, the older woman who knows herself and clearly wants her baby can manifest phenomenal endurance, more than enough to see her through delivery. The greatest benefit of working with women in their late thirties or early forties is their accumulated life experience and resulting self-assurance; they generally relate to pregnancy deliberately and responsibly. With adolescence far behind them, they are less apt to project maturation issues onto the experience of pregnancy than are younger mothers. They have learned quite well how to care for themselves; they are open to suggestion and respond with initiative.

On the other hand, some have focused so intensely on their own development that the idea of modifying established routines to meet a newborn's needs is rather unappealing. If conception has been by default, i.e., the woman fears her biological clock is running down and it's her last chance to have a baby, the anticipation of disrupted schedules, unwashed dishes, and hurried meals (along with general self-abnegation) may make her feel somewhat panicked or depressed.

You can help by emphasizing that her maturity provides the emotional scope and stability to make her a thoroughly capable parent. Let her know that the most effective mothering techniques depend on integrity and forthright communication. Urge her to connect with other mothers for support, especially if her social circle is comprised mostly of childless women or couples. Appeal to her greatest asset—a well-seasoned sense of humor—with anecdotes that illustrate how levity can mediate the toughest trials of parenthood. A woman of experience is quick to appreciate that which it takes a less mature, younger mother much longer to comprehend, i.e., her child is his/her own person, right from the start.

What about the older woman having another child? I once assisted a 45-year-old woman having a third baby; her others were already in their teens. Her physical condition was that of a woman ten years younger; she was well toned, and had great flexibility and an excellent diet. Recent physical examination showed her to be completely healthy; her heart was fine and blood pressure lower than average. She had a four-hour, problem-free labor. And her recovery was perfect; she had plenty of energy postpartum.

Attitudes have also changed with regard to the grand multipara, i.e., a woman who has given birth five times or more. Long considered at risk for postpartum hemorrhage or fetal malpresentation due to lax muscle tone, research has shown no additional risk for the parturient mother based on multiparity alone. With attention to nutrition,

exercise, and rest, a woman's physical condition can be optimal regardless of age or previous childbearing.

PROBLEMS OF ESTRANGED COUPLES

Working with an estranged couple in pregnancy is complex; you strive to reconcile differences between partners as best you can, at the same time supporting the expectant mother in being autonomous should reconciliation prove impossible. The latter is important regardless of what transpires during pregnancy. Help the expectant mother articulate her vital needs, and identify those not being met in the relationship. Reaffirm her ability to single-parent if she must, while encouraging her to communicate assertively with her partner.

There are many variations on the theme of estrangement during pregnancy. Perhaps the couple has been together for a while but has not stabilized, with parties vacillating on whether to define their relationship as long-term or let it go. Be prepared for tearful prenatal sessions, and continued repetition of problems. Your own counsel will repeat itself too, and you may decide to refer the couple to a specialist who can work with them more intensively.

And how best to deal with the expectant partner? Seldom does an estranged partner request advice or assistance; more often than not, he/she simply drops out of the picture. On several occasions, I've received middle-of-the-night, drunken phone calls from distraught fathers. These contacts were ultimately unproductive, and more than a little disturbing. Should this happen to you, tell the expectant father you will speak to him during normal business hours only, unless his partner has some physical emergency. Above all, take care to be entirely platonic in your tone of voice and manner of speaking—men can read strange meaning into the midwife's compassionate ways. Refer the couple to counseling, and reassert your primary commitment to caring for the expectant mother.

Hopefully, the couple in distress will decide well in advance of labor whether they will stay together. If they remain undecided late in pregnancy, it is important to advise them of the difficulties emotional ambivalence can create during birth. If they can't work out their differences, you may suggest the expectant mother prepare to labor without her partner. Make clear that she is the center of the event, and thus must feel fully at ease and supported in order to give birth naturally and safely. Contemplation of this fact may make partners decide to reconcile, or cause them to see that it's simply impossible.

If it seems like the woman's partner is destined to depart, have her take a close friend or other support person to classes. And begin to broach the same topics for discussion as you would with an expectant single mother.

If the couple does reunite for the birth, go out of your way to encourage partner involvement. Little details of participation, like supporting the mother in difficult positions, assisting with perineal massage/support, or feeling the baby's head as it crowns, are intrinsic to the bonding experience and therefore make a tremendous difference for the tenuous couple.

Yet another situation you may encounter is that of the expectant mother no longer with her original partner, but with a new love who is interested in sharing the pregnancy and attending the birth. This newcomer may be very curious about the mystery of birth, but is also apt to suffer intensely from postpartum blues. Passionate, fledgling couples approaching parenthood must be briefed on the difficulties of the early weeks with a newborn, and you must persist through their joking affection to get at the thorniest issues. Have they discussed their respective roles after the birth? How are they prepared to deal with sleepless nights, hours of baby-crying, loss of privacy, etc.? Do they understand how volatile the postpartum period can be, and how lack of privacy/breastfeeding may temper sexual activity for quite some time?

At some point, plan to see this expectant mother alone in order to discuss the prospect of single parenting. Ask her how she would cope if she and her new love grew apart after the birth, and whether or not she has any backup plan as per living quarters, financial support, etc. Remind her of her former self-reliance, and suggest she not lose sight of it if the relationship becomes troubled.

CHALLENGES FACING LESBIAN MOTHERS

In the past, lesbian women contemplating motherhood were met with ridicule and/or hostility. Fortunately, these antiquated reactions are falling by the wayside in large segments of our society, as same-sex couples are more openly and positively portrayed in mass media. The notion that lesbian mothers are somehow unfit to be parents is being replaced with an understanding of how much their children benefit from being carefully prepared for, and very much wanted.

Artificial insemination is available through both physicians and midwives. Sperm is obtained from sperm banks for 94 percent of inseminations. Otherwise, fresh sperm is secured from known or unknown donors, after careful screening for HIV and other diseases. (Sperm banks also screen donors for HIV, which is critical since the virus can survive freezing.)

Rarely, the donor may want some knowledge of the child or may wish to co-parent. But because the relationship between mother and donor is usually tentative, legal contracts are advisable to delineate these agreements and prevent future custody battles. In numerous states, the donor surrenders all claim to the child if insemination is done through a physician.

Offer the lesbian couple the same guidance and support as a heterosexual couple for handling the stresses of pregnancy and early parenting. Occasionally, the lesbian mother is treated like a single parent in childbirth classes, even though her partner is present! Speak to the instructor on behalf of the couple, or refer them to another educator who will respect their relationship.

Some of your lesbian clients may want to be closeted, while others will definitely be "out." Should consultative visits or transport become necessary, be sure you understand how the expectant mother and her partner want their relationship presented to the backup physician and medical staff.

The birth certificate poses a special problem. If the new mother indicates that she was artificially inseminated, the state may try to track the father if she later applies for aid. Better to leave the space for father's name blank, or write "unknown." Only the mother can be listed on the certificate in the capacity of legal guardian; her lesbian partner cannot. In most states, her partner cannot adopt the child either, although states where this is allowed may grant reciprocity to others. And if anything were to happen to the mother during delivery that rendered her disabled or incompetent, her partner would have no authority unless she established power of attorney in advance; then she would be treated as next of kin.

The actual insemination process often takes many months and is quite costly. The success rate quoted by most sperm banks is only about 19 percent. If two inseminations are performed monthly, it takes an average of six to nine months to conceive. This gets expensive, at $50 to $100 per insemination. Again, this points to the fact that lesbian women desiring motherhood must be thoroughly committed to their decision.

Encourage lesbian mothers to find others in their community for support. It is a sobering fact that some lesbian mothers do not tell their midwives the truth, but pose as single mothers. Check yourself for homophobia, and if you personally feel you cannot serve lesbian mothers lovingly and well, refer them to midwives who can.

ISSUES IN FAMILY RELATIONSHIPS

The family in today's world has taken a bit of a beating. As family members commonly live at a distance from one another and communicate infrequently, it's no wonder that most expectant parents think little of how their feelings for their own parents might affect childbearing. Many women are quite surprised to find memories of childhood, particularly unsettling emotional configurations, surfacing as pregnancy progresses. Not every expectant woman will choose to delve into the past, but many feel the urge to talk with their mothers about birth and baby care.

This desire to reanimate family ties links to the power of bonding, which may remain unconscious until maternal and paternal surges turn the wheel and complete the cycle of biological relatedness. With a first pregnancy, expectant parents often express some negativity about how they were

raised, and resolve to do a better job than their parents did. Ultimately, becoming a parent is a process of defining oneself as an individual, while culling the best techniques and greatest wisdom from one's own upbringing. This requires letting go of anger and resentment—reactions of attachment—towards one's own parents.

When the expectant mother and/or her partner have trouble with this, help them find ways to forgive their parents for any wrong doing (whether real or imagined). If still fairly young, expectant parents may confuse bitter memories of adolescence with otherwise happy childhood experiences. Help them recall positive early memories, and guide them to incorporate these in their own approach to childrearing. The most difficult (and profound) aspect of first-time parenting is reckoning one's ideals with one's limitations. Stress that parenting is about process, not perfection; about receptivity, not mastery; about flexibility, not control.

Prospective parents may also have different levels of idealism as regards raising a child. One parent may have many preconceived notions of what is best, while the other maintains a more pragmatic, "wait and see" approach. It's best to treat any disagreements that arise in your presence lightly, as ultimately, time will tell. You don't need to squelch expectant parents' idealism, but a few examples of times in your own experience when compromise was necessary, or the graceful, tactful thing to do, may be beneficial. Frequently, women/couples with rigid ideals about parenting are likewise fanatic about the forthcoming birth, and need to broaden their perspective.

Some men and women with decidedly unpleasant childhood experiences may confide to you that they don't really like children, and wonder how in the world they will be able to parent with such feelings. Even those blessed with happy memories may suffer from our cultural bias towards young-adultism; with little or no exposure to the world of infants and toddlers, they fear their enthusiasm is far less than it should be. The hardest thing for prospective parents to grasp is that their baby will be *their own*—not just some abstract, alien little infant like everyone else has!

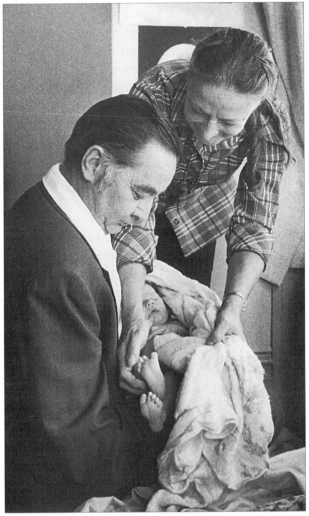

Grandparents thrill to the miracle of birth.

woman, the average man will either withdraw or become defensive.

For their part, expectant mothers may struggle with conflicting images of self-sacrificing madonna and self-determined free spirit. The hormones of pregnancy complicate matters by stirring up the emotions, to the point that women may wonder how they will ever be stable enough to handle a baby and have anything left for themselves. Sometimes, a damaging cycle of self-doubt, fear, and repression sets in long before the birth. Don't let this slip by unattended, or the mother may suffer terribly from postpartum depression.

In lesbian relationships, the non-pregnant partner may feel alternately oppressed by impending responsibilities, or compelled to reach new heights of sensitivity and perfection. Whatever their situation, expectant parents need to be told that it is possible to be a parent and be human at the same time, and that it is infinitely better to express emotions with spontaneous intensity than to vent them later as distorted or violent outbursts. Explain that parenting operates on the same principles of honesty and assertiveness that work in adult relationships. The more they can relax and trust their instincts, the better they will deal with the expectations and desires of other family members and society at large.

SEXUAL PROBLEMS

Problems with sexuality often stem from mistaken concepts of proper masculine or feminine behavior. Heavily polarized gender roles have been typical of our society since its inception, and even now, while subscribing to sexual equality, the feminine aspect is little expressed in our culture. Women struggle to retain their femininity as they work and play in a man's world, while men feel both resentment and fascination at finding their gender-based superiority increasingly swept aside.

As regards sexual intimacy, most problems spring from an inability to communicate personal needs and desires. Broach the subject of sexual satisfaction by explaining physical and emotional changes trimester-by-trimester, including various sexual positions and other adaptations appropriate for different phases of pregnancy. This can help

Much anxiety over having children has to do with fear of perpetuating negative role models. Some men remember Dad as a rigid, unfeeling authority figure, and imagine that becoming a father means playing this part. Thus pregnancy may be viewed as a sobering event concomitant to the loss of freedom. Expectant fathers caught up in this may react with rounds of heavy drinking or other substance abuse, overwork, promiscuity, breaking time-related agreements, or fits of depression. If the expectant mother reports such behavior in her partner, ask her to bring him to your office, or you may want to make a special home visit. Deal tactfully with the male ego in this state of polarization by discussing the matter intellectually, taking a simple, objective look at relevant social patterning. If you delve emotionally as is so easy and stimulating when counseling a the expectant mother articulate what she desires from her partner, and vice versa. In this respect, discussion with other expectant couples is ideal, because all are undergoing similar changes and adjustments.

A woman's desire for sex will vary considerably during pregnancy. At no other time will the emotional component have so strong an influence on her response. In turn, her emotions are influenced by the stage of pregnancy through which she is passing. The first trimester is often a time of all-barriers-down intimacy and tenderness. If she has a male partner, this may be partly due to relief from worries about birth control—but there is also a special intimacy that flows from conception itself, from the knowledge that she and the father have truly become one and that the fruit of their union is living inside her. Of course, these feelings will be modified by any ambivalence regarding the pregnancy or her partner. And sometimes, normal nausea and fatigue interfere with sexual response at this stage.

Once movement is felt, the expectant mother may sometimes withdraw to focus on her relationship with the baby. Still, increased pelvic circulation plus high levels of estrogen, progesterone, and oxytocin—the "love hormone" released with sexual arousal, nipple stimulation, and orgasm—generally serve to boost sexual desire in the latter part of pregnancy. As the baby grows, the mother may be hindered in certain positions, and may feel most comfortable being on top or on her side.

As the birth becomes imminent, she may once again withdraw to focus on her baby and impending labor. In order for sex to seem right at this point, she must never feel that her partner is trying to turn her attention away from the baby, but rather, is making love to both her and the baby. This is a very vulnerable time for the expectant mother, and it is perfectly all right for her to be selective regarding the nature of her sexual encounters.

It is important, though, that she try to keep her sexual circuits open, as this has great bearing on the sensual scope of her labor. The compelling intensity of birth necessitates the same kind of free expression that happens when she is about to reach

orgasm. How can the midwife help with this? A graphic demonstration may serve to convey the idea. Start with intense breathing like that at the end of first stage, combine with an attitude of physical surrender, add a few moans or urgent demands, e.g., "Squeeze my shoulders . . . mmm," or "There . . . push harder," and you will have made your point. This dramatization may move expectant parents to embarrassed laughter, but you will have imparted more truth about the psycho-sexual nature of birth than any amount of technical training can provide.

Sometimes the expectant mother complains that her partner is sexually insensitive to her slower, more sensual pregnant pace, and either skimps on foreplay or progresses too quickly altogether. Suggest she take more initiative, and explicitly show her partner what she wants to feel, and how to go about it. If intercourse begins with her on top, she can more readily control the tone and timing of the encounter and make sure her needs are met.

Shy women afraid of their own passions may recoil at these suggestions. Make clear that labor is a body-centered experience which will call on her to take the lead. Help her redefine her sexuality as a sharing of her power, rather than her skill in submitting to or pleasing her partner. Encourage her to take sensual pleasure in hot baths, relaxed meals, massage, etc. Physical practices of yoga or dance may help her get in touch with her rhythms, release tension, and find her own resources for feeling good. Many pregnant women report masturbating more than ever before, perhaps several times daily.

The expectant mother's ease with her own sexuality will influence not only her response to labor but her handling of the baby, her ease of recuperation postpartum, and her continued commitment to breastfeeding. Help her explore and celebrate her sexuality as much as she can.

ABUSE ISSUES

Childhood sexual abuse can be defined as contact or interaction in which a child or adolescent is used for the sexual gratification of an adult. The incidence is estimated to be 33 percent of women, and 20 percent of men. One study in

Washington state showed that over 66 percent of pregnant teens had experienced sexual abuse. Repressed memories of sexual abuse are most likely to arise: 1) when a woman gets married or commits to a monogamous relationship; 2) when her own daughter reaches the age when she herself was first molested; 3) when her perpetrator dies; or 4) during the perinatal cycle. If the expectant mother responds to questions on the medical history form with some uncertainty but is willing to discuss her experience, ask the following questions:

1. Have you ever been tricked into an intimate situation you did not desire?
2. Has anyone ever touched you intimately against your will?
3. Have you ever been forced to have sex when you didn't want to?
4. Have you ever been forcibly held down or restrained for sex when clearly indicating you wanted to be free?

A woman with history of sexual abuse may be plagued with chronic health problems, such as extreme PMS, pelvic pain, constipation, pain with intercourse, and eating disorders. There may be history of habitual abortion, hyperemesis gravidarium, or premature labor with this or a previous pregnancy. She may also have strong reactions to internal exam, speculum exam, breast exam, even venipuncture. She may suffer from **vaginismus**, an involuntary contraction of the vaginal muscles if any attempt is made at penetration.

Sometimes an abuse survivor suffering from a disassociative disorder manifests the opposite behavior. She may be sexually demonstrative, e.g., may splay her legs extra wide or open her labia far apart, but emotionally she remains detached, checked out, not there with you. In the extreme, a woman who has suffered severe prolonged sexual abuse may suffer from multiple personality disorder. Here is a list of characteristics or behaviors common in women who have been abused:

- Describes self as never having been a child
- Extremely concerned with control
- Overly willing to expose genitals to others
- Unexplained pain with intercourse
- Extreme ideas about sexuality
- Hypersensitive to touch
- Repeatedly exploited by others in relationships
- Deeply estranged from family
- General feeling of being "under it"
- Detaches from self and others
- Nothing ever wrong with life, always neutral
- Childlike behavior, dress, or appearance
- Unkempt personal appearance
- Chaotic surroundings or habits
- Overly controlled surroundings and habits
- No personal boundaries
- No trust
- Anger inappropriate or out of proportion to the situation
- Inability to appreciate others
- Blind adoration of others
- Fanatic religious or philosophical beliefs
- Jumps into situations or to conclusions
- Difficulty with decision-making

With regard to the birth, certain effects of sexual abuse are classic. There is tremendous fear of losing control. Survivors of abuse cannot tolerate the thought of grunting, trembling, crying out, or feeling helpless in labor. They are terrified of being "ripped apart" by delivery. cesarean birth is common. Typically, labor arrests around four or five centimeters, the woman is given pitocin and proceeds to labor "beautifully," but never progresses further. Once postpartum, an abuse survivor may have great difficulty with breastfeeding, particularly when her baby reaches an age where it begins to fondle the nipple or play at the breast.

Experts Penny Simpkin and Phyllis Klaus suggest that working with sexually abused women can be difficult because they are almost always needy, controlling, and angry. Even if the midwife is doing everything in her power to be of assistance, an imagined slight may rapidly snowball into litigation if the midwife is unaware of what she is dealing with. Keys to coping are:

1. *Don't withdraw*—even if the mother is critical, or behaves in a childlike way, stay present in a state of active listening.
2. *Validate the mother's perceptions*—even though they may seem far afield or wildly inaccurate, you would do well to concur with her views. This diffuses her anger, which might otherwise be directed at you, at her baby, or at herself.

3. *Once trust is established, negotiate*—if you are able to be patient with the mother and can win her trust, you can work to settle any disagreements or field any disappointments she has regarding her care.

A woman who is a victim of **rape** may have striking similarities to the woman described above, depending on how well she has healed from her trauma. She may also be needy and angry, and may likewise struggle with labor unless she receives intensive counseling during pregnancy. As you take her history, do your best to validate any residual feelings of fear or embarrassment.

A victim of **physical abuse** needs special care. First and foremost, she must be apprised of her legal situation. Increasingly, if a woman shows physical evidence of abuse, her abuser will be automatically charged and arrested. In many parts of the country, healthcare providers are obligated by law to report cases of physical abuse to the proper authorities.

More worrisome are the emotional ramifications of physical abuse. If your pregnant client is still with her abuser, you may set whatever limits you consider feasible or appropriate. Be aware of support resources in your area. Group therapy for abusive partners and their survivors is increasingly available.

With any history of abuse, the laboring mother tends to be highly protective, which often means keeping the baby inside her as long as possible. Even though her partner may wish to be present for the birth, you must separate the mother's needs for support from her partner's presence. In many ways, you must treat her as you would an estranged or single mother.

Emotional liabilities of the physically abused woman are considerable in the postpartum period. She will tend to self-abnegation, repression, frustration, and most unfortunately, child abuse. Recognize her right to self-determination, but know where to draw the line both for her well-being and that of her child. Get expert consultation or refer her to counseling as needed.

PSYCHOLOGICAL SCREENING OUT

Despite your best efforts, sometimes a client continues to have serious emotional problems that cause you to question the wisdom of assisting her birth at home. Be sure to discuss your concerns with your midwifery partner or other associate familiar with the expectant mother, who may see signs of improvement that you have overlooked. On the other hand, guard against excessive optimism. Give credence to the emotional aftertaste of working with a troubled client, and take pains to distinguish the exhilaration of extending yourself as counsel from her actual responsiveness.

If you've exhausted every personal and professional resource and still feel her progress to be inadequate, it's a sign of wisdom to excuse yourself from her care and appropriately refer her. Provide a list of alternative caregivers, including contacts for hospital birth. Not uncommonly, the expectant mother and her supporters are relieved at your decision, and it quickly becomes evident that her lack of comfort with you (or perhaps with the prospect of birthing at home) was part of the problem all along. This amounts to psychological screening out.

Sometimes the shock of being screened out may prompt a woman to rally her resources and make long overdue changes in her situation. Therefore, an expectant mother determined by one midwife to be psychologically at risk may be cared for by another and do just fine. This doesn't work in every case, however. If the expectant mother's emotions remain jumbled regardless of a changed situation, her chances of developing complications are dramatically increased, and it's best for her to birth in hospital.

The only way to learn psychological screening is by experience. I cannot remember a single workshop on this subject where a midwife has not presented a hair-raising case history capped with the final lament, "I knew from the very start I shouldn't have worked with her." Those who have endured malpractice proceedings will tell you that initial feelings of ambivalence are a warning every midwife should heed.

Once you have made a decision to risk-out, by all means hold firm. If you agree to continue care and assist the woman in hospital, remember that seeming last-minute improvements are probably due to increased security with more conventional plans. Don't be tempted to reverse yourself just because things are looking better. This takes the wisdom to let things be, and to forego your desire for a certain kind of personal experience or involvement.

Keep in mind that hospital birth under these circumstances may require an incredible amount of coaching and postpartum support. The birth may not be any easier in the hospital than it would have been at home, but at least some of the weight is off your shoulders. You may vow to screen more stringently after an experience like this, but chances are you will find yourself in dubious situations from time to time. Just take responsibility for your choices, keep abreast of your personal limitations, and try to stay free of illusion.

Do make an effort to discuss any borderline cases with your backup physician before the birth is imminent. This will render any problems arising in labor more comprehensible in the event of transport.

DANGER SIGNS IN PREGNANCY

Report to your midwife immediately if you notice:

1. **Vaginal bleeding.** In the first trimester, bleeding may indicate threatened, spontaneous, or missed abortion (miscarriage), molar pregnancy, or ectopic pregnancy. In the second or third trimesters, it may indicate placenta praevia, placental abruption, ruptured cervical polyp, or other causes.

2. **Initial outbreak of blisters in the perineal or anal area during the first trimester.** This may be herpes virus; contact midwife at once so culture can be taken.

3. **Severe pelvic or abdominal pain.** In first trimester, this may indicate tubal pregnancy. In last trimester, it may indicate placental abruption. Both are emergencies; contact midwife at once.

4. **Persistent and severe mid-back pain.** May indicate kidney infection/pyelonephritis; contact midwife at once.

5. **Swelling of hands and face.** Particularly if face looks puffy or features coarse, notify midwife immediately. May indicate preeclampsia.

6. **Severe headaches, blurry vision, or epigastric pain (under ribcage).** May indicate preeclamptic condition becoming critical. Notify midwife immediately.

7. **Gush of fluid from vagina.** If in first or second trimester, may indicate miscarriage. If in late second or third trimester, may indicate premature delivery. Contact midwife at once.

8. **Regular uterine contractions before 37 weeks.** May indicate impending premature birth. Don't wait to see if they will abate; lie down and call midwife immediately.

9. **Cessation of fetal movement.** May indicate fetal demise. The baby should move several times per hour, more after you've eaten a meal. If less than this, or less than usual, report to midwife at once.

CHAPTER 4

Assisting at Births

The first principle of attending births is to maintain an open mind and pay good attention to what's happening in the present. Regardless of any turmoil or conflict that existed prenatally and perhaps remains unresolved, the birth is the main event and every effort must be made to come to it clear and clean of preconceptions. This quality of freshness will be well appreciated by the birthing woman and her partner; it's the spark for getting things off to a good start.

EARLY LABOR

Every woman should be taught signs of early labor towards the end of her pregnancy. Encourage her to call you at the first indication. Once you know labor is impending, you can get your personal life in order and prepare yourself for the birth, even if it doesn't happen for several days. Most women are eager to discuss their warm-up signals, which gives you an opportunity to allude to labor's forthcoming intensity. Even if contractions are extremely light, remind her to breathe and relax completely with each one. And don't hesitate to tell her how very much stronger her sensations will become.

Obvious signs that labor is impending include **the show** (mucous plug coming away), **spontaneous rupture of the membranes/SROM** (water bag breaking), or **regular contractions**.

Many women lose globs of mucus in the last week or so, but only if secretions are blood-tinged can you assume that cervical changes are actually occurring. Sometimes the plug is lost and labor takes a day or two to commence. Be sure that a woman knows the difference between normal, pink-tinged mucus, and abnormal, excessive bleeding which might be related to placental problems.

If a woman has lost her mucous plug and is not having contractions, suggest she go about her normal routine, eat high quality, nonconstipating foods, and get plenty of rest. Explain that she does not have to try to get labor going. What matters most is that she take the best possible care of herself, and let flow her sensitivities. If she is experiencing the usual pre-labor burst of energy, encourage her to sleep so she has energy for her work later on. But

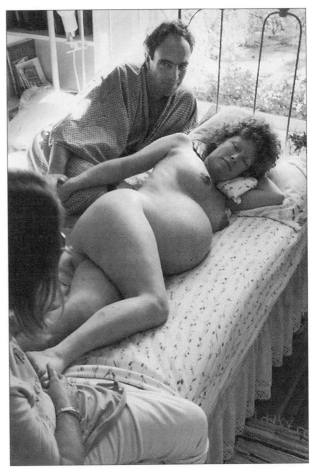

The midwife makes her presence felt by holding the woman's feet without intruding on the couple's privacy.

share in her elation too, as this will help her release nervous tension and get down to business.

Less commonly, labor begins with the amniotic fluid leaking, or gushing out completely. It may be difficult to be certain that what appears to be a slow leak isn't just a bit of urine the woman is losing involuntarily due to constant pressure from the baby's head on her bladder. Time will tell, and it is better not to place a speculum (or anything else) in the vagina if you suspect SROM, at the risk of precipitating uterine infection.

If the woman reports a gush of water followed by little else, we refer to this as a **hind leak**, caused by a tear high in the membranes. This commonly releases just enough intrauterine pressure to allow the baby to settle snugly in the pelvis, effectively sealing off any further flow of fluid. But sometimes a bit of amniotic fluid does filter down and is trapped behind the intact membranes still encasing the baby's head; these are the **forewaters**, which feel like an intact water bag.

Once the membranes are ruptured, serious considerations arise. There is a definite possibility of infection if germs from the vagina or outside enter the sterile uterine environment. On the other hand, if the woman drinks a sufficient amount of liquid at regular intervals, her body will defend itself by increasing the production of amniotic fluid, which flushes the vagina and discourages bacteria from migrating upwards. She must be meticulous in her toileting, avoid tub baths and put nothing in the vagina. To ward off infection, 250 mg. vitamin C can be taken every few hours. If you are not yet with the mother, have her check her temperature periodically and note the odor on her pad—it should smell clean and fresh. Ask her to report any changes immediately.

Although not directly related to infection, also have her contact you at once if she notes a green or yellow tinge to the amniotic fluid, indicating that the baby has passed **meconium**, i.e, epithelial cells lining the intestines. This is due to relaxation of its anal sphincter, which may be caused by a lack of oxygen, or period of fetal **hypoxia**. As meconium in the waters is suggestive of fetal distress, you must immediately attend the mother and check fetal heart tones.

There is quite a debate concerning the maximum time membranes can be ruptured before infection becomes a real possibility. This subject will be thoroughly covered in Chapter Five; just remember that women reporting ruptured membranes at term should always be acknowledged as being in labor. Explain that the bag was broken by contractions; they may not yet be strong enough for her to feel, but more are on the way. *In managing ruptured membranes, place primary importance on helping the mother conserve her resources for the hard work ahead. Don't make the mistake of trying to get labor going if she is not having regular contractions.* If it is near bedtime or in the middle of the night, suggest that she have a strong cup of relaxant herb tea (such as hops or valerian) or a glass of wine (barring history of alcoholism) and get to sleep. Her partner might want to give her a massage, but no intercourse, finger-genital, or mouth-genital contact.

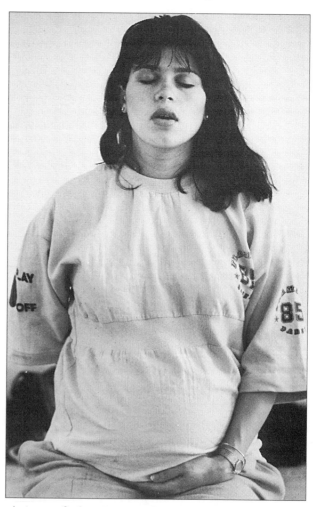

A picture of relaxation: note the loose mouth and easy jaw.

A labor beginning with contractions alone is a bit harder to confirm, as many women have warm-up rounds of contractions for weeks before actual labor. Typically called **false labor**, this negative terminology only serves to make the frustration of starting and stopping worse. Explain that incoordinate uterine action is at play, and even though these contractions may not dilate the cervix, they nevertheless tone and strengthen uterine muscle, and may facilitate effacement and/or fetal descent. We may more accurately term this sort of uterine activity **warm-up labor**.

There are several classic warm-up labor patterns. One typically occurs when the baby is large and unengaged. As the baby descends, the mother experiences **lightening** or **dropping**, with considerable stretching of the lower uterine segment. This may cause some cervical effacement, but little or no dilation. What this mother calls contractions are usually just twinges associated with descent, with no particular pattern of dispersal or duration. Suggest that she take a hot bath, do deep relaxation, and rest up.

The other type of warm-up labor is more like the real thing, with some pulling discomfort or cramping in the cervix or back. Contractions come every ten minutes or so, sometimes as often as every three minutes, but generally last less than 40 seconds and never form a consistent pattern. The sensations are often spastic and quite uncomfortable. This is typical **incoordinate uterine action**—nothing to worry about, though rather distressing for the mother. Suggest a glass or two of wine, which will slow or stop things altogether if the time is not really ripe.

True labor is characterized by contractions which gradually become more intense and fall closer together. It's hard to lay down firm guidelines for determining true labor; it's more a matter of wait and see. Contractions may remain erratic in spacing and duration for many hours, but if there is cervical (menstrual-like) cramping, chances are it's the real thing.

Patterns of early labor vary dramatically. As a general rule, women who commence with close-set contractions will deliver sooner than those whose early contractions come every 20 minutes. But never forget that a woman can shift gears to active labor very suddenly, so be conscientious about staying in touch, and be sure to explain signs of active labor so she or her partner knows when to contact you. If she is able to make a smooth transition from early to active labor on her own, she may very well call too late for you to make it on time. *In general, contractions a minute long, coming every five minutes, signal the onset of active labor.*

This brings up the question of when to go to the birth. Once she has spoken to you initially, the mother will want to know when next to be in touch. The best answer is, "Whenever you feel the need for company, or if anything changes." It's important to let her know you are there to help her through any rough periods, regardless of dilation/ progress. Explain your willingness to come and go, and reassure her that there is no such thing as calling too soon.

There are certain indications to attend the birth at the outset. If the baby was high at the last prenatal exam and the mother calls to report that her water bag has ruptured, you should immediately go and check fetal heart tones to rule out cord prolapse. Or if you have any question concerning the baby's ability to handle labor due to an SGA or postdates condition, you should be there from the beginning to monitor fetal response. A report of meconium-tinged waters or decreased fetal movement necessitates your immediate presence to rule out fetal distress. And maternal conditions such as borderline hypertension or polyhydramnios need to be monitored right from the start. In general, any marginal findings in the final weeks of pregnancy require earlier involvement and more diligent assessment during labor.

Otherwise, leave it up to the mother and her partner. Those with emotional issues may want an early visit for reassurance. Commonly, women call at about two centimeters dilation to report some "really intense" contractions, aware they are still early in the process and fearful they will never be able to handle it near the end. This is a fairly universal response, this reckoning with the forces. Explain how, as labor progresses, the body releases endorphins (nature's pain relief) that make the pain easier to bear. As long as she surrenders and lets this happen, her body will labor automatically, and she'll find resources for coping that she doesn't even realize she has. You might suggest a hot bath to help her get used to her sensations, as long as her water bag is intact. And remind her of the importance of relaxation; women often forget to use their relaxation techniques in early labor. Recommend that she go about her usual activities, leaning against something when contractions come and releasing her pelvis and hips completely. Maintain good phone communication, and you may be able to guide her through early labor without having to make a visit. This can be of crucial importance if you are doing many births, or are tired from a recent delivery.

Aspiring midwives sometimes have difficulty with the concept of anything less than start-to-finish involvement in labor. Isn't this what being a midwife is all about? No, that is the role of a birth assistant, or labor coach, whose participation culminates with the birth of the baby. The midwife's responsibility continues on, and may not reach a peak until after delivery. Last-minute complications may require her to handle a shoulder dystocia, or resuscitate a baby, or manually remove a placenta, or attend to persistent bleeding, or repair a torn perineum precisely at the point when parents and labor coach are finished with their part. Since the midwife's participation curve is weighted to the latter part of the birth process, conserving her energy in early labor is essential. But this is only possible if she methodically attends to her clients' needs for support and information prior to the birth, in the context of prenatal caregiving.

When an expectant mother calls to report uterine activity, keep her on the phone for a few contractions and listen to her breathing. You can usually gauge the intensity of her contractions by how long it takes her to recover. A definite pause, lasting some time after breathing stops and before conversation resumes, may be indicative of active labor. If she seems to be going deeper with each contraction, or the pause period before she speaks is increasing, you should go and attend her regardless of her or her partner's subjective evaluation of labor's intensity.

Complaints about environment also deserve attention. It's impossible for a woman to relax and dilate if her home is chaotic; beware of loud partying noises in the background. You may need to help her clear the house of distractions, by explaining to well-meaning friends that it will be a while yet and she needs a chance to concentrate. Friends can also be sent on last-minute food runs, or can do a bit of cooking if the expectant mother is still hungry, or for after the birth. The birth room itself should be neat, well-ventilated and aesthetically pleasing, with ample fluids by the bed, massage oil, towels, heating pad, etc., all laid out and ready for use. Many women use their natural nesting instincts to take care of this in early labor, but those who feel frightened may need help getting organized.

Encourage the expectant mother to keep eating as long as she possibly can. Emphasize high calcium foods to raise the pain threshold, and complex carbohydrates for energy. And remind her to

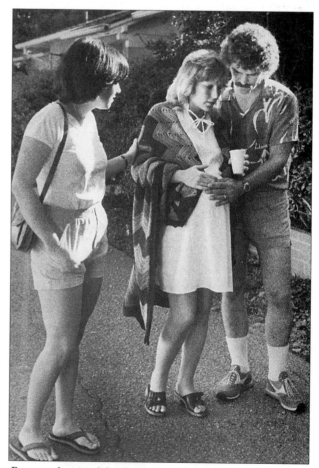

Pep up a lagging labor by getting out in the fresh air.

keep drinking—juice or tea with honey is better than water—and to urinate frequently. Suggestions for activity depend on the time of day; if it's morning, she can do whatever suits her, if it's late in the day, she must try to rest, and if it's nighttime, she should drink a cup of herb tea or a glass of wine and get some sleep.

THE MIDWIFE'S ROLE IN EARLY LABOR

If you attend the mother in early labor, start your labor record (see Appendix E) with notes on how labor began and how it is progressing. Take and chart initial vital assessments of maternal blood pressure, pulse, and urinalysis. Palpate the baby for position, take fetal heart tones, and chart. Do these assessments between contractions so as not to disturb the mother, all except the FHT. Listen to the fetal heart during and immediately after a contraction to accurately gauge fetal response (more on this in the next few pages). You may also wish to palpate the uterus during a contraction to assess the intensity of uterine activity.

Vaginal exams are optional in early labor, but useful for establishing a baseline and letting everyone on the birth team know exactly what's going on. Some women react very intensely to early labor, and appear to be further along than they are. Check whenever in doubt.

Your goal in doing vaginal exams during labor is to be as gentle and undisruptive as possible, while quickly obtaining as much information as you can. Use sterile gloves with lubricating jelly (or a squirt of Betadine or other antiseptic if the membranes are ruptured and labor has progressed). Start the exam the moment a contraction ends and you have the woman's consent to proceed. Begin by checking **dilation**, being careful not to stretch the cervical opening when you spread your fingers open to make your assessment, and record in centimeters. Then note the **placement of the cervix**: is it central, anterior, or posterior? The cervix is usually posterior if the head is above - 1 station, then swings forward as the baby descends. Check for **effacement** by estimating the percentage of cervix that has thinned away into the lower uterine segment. Note the **quality of the cervical opening**: is it stretchy and yielding or tight-rimmed? Also note **how well the cervix is applied to the head**; it should feel smooth against it. If it is loose like an empty sleeve, the head is either malpresenting or not fitting well into the pelvis (see Chapter Five, Cephalo-Pelvic Disproportion).

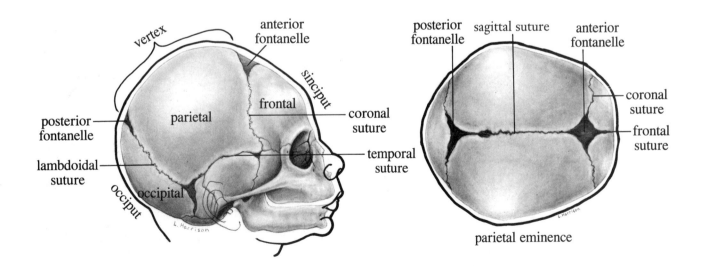

Fetal Skull

Next, estimate the **station** of the head, and note how evenly it fills the pelvic cavity. Finally, if the cervix is effaced or dilated enough, **identify fetal position** by feeling for landmarks of the baby's head, i.e., the sutures and fontanelles. Of these, the sagittal suture is generally most prominent as it is most subject to molding; when you sweep your fingers across the surface of the head, it feels like a bony ridge. Follow the suture line, and feel for fontanelles at either end. If you know the head to be well-flexed by palpation, you're likely to find only the posterior fontanelle—it's the smaller of the two, triangular and about the size of a fingernail, whereas the anterior is diamond shaped and more like a thumbnail. By noting the location of fontanelles and the direction in which the sagittal suture is running, you'll discover the exact position of the baby's head.

You may not be able to get all of this information in one exam. Check again after the next contraction, starting over with a fresh glove.

Interpreting your findings depends on how labor is progressing and how the mother is responding. At this stage, the most crucial assessments are of dilation and station, which serve to indicate an appropriate course of action. If the mother is losing control at only two centimeters, with cervix still long and firm, she needs a change of scene and new input in order to relieve tension and smooth out her labor. If it is late at night, her contractions are not particularly compelling, and she is dilated just two or three centimeters with baby high in the pelvis (-2 or above), rest and/or sleep is best for everyone involved.

If the latent phase is prolonged or there seems to be a lull in progress, determining the baby's position is important. For example, in posterior positions, the baby's head may be deflexed and poorly applied to the cervix, and without adequate pressure on the cervix, contractions will wane and progress will cease. You can attempt to reposition the head, but if the baby is too high to reach, encourage upright positions to promote descent, with squatting to open the pelvis. (More on this in Chapter Five.)

ACTIVE LABOR

Sometimes you'll get the feeling that stronger contractions and hard labor are impending, but the woman is keeping them at bay. Up to about four or five centimeters (and sometimes beyond), women have the power to control labor's ebb and flow, and can choose the time when they let the forces of birth take over. Difficulties occur if the uterus has worked up to a certain intensity and the mother begins to fight against it. This is often the case when a woman is groaning and rocking at only two or three centimeters of dilation.

Women often need special guidance at this point. To move into active labor, the mother must give up notions of how labor is "supposed to be." She may no longer find slow, deep breathing effective; if her breathing sounds ragged or jerky, introduce slightly more accelerated but relaxed chest breathing. Movement during contractions (even pelvic rocking) can create muscular tension; show her how to be still and let her body "melt" while focusing on the rhythm of her breath. Enable the mother to make this shift, and frantic agitation will be replaced with peaceful resignation that permeates the environment, and sets a tone of readiness for harder labor.

Touch is very important. If the mother is restless, offer to rub her lower back—most women welcome this. Use olive oil, and let your strokes be strong, smooth, and sensual, timed to the rhythm of her breathing. Transmit reassurance through your hands; it will ground her and give her focus.

The mother's position can make a big difference in her comfort; what works best depends on the position of the baby and what the woman prefers. If the baby is well down in the pelvis, she may like lying on her side with pillow support and lower back massage. If the baby is not yet engaged, a more upright position will maximize the effects of gravity, and will increase pressure on the cervix to keep the contractions coming. Walking serves the same purpose. If the baby is really high (-2 or -3 station), squatting down with each contraction and walking in between is good for progress. But this routine can be tiring, and should thus be interspersed with periods of sitting or reclining (with pillow support).

Some women feel vulnerable lying down, particularly those who like being in control. Sitting cross-legged, with shoulders and hands loose, can give the mother a sense of steering herself through contractions, and a straight spine can keep tension from stacking up her back. Have someone sit behind her and squeeze her shoulders or push on her lower back periodically, to help her stay loose in this position.

If the baby is posterior and not yet descended, the mother can try the hands-and-knees position, with pelvic rocks to encourage rotation. If she likes, you can massage her buttocks using long, downward strokes. This helps her focus low in her body, and encourages her to relax her breathing.

If the woman's partner is ready and willing to get involved but at a loss for what to do, first help the mother figure out what is most comfortable for her, then show her partner how to support and/or facilitate this. You must be sensitive to what her partner is feeling; perhaps he/she's a bit shocked by the intensity of labor and needs to observe a while before participating. Men overly concerned with performance may be more than a little hesitant, and, if partnered with a woman unused to being assertive, may need extra help getting started. Just give the couple privacy as soon as you are sure they are working well together. Letting them labor alone can foster trust and intimacy between them, which better prepares them to parent and makes your job easier in the long run.

PHYSICAL ASSESSMENTS DURING ACTIVE LABOR

What are the midwife's medical duties during active labor? She must keep a closer eye on the mother's condition, and **check blood pressure** hourly if it was normal in pregnancy, or every 20 minutes if it was, or remains, borderline high. She must also **see that the mother is well hydrated and urinates hourly**. In fact, encourage the mother to eat as long as possible, or take an occasional tablespoon of honey to help prevent clinical exhaustion.

If labor has been long in the active phase, i.e., three hours or so without much progress, **do a urinalysis to check for ketones**. Ketoneuria indicates that the mother is dipping into her fat reserves for energy. A trace reading is fairly normal in labor, but higher levels indicate a disrupted electrolyte balance and the need for more fluid and calories. An intravenous solution of Ringer's lactate might be given in the hospital; at home, you can replicate this formula with something called **labor-aide**. Here is the recipe: 1 quart fluid (water); 1/3 c. honey; 1/3 c. lemon juice; 1/2 t. salt; 1/4 t. baking soda; 2 crushed calcium tablets. Better yet, have the mother eat whatever she can; even a piece of toast will help immensely. **Take her pulse** every few hours; it should stay within 10 to 15 points of normal range. If it rises, **check her temperature** as well. Elevation of all three vital signs indicates a level of exhaustion threatening to both mother and baby, for which transport to the hospital is advisable. Exhaustion is most often a problem if the mother has been vomiting and is unable to keep anything down.

Take fetal heart tones with increasing frequency, at least every half hour. If anything unusual arises, listen continually until the problem resolves spontaneously or a decision is made regarding appropriate response. For routine monitoring, listen throughout a contraction and for 15 to 30 seconds after it ends, in order to get a fully accurate

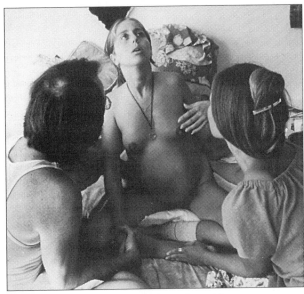

Moment of reckoning as labor forces intensify.

sense of fetal response. It is normal for the heart rate to accelerate slightly with a contraction. The heart should retain a steady beat, with no thready or erratic tonality.

Heart rate over 170 BPM is called **tachycardia**. This is cause for concern, as it may indicate maternal exhaustion and/or fetal infection. The baby's baseline has some bearing on determining tachycardia, as a rise to 170 BPM is considered serious for a baby normally at 130 BPM, but is not an issue for the baby averaging 160 BPM.

Sometimes the FHT dips and bobs dramatically during a contraction, with highs to 160 BPM and lows below 80 BPM, in a pattern of **variable decelerations.** This is caused by cord entanglement or compression, the degree of which varies according to the strength of the contraction and resulting pressure from the baby's head. Although not an immediate emergency, if variable decelerations are unaddressed they may progress to serious fetal distress. The solution is simple—*have the mother try a new position.* This often relieves pressure or traction on the cord and brings the FHT back to normal.

There are several more ominous patterns; one is **flat baseline with no variability**, and the other is **late decelerations**. With the latter, the FHT is normal at the beginning of a contraction but dips at the peak, and does not return to baseline until the contraction ends. If the baby is really compromised, you will notice **poor recovery** as the period of deceleration extends past the end of the contraction. Late decelerations may be correlated to placental insufficiency or fetal acidosis; in either case, the amount of oxygen reaching the baby is not adequate to see it all the way through a contraction. Flat baseline indicates a baby more or less on automatic pilot—no fluctuation in heart tones indicates hypoxia so severe that the baby's autonomic nervous system is unable to adjust its heart rate to its environment. The presence of variability is currently considered the most important indicator of fetal well-being. The midwife can usually tell if variability is absent without even timing the heart beat—as one explains, "When the FHT sounds like a metronome, you

get an unnatural, creepy sensation." If you pick up either flat baseline or late decelerations during first stage, you should give the mother oxygen and transport.

One of the most important things a midwife can do at this stage of labor is **pay attention**, keeping a constant eye on maternal and fetal well-being while discreetly facilitating progress. Some midwives are too little involved, and in the name of non-intervention, allow a woman to languish in an ineffectual position or with unresolved tensions that negatively affect both her strength and her confidence.

Occasionally, though, a mother needs to slow her labor temporarily in order to integrate herself enough to go on. This is the **plateau phenomenon**, which may occur at four centimeters, seven centimeters, or again at nine-plus centimeters. It is helpful to note that each of these is a turning point in terms of new sensation. Four centimeters marks the challenging transition from control to surrender. From seven centimeters to full dilation, transition-like contractions may be surprisingly long and overwhelming. Difficulties at the very end of first stage are linked to the confusion of fielding bearing-down urges with the continued need to relax and finish dilating. You can help the mother master these plateau points by understanding their nature, but no harm will be done if she holds back a bit to collect herself. An arrest of several hours is fine as long as the baby is OK, and the mother's condition is good/her morale is high. On the other hand, if she repeatedly chooses non-dynamic positions in an effort to keep sensations manageable, remind her with humor that labor is not always comfortable, stronger contractions get the baby born, and she should go on while she still has the energy.

Sometimes the atmosphere in the room becomes stale, and a walk outside is in order. A room full of dozing friends and tired birth attendants is especially depressing for the laboring woman. Clear people out to sleep elsewhere, open windows, turn up the lights, get out the ice chips, or serve up some food—all these are good catalysts for stimulating progress.

CARDINAL MOVEMENTS OF THE FETUS DURING LABOR

It is crucial to understand that the fetus, the baby, is an active participant in the birth process. We have only recently dispelled the notion that the fetus is unconscious during pregnancy, and most of us do not appreciate how significant fetal movements are to progress in labor.

There are seven cardinal movements made by the fetus during the birth process:

1. **Descent/engagement:** the baby descends into the pelvis, and as the widest part of its head clears the pelvic inlet and engages at the ischial spines, increased pressure on the cervix stimulates labor;

2. **Flexion:** descent continues throughout labor due to decreased intrauterine space and pressure exerted at the fundus, while counter-resistance from pelvic musculature and bony structures prompt the baby to flex and present the smallest diameter of its head;

3. **Internal rotation:** in order to negotiate the ischial spines, the baby turns at the neck and rotates its head to OA or OP (the body must remain in its original position for the shoulders to descend);

4. **Extension:** pelvic floor muscles hold sinciput and face back as the occiput crowns, then pivots under the pubic bone and extends upwards, facilitating birth of the head;

5. **Restitution:** the neck untwists, and the head realigns with the shoulders;

6. **External rotation:** the shoulders rotate to align with the anteroposterior diameter of the pelvis;

7. **Birth of the shoulders/delivery:** the anterior shoulder delivers under the pubic bone and the posterior shoulder lifts up by lateral flexion, facilitating delivery of the body.

PREPARATION FOR WATER BIRTH

If parents intend to have a water birth, they will need an ample sized tub and some help preparing it. It is generally agreed that a mild saline solution can help discourage the growth of microorganisms and keep the birth environment similar to that which the baby has known in utero. The tub should be scrubbed with iodine and rinsed thoroughly before it is filled with water. Parents should shower before entering the tub. Be aware that it is difficult to utilize universal precautions when assisting water birth.

Benefits of water birth include increased relaxation and comfort for the mother, and possibly, a smoother transition for the baby. Water birth can also ease delivery if labor has been painful or tumultuous. Parents' most common concern regarding water birth is for their baby's safety—what if it tries to breathe while still underwater? This fear is unfounded, as the baby will not attempt to take a breath unless its body is exposed to air, or it has been depressed immediately before delivery. It is nevertheless wise to bring the baby out of the water as soon as it is born.

Monitoring labor is a bit challenging, but not impossible. You can auscultate fetal heart tones under water by placing the fetascope or Doppler in a plastic bag (waterproof Dopplers are also on the market now). Just advise the mother to stay flexible, and see how she feels as labor progresses. Midwives in my area estimate that less than 30 percent of their clients intending to birth in the water actually do so. The rest report feeling claustrophobic in the tub, and/or unable to exert enough effort or get enough leverage to bear down without the benefit of gravity.

Definitely have the mother come out of the water if there is any sign of fetal distress, meconium, or blood loss during labor. If labor is prolonged and the mother is at risk for postpartum hemorrhage or the baby may be slow to start, have her leave the tub immediately as transition ends.

HEAVY LABOR/TRANSITION

Heavy labor ensues once a woman has made the shift to stronger sensation, and has reached a deeper level of surrender. The phase from six to eight centimeters is often characterized by great concentration and quietude, creating the illusion that time has stopped. If labor has been long thus far, it may be difficult for attendants to stay alert because the rhythm of the contractions is so hypnotic. This is generally a good time for the mother's partner to take a break, and for the midwives to alternate periods of rest and participation with one another. The mother will be so immersed in her work that she will hardly notice these comings and goings, as long as there's a hand on her lower back and a comforting voice nearby.

Transition, which occurs from approximately eight to ten centimeters, is the phase of labor that women later relate intimated the experience of dying. As the mother yields her body up completely, the rhythm of her breathing and sheer force of energy sweep her to the outer reaches with every contraction. To observe women at this time is a privilege; most have a softness and beauty about them as social masks fall away and their true nature emerges. The sleepy, far-away quality we observe between contractions is reported by many women to be blissful and renewing. Birth attendants must respect this phase of labor for what it is; a peak, out-of-body experience which prepares and rejuvenates the mother for the back-in-the-body, re-entry phase of pushing and delivery.

By now, the laboring woman has few demands to make. Having learned to work with her sensations, she wants only to concentrate on staying as open as possible. If ever you notice that her breathing is faltering, a word or two, or gentle touch will usually guide her to focus.

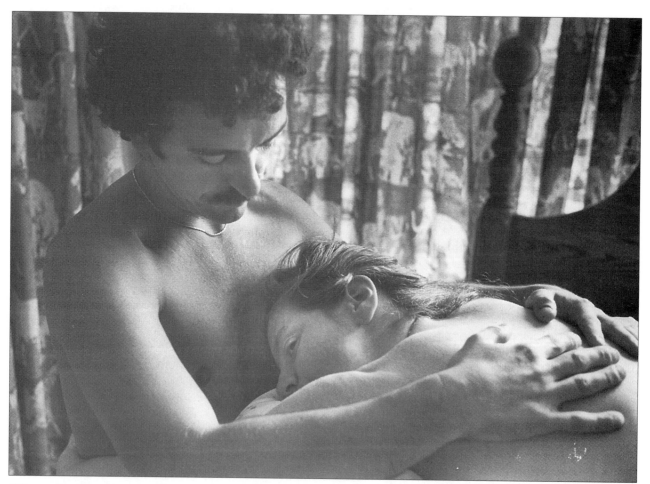

Skin-to-skin contact is tremendously reassuring to the laboring woman.

Whenever there is a marked shift in the strength of contractions, check fetal heart tones more frequently to see how the baby is adjusting. The FHT should be assessed every 20 minutes now; otherwise, your surveillance of the mother remains about the same, with attention to her fluid intake and elimination. Help her get a sip of tea or water as each contraction ends (bendable straws make this easier). Your most challenging task at this point is to avoid disrupting her comfort and concentration. She may have to lean back slightly in order for you to obtain clear fetal heart tones, so be quick and efficient. If you have a Doppler, you may wish to use it now.

The membranes often rupture spontaneously as contractions intensify. What should you do if you find the fluid stained with meconium? This depends on the color and consistency of the fluid: **old meconium** creates a yellow tinge, and is evidence of some brief episode of hypoxia much earlier in labor or in the days preceding it; **new meconium** is particulate and green/brown like pea soup, indicative of recent or current fetal compromise. If you find fresh meconium, immediately listen to fetal heart tones for several contractions, tracking even the slightest deviation from normal. Unless the baby sounds absolutely perfect, with a healthy acceleration response to each and every contraction, consider transport. Particularly if this is a first baby, the mother's second stage may be somewhat prolonged, which will tend to exacerbate any underlying causes of fetal distress and resulting meconium in the water.

Don't forget the importance of vaginal exams. With the unrelenting rhythm of contractions, it's possible to forget to assess the mother's progress. If you can tell by her posture, breathing, and expression that she's moving ahead, there is no need to check, but if you're uncertain, do an exam. If you find no change in dilation, suggest lighter breathing, and upright positioning to facilitate progress and help her conserve energy for the final stages of labor.

Vaginal exam is often prompted by transition symptoms of restlessness, complaining, shift of focus, or loss of control. If the mother has reached eight or nine centimeters, she should be helped to

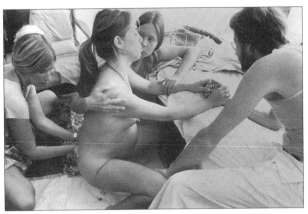

Perfect support for a woman in transition: one midwife holds the mother from behind, the other does coaching and the father gives his total attention.

an upright position to get maximum pressure on her cervix and speed the last bit of dilation. There seems to be a tendency for the cervix to become edematous at this point if deprived of this pressure. The squatting position is perfect, although it often causes quite a bolt of new and stronger sensation for the mother. (*A hint: taking fetal heart tones in this position is difficult, so take them immediately before squatting is begun.*) If she is feeling a strong urge to push with yet a few centimeters to go, squatting may be tough to integrate. Still, give it a try, while coaching her to blow out her breath whenever the urge becomes overwhelming. On the other hand, if she is pushing involuntarily, try a less compelling position like kneeling, or standing with forward leaning.

Understand that transition sensations are often difficult or impossible to integrate. Transition means turning point, change—this is not a time of having it all together! Convey your understanding and acceptance of this to the mother, and she may feel easier about expressing powerful, explosive, or awkward emotions. On the physical level, there are conflicting sensations and messages from the body, one being "Hold and bear down," the other, "No, it hurts, let go and open." Psychologically, there is a return from universal to personal awareness, a beckon back into the body. All this serves to bring delivery into focus.

It's especially important now to watch the woman's body language. Make sure her shoulders and neck are loose and relaxed and that her focus is low in her body. Sometimes women are confused when told not to push and think they must hold the baby back, but such tension impedes final dilation. "Be really open and let that force move through you, just let it be, let it down," is a phrase that sometimes works. Look into the mother's eyes, squeeze her shoulders, and breathe with her.

If this is a woman's second or subsequent baby, she will probably give birth soon after reaching ten centimeters, or complete dilation. Prepare for delivery by straightening up the room a bit and clearing the floor area. This is critical in case of emergency. Make sure there are no open flames or candles lit, in case you need to run your oxygen. Remove the blankets from the bed and set them aside so they don't get bloodied or wet. And here's a tip from a very experienced midwife: place several strips of masking tape on your pants legs to make notes in case of emergency. This saves you from having to fumble with the chart or worry about getting it dirty.

Scrub up well with Betadine or other soapy antiseptic, using a nail brush and working well up your forearms. Then set up for delivery, laying out a disposable underpad or toweling on which you place your tray of instruments, bulb syringe and DeLee suction device, extra pairs of long cuffed gloves, 4x4 sterile pads, and a bowl of hot water (with a squirt of Betadine added) for giving perineal compresses. Have syringes and drugs for controlling hemorrhage (pitocin and methergine) readily accessible, herbal and homeopathic remedies near at hand. Tear off the tops of the gauze pads. Have parents' supplies (washcloths, baby blankets, and towels) close by, along with a bowl for the placenta. Open your bottle of olive oil, and voilà—you are all ready to check the mother whenever she manifests her first irresistible bearing-down urge, and can devote your energy to protecting the perineum and assisting delivery.

Setting up during transition is also wise if the mother has a small baby and ample pelvis, or if either the current or previous labors have been precipitous.

One last point: *make certain that the mother urinates before entering second stage.* A full bladder can hinder descent, and may lead to postpartum hemorrhage.

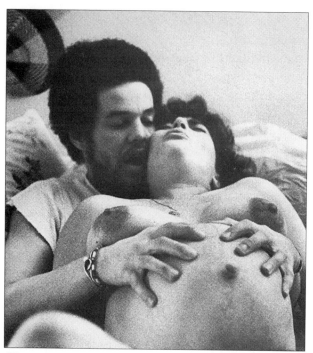

The uterus rises tall with a strong contraction, and the parents feel the passion of the second stage.

SECOND STAGE

Second stage begins when the cervix is finally out of the way—fully dilated, at last! Almost every woman feels some relief and excitement at this point, as she shifts from passive surrender to active participation with bearing-down urges. This is the most striking turning point in labor, the time when the mother's identity and body consciousness return anew, accompanied by a burst of energy and enthusiasm.

Debate regarding the proper style of working with second stage contractions should be over and done with by now. The old school method advocates strong, sustained pushing with every contraction and is at odds with a more natural approach involving sensitive, variable efforts according to what each contraction demands. There is also the breathe-through style of non-pushing, purported to conserve energy and assure maximum oxygen flow to the baby. The truth is that all these techniques have their place, according to what labor requires. It depends on the position and size of the baby, the mother's pelvic dimensions and internal muscle tone, and whether this is a first or subsequent delivery. Adaptability is the key; it's no exaggeration to say that some con-tractions are so powerful and compelling as to be totally obliterating, enough to leave a woman des-perately gasping for air unless she has a good deep breath held in advance. Then again, second stage contractions may be so mild that breathing through them is more than sufficient. In general, contrac-tions of varying intensity persist only until the head reaches + 1 station; as it moves lower and presses on the pelvic floor muscles, the urge to push becomes established and remains consistent from contraction to contraction. Urges of varying inten-sity may recur, however, as the perineum begins to stretch and the mother receives distinct messages from her body on how much to push, and when.

With this uniquely evolving sequence of events, it's obvious that the mother should be the judge of what to do, as long as there is no undue arrest of progress or any sign of fetal distress (cov-ered later in this section). Your role is to offer sup-port and guidance as needed. If the mother sud-denly experiences an overwhelming urge to push

and is floundering, help her get a breath, then have her center her energy and guide it downwards. Massaging her shoulders will keep her from trap-ping energy in her chest and throat. Encourage her to make sounds—some women make loud, moose-like bellowing noises with each exhale—but whatever sound she makes, suggest she keep her throat open. She may well scream out with her first involuntary pushing urge, as the onset of second stage is generally accompanied by a rush of adrenaline. However, continued screaming can cause tightening of the throat muscles with corre-sponding tension in the pelvic floor. Remind her to relax, and show her how to bear down with a released jaw and smooth brow. And remember that the feeling of a baby's head pushing through the vagina is some incredible stimulation! Give her your gutsy appreciation, and do your best to help her settle down into her sensation.

Vaginal and perineal massage can be very help-ful at this point. With the mother's consent, do a bit of massage fairly early in second stage to help

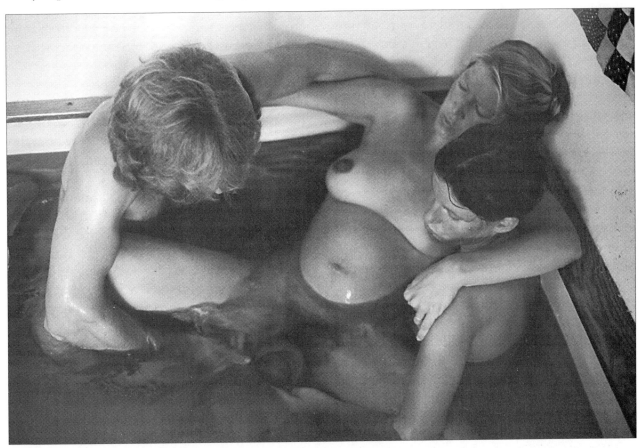

Midwife (right) gently controls the rate of expulsion in this lovely water birth.

her focus low in her body, as you identify any specific areas of tension. Olive oil is a good viscous oil, and will provide a smooth continuous coating over vaginal secretions. Pour a freshly opened bottle into a squeeze-type container for easy application.

Start your massage slowly, and be sensitive to the mother's response. If she finds it annoying or distracting, discontinue at once. Otherwise, do it only between contractions so as not to interfere with her efforts to interpret her sensations and establish a rhythm. Concentrate on the areas nearest the head, and work your way downwards as the baby descends. (Some women request clitoral massage at this point, or may do it themselves.)

For working on tight internal muscle bands, the best strokes are either smooth sweeps of the entire band, or else deep pressure penetration on the tightest areas. Both are good; the first thins out and stretches, the second breaks up and unknots tension. Often, only one side of the musculature is tight. Work gently, and take your cues from the mother's response. It's very important to continuously verbalize your findings. So strongly do most women want to avoid tearing that the response to a comment like, "You're a little tight right here, now just try to let go," can be rather miraculous. Every woman should be taught techniques while pregnant for releasing internal tension, using images like breathing out or exhaling from the vagina, and should develop an ability to release vaginal muscles at will. These skills facilitate progress in second stage, and spontaneous, tear-free delivery.

Ultimately, vaginal/perineal massage is less critical in preventing tears than the mother's attunement to her own sensations. And if ever you notice perineal swelling with massage, you should definitely stop. This is rare, but could actual contribute to a significant laceration.

If the mother is tightening up with pushing (her muscles draw closed or remain rigid as she bears down), it's probably because she's not sure of where to direct her energy. Remember, there is no hurry. Have her sit on the toilet for a while, or try a heating pad between her legs. If problems persist and she is growing weary, try the following technique: place two fingers pad-side down in the

vagina, and press firmly down against the rectum. This will stimulate her to bear all the way down through her vagina. You might also find this technique useful for facilitating the descent of very large babies, particularly if stuck at or above 0 station. Artificially stimulating the mother's pushing urge can help her bring the baby low enough to activate her own bearing-down response.

If the mother is planning to have her partner assist with delivery, she may wish to have him/her feel the baby's head as it descends, or do a bit of massage. Touching the baby internally and feeling it come down with a push will awaken even the most tentative partner to the fact that birth is impending.

Some fathers get quite nervous at this first touch of the baby, and may need to be steadied with an arm around the shoulders and very clear instructions on what to do. If he is going to do massage, have him place his fingers next to yours as you demonstrate pace and technique. He may tend to overdo it at first—just give positive feedback while encouraging him to be gentle, and he'll probably relax and start to enjoy it. Check from time to time to see how well tense areas have responded to his touch, and assist as necessary.

PHYSICAL ASSESSMENTS DURING SECOND STAGE

What are the vital duties of the midwife at this time? Second stage is a rather trying one for the baby, especially if contractions are consistently strong and unrelenting. Your top priority is to listen to fetal heart tones with every other contraction, both during and immediately after each ends. Once the head is on the pelvic floor, listen with every contraction. The baby's condition determines whether the mother needs to accelerate her efforts to get him/her born. Strong pushing is not always the answer—change in position, deeper breathing, or greater relaxation may be the key. Babies definitely have their limits if subjected to hours of strong pushing and/or extreme head compression, so listen well and often, and stay focused on facilitating, not forcing, progress.

Fortunately, the fetal skull is generally capable of molding and adapting to the musculature and bones of the pelvis. This may be less true of post-mature, very large, or malpresenting babies who can give only so much in relation to their mother's internal structures. In these cases, increased head compression may result in **early decelerations**. With this pattern, fetal heart tones start decelerating as a contraction begins, reach a low point as it peaks, then return to baseline as it ends. Dips of ten points are normal in the early part of second stage; dips of 20 points are considered acceptable during perineal dilation. Occasional dips to 100 BPM are not unusual, nor are dips to 80 BPM as delivery approaches. But dips to 60 BPM will render the baby hypoxic before long, and require either immediate delivery or transport if birth is not imminent.

More important than the severity of the dip is recovery as the contraction ends; if the heart rate bounces back to baseline immediately, there is less cause for concern. A pattern of fetal heart tones consistently below 120 BPM is termed **bradycardia**, considered to be moderate if above 100 BPM, severe if below 100 BPM. In any case, bradycardia indicates fetal distress necessitating quick delivery or immediate transport.

It is unusual to hear a pattern of early decelerations before the head has reached the pelvic floor. This may be a sign of pelvic tension, or some disproportion between the size of the baby's head and the mother's midpelvic dimensions. It may be that the mother has a prominent sacral vertebra or sharp ischial spine obstructing a particular plane of the pelvis, and once the head is past that point, pressure will diminish and heart tones will return to normal. In this case, your goal is either to reduce head compression by creating more space for the baby, or else shorten the period of head compression by hastening the delivery (see Chapter Five, Cephalopelvic Disproportion). Formidable pushing efforts may be required of the mother, but she can compensate by breathing deeply between contractions. Communicate your findings to her, and listen to her instincts regarding movement or a change of position she thinks might assist her with pelvic relaxation.

Oxygen therapy is not usually recommended for early decelerations as most head compression is physiologic, but it may be warranted as a secondary treatment if decelerations become extreme. If so, give the mother oxygen by mask, at a flow of six litres per minute.

You may also pick up variable decelerations in second stage, indicating cord nipping, pinching, or entanglement. Occasionally, cord sounds are heard in the vicinity of the heart tones—these have a swishing sound, at the baby's rhythm. If the head is still high, try reversing or changing the mom's position to relieve pressure on the cord. But if the head is well down, listen constantly and be prepared for cord around the neck at delivery by having clamps and scissors open and readily accessible.

The water bag sometimes breaks with the first strong pushes. If you find the water stained with meconium but heart tones are normal, there is no need for panic. Be ready to do a gentle but thorough suctioning of the baby's mouth and throat with a DeLee trap (plastic tubing with catch compartment) as soon as the head is born and before the baby begins breathing (see page 105). Meconium aspiration is a serious matter which can cause neonatal pneumonia.

In case of **prolonged second stage**, have the mother drink ample fluids and take tablespoons of honey to boost her energy level. She may become very tired if second stage lasts more than two hours, and must be encouraged to rest completely between contractions. Her position makes a big difference; those which employ gravity, like squatting or standing, work best. Yet she may refuse the most effective positions because sensation is so intense, and get lost in the rigor of her work, fearing it will never end. Remind her that the baby is almost born, and soon she will be holding it in her arms.

The other extreme of second stage is **precipitous delivery**. Particularly for women who have had three babies or more, one push may bring the head all the way down to the perineum; the next, the entire baby, head to toe! Any mother with a history of precipitous second stage (20 minutes or less) is apt to birth even more quickly with a subsequent delivery. Far from being the boon it appears, a short and vigorous second stage can lead to postpartum hemorrhage. Women who have birthed precipitously often complain that they missed the satisfaction of pushing, and greeted their baby in a state of emotional shock. Suggest a semi-reclining or side-lying delivery position to minimize the effects of gravity. Or, if you anticipate a very quick descent, position the mother on hands and knees during transition so she commences second stage more slowly. This may give her a few extra moments to integrate her sensations, and you, a bit more time to prepare for the birth.

ASSISTING DELIVERY

Delivery positions should be discussed prenatally, as many women have definite ideas and preferences. The most popular positions are semi-sit, kneeling, or hands-and-knees, followed by squatting or standing. Reclining is contrary to the laws of gravity and bad for the baby, due to compression of the maternal vena cava and resulting oxygen deprivation. Lying on one side with leg raised has an unbalanced, passive quality that may affect the mother's feeling of active participation, although it does reduce strain on the perineum and can be helpful when there is history of perineal scarring, or precipitous delivery. Most women prefer the semi-sit position because it allows them to see what's going on, and facilitates touching and/or lifting the baby up as it is coming out. This position also makes the midwife's job easier, as she has ready access to fetal heart tones. The parents experience an emotional benefit if the mother's partner sits behind her so they are completely in touch and united as they witness the miracle of birth.

Hands-and-knees position does have some strong points, particularly for women birthing large babies, or for those who have pushed for a long time with the head low (which may indicate some degree of disproportion in the midpelvic and/or outlet dimensions). Hands-and-knees is effective in these cases because it opens the pelvis to its greatest capacity, and promotes good muscular release. This position is a well-known remedy for delayed delivery of the shoulders; simply having the mother turn to hands-and-knees will often bring the baby spontaneously, without any need for further maneuvering.

Many women find a delivery position instinctively just as the birth is about to occur, so it's best to be ready for anything. One mother recalled pushing happily in hands-and-knees throughout second stage, until her midwife insisted she switch to semi-sit for delivery. Perhaps the midwife had never assisted a woman in hands-and-knees, but the mother felt quite disoriented by the change, and believed that her subsequent loss of control and extensive tearing with delivery were due to this last-minute shuffle. Every midwife should visualize and prepare to assist birth in a variety of positions, so she can comfortably follow the mother's lead in this regard.

Once delivery is imminent, the time of utmost concentration has arrived. No matter how many birthings a midwife has assisted, there can be nothing matter-of-fact about assisting delivery, especially if she is close to the mother and is willing to let her participation be guided by love. *Every delivery is unique!* There are particular skills for making it run smoothly, but the midwife's main responsibility is to concentrate and respond on all pertinent

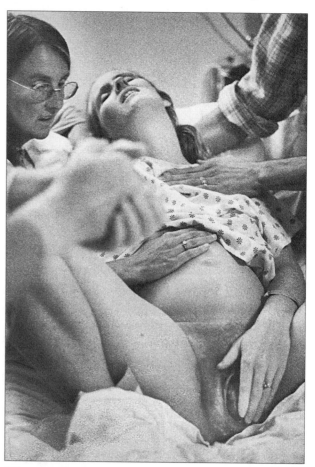

The magical wonder of touching your baby for the first time.

levels with an *attitude of devotion*. This is the essence of midwifery care; not only are you an assistant to the mother and her supporters, but a handmaiden to the forces of creation.

Now for the **specifics of preventing tears**. One of the most helpful and appreciated techniques is the application of **hot compresses to the perineum**. These stimulate good circulation, promote relaxation and provide relief from burning, tingling sensations. Use a sterile gauze pad, sanitary napkin, or clean washcloth soaked in a solution of hot water with a squeeze of Betadine or other antiseptic. Hot compresses are especially crucial if the perineum blanches with distension. They are also a help for mothers who involuntarily contract their outlet muscles. If delivery is precipitous and you can't find time for compresses, have your apprentice or assistant apply them while you concentrate on your other responsibilities.

As the head moves toward the outlet, massage any muscle bands inhibiting it, beginning at the start of the contraction and easing up at the peak to allow the head to stretch through the area on which you've been working. Use plenty of oil! If there is a prolonged delay of progress due to excess fatty padding or muscle tissue, place two fingers of each hand inside the mother and pull down and outward at points four and eight o'clock, literally making room for the head to descend. Whenever you work on thick or rigid tissue, freshen and reapply hot compresses after each contraction. (And remember to desist in the event of swelling.)

As you attend to the mother's perineum, remember to check the baby's condition. This factor determines how much time you have to work on keeping the perineum intact. For convenience, keep your fetascope hanging around your neck. The forehead rest allows you to listen to the baby during a contraction and continue to support the perineum at the same time. However, midwives in partnership may wish to divide these tasks, so that each has a chance to rest occasionally or to focus on the emotional needs of the mother and her partner.

At this time of maximum head compression, early decelerations to 100 BPM should not cause concern. Most worrisome are decelerations with poor recovery or persistent bradycardia. Oxygen for the mother can help, but if the heart rate remains below 100 and the head is on the perineum, the baby should be born at once. Inform the mother that she must get the baby out quickly, and that you need her full attention and cooperation. Tell her to let go completely, and you'll cue her when to push. Sometimes this advice is enough to dissolve the last bit of resistance, and the baby births spontaneously with the next contraction. Otherwise, you may need to do an episiotomy. If so, you must first obtain the mother's consent. Injecting lidocaine is optional due to the high degree of numbness in the perineum by this point, but you may wish to infiltrate the area if you have time. Position two fingers inside the perineum to protect the head, and have your scissors inserted between them and ready to cut as the head comes down the next contraction. Episiotomy may cause some bleeding; apply pressure with a gauze pad if necessary. The tissues will be also be vulnerable to tearing beyond the apex. It is crucial to prevent this by supporting and applying counterpressure to the base of the wound, just as you would the midline of the perineum.

Sometimes it becomes difficult to hear heart tones during second stage. Eventually your fetascope will rest at the edge of the pubic bone, and as the baby moves lower still, heart tones may become inaudible. This coincides with the phase of perineal stretching, which generally lasts for only a few contractions but may occasionally take longer. So the problem presents itself: how can you justify taking time to ease delivery if you have no clue to the baby's condition? Fortunately, there is another indicator you can use—**the color of the baby's scalp**. Also significant is the rate of venous return when the scalp is gently depressed. These assessments indicate how much oxygen the baby is getting. Once, while attending a hospital delivery, I heard the obstetrician say, "I'll hang my hat on pink scalps." Color assessment must be modified somewhat for babies of African-American parentage due to slightly dusky skin tones, but you can still check the rate of venous return, and pay attention to the shade appearing immediately after depressing the skin. Pinkish-blue is good, blue is less favorable, and white-blue is ominous.

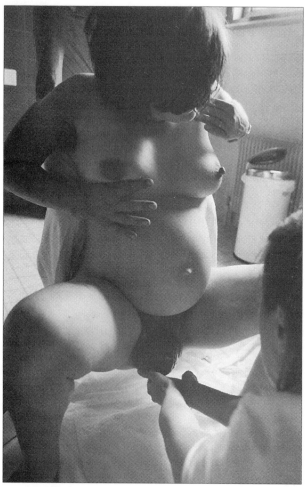

Upright delivery positions are tremendously empowering for the mother.

Now, back to the mother and her distending perineum. If the baby is doing well, its heart tones are fine and/or scalp color reassuring, you can afford to relax and take your time slowly easing the birth. Most important at this point is to **engage the mother in sensitive breathing**. As soon as the head is bulging forward, have her pant, and show her how to stay with it without tightening up or holding back. Although prenatal classes (and some popular texts) suggest that panting be used only for the moments of crowning, experience teaches that if the baby is coming down quickly, it ought to be started much sooner. Anyway, there is nothing to lose by having the mother pant through one contraction, as this gives you a chance to see how much force her body is exerting on its own so you can assess how rapidly delivery is approaching. And by getting her accustomed to panting before her sensations are

entirely overwhelming, you give her the power to ease up or come on according to what she feels. If she pants through one contraction and there's no descent, have her resume pushing as before. But if ever she complains of the burning or tingling characteristic of extreme stretching, it's time to have her pant.

And what about perineal massage? Your emphasis changes to support, because by now, the head has nearly filled the vagina. This brings us to the most critical maneuver for avoiding tears—**maintaining flexion of the fetal head.** As soon as the head begins to bulge forward, apply counterpressure to the perineum with a compress or gauze pad. In so doing, you hold back the forehead and promote flexion, so that the smallest possible diameter of the head presents. With final descent, pressure on the rectum may cause the mother to pass fecal matter. If your gauze pad or compress becomes contaminated, discard it for another.

As the head approaches crowning, apply some oil to the entire outlet, gently restroking any whitened areas. Once the head begins to work its way outward, keep one hand on the perineum while the other guards the urethral area and controls the rate of expulsion. By positioning the wrist of this hand at the top of the outlet and extending your fingers downward, you can simultaneously ease the head under the pubic bone and keep it from birthing too quickly. Maintain counterpressure with the other hand, so the parietal bones clear the upper part of the outlet before the face begins to emerge.

This two-handed juggling act of easing the birth of the head is obviously best learned by experience. Here is a general guideline, though: if you feel that a tear is unavoidable and something has got to give, let it be the perineum. Never let up on your upper hand control; many novices make the mistake of over-guarding the perineum so that periurethral tears result, which are extremely painful and difficult to repair. *And hold on to the perineum as the head is born over it—don't let go!*

Occasionally an arrest occurs in the perineal phase. Although the head has been near crowning for a number of contractions, and the mother is panting and relaxing well, no progress occurs. This arrest may be due to tension in maternal tissues, a large or deflexed head, or unconscious resistance caused, ironically enough, by fear of tearing!

Encourage the mother to feel her baby's head. This often brings a sigh or moan of surrender as she more deeply connects with the baby, and delivery soon follows. If this doesn't work, try having her **push between contractions**—she will feel more in control, and your efforts to prevent tears will be more successful without any additional pressure from her uterus. This approach is almost always effective. If not, and/or the perineum is becoming edematous, it's probably best to have the mother side-lying during delivery to minimize tearing.

As soon as the baby's head is out, do a quick appraisal of color and presence. Note how energized, vital, and physically alert the baby appears to be. Look for signs of stress: white-blue head with clenched mouth usually indicates a baby that needs to be birthed quickly, and one that may need some

help getting started. Wipe excessive amounts of blood and mucus or meconium away from the eyes, nose, and mouth, and suction as indicated. A large rubber ear syringe (three oz.) should be used for moderate secretions. Be sure to squeeze all the air out before inserting it into the baby's mouth, or you will force mucus and fluids further down the throat and possibly into the lungs. And don't insert it any further than a few inches, or you will stimulate the gag reflex at the back of the baby's throat, which can suppress its respiratory efforts.

The DeLee trap provides deep suction essential for thick mucus or meconium. Check to see that the lid is screwed on tightly so the device will work properly, then insert the tubing about four and a half inches into the baby's mouth. Withdraw slowly while sucking sharply and repeatedly (see illustration, below). Tell the mother not to push, and have your assistant hold the baby's shoulders back until you are finished. If you are still bringing up meconium as you remove the tubing, repeat

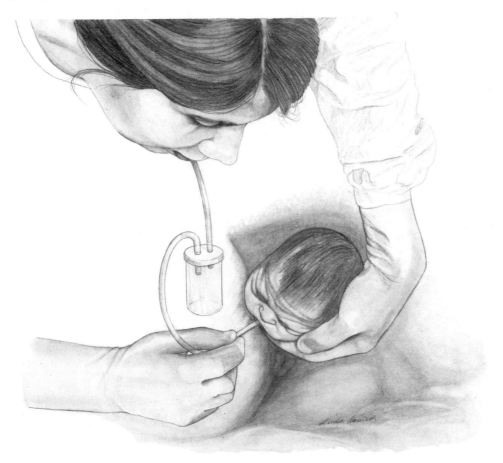

Using the DeLee Mucus Trap

the procedure until the fluid is clear. But work quickly, particularly if it appears that the baby may require resuscitation. If the baby has no fluids bubbling at its mouth and its color is good, there is no reason to do anything. Suction need not be done routinely.

Next, check around the neck for any loops of umbilical cord. Slip your finger along the back of the baby's neck, and if you find any cord, simply pull it over the head. Remember, any suction and/or cord maneuvers must be completed before the next contraction! If you find you cannot pull the cord free or there is not quite enough slack to slip it over the head, perhaps you can create a loop large enough for the shoulders and body to birth through. As a last resort, quickly clamp the cord twice with curved hemostats placed several inches apart, cut between them with blunt scissors, and unwind the cord away.

It is crucial when the cord is tight that you remind the mother to keep panting, and tell her firmly not to push until you let her know that it's all right. You might also announce "tight cord" as soon as you discover it, so your assistant can hand you the necessary instruments. If you must cut the cord at this point, you are literally cutting off the baby's oxygen supply, thus it must be born immediately. Then again, if the shoulders cannot be held back, tuck the baby's face against the mother's thigh and let its body "somersault" out.

Unless you've cut the cord, there is no need to hurry delivery of the shoulders as long as the baby's color is good. But if the head becomes suffused with blood and is turning purplish, encourage the mother to push her baby out right away. Don't wait on this—as long as the baby's chest is compressed inside the mother's vagina and venous return is impaired, intercranial pressure can build to dangerous levels.

In any event, have your assistant support the perineum as you deliver the shoulders, or do it yourself if her partner is catching the baby. The head should be gently grasped on either side, guided downward until the first shoulder appears, then immediately lifted up and outward at a 45-degree angle so the lower shoulder will not drag and cause a tear. Once the shoulders are out, turn the baby so it faces the mother, and encourage her to reach down and bring it out the rest of the way. Or simply catch the baby and lay it gently on the mom's belly. Cover the baby immediately with three flannel blankets (preferably oven-warmed) to help maintain its temperature.

Keep an eye on the baby, and do Apgar scoring at one and five minutes (see Appendix H). *The two most critical factors in stabilizing the newborn are warmth and a clear airway.* Make certain it is breathing well—if so, its color will be good, or if not, give suction and stimulation. Keep the baby warm by promptly changing its first set of blankets, which are usually dampened by fluid. Once the baby is stable, help the mother get comfortably positioned so that she and the baby can both relax. See that she is warm enough and has something sweet to drink, then ease back to your tasks and give the new family a chance to bond.

These are the mechanics of normal delivery; at least 90 percent of your clients will follow this basic pattern. But every delivery is unique emotionally, depending on how passionately the mother has labored, how alert or tired she feels, and in general, how happy she is to be having a baby. For the woman who has really found her way with labor, the moments of delivery are a time of complete concentration and inner focus. Intensity builds in second stage until the baby's head puts constant pressure on vaginal nerve endings. So overwhelming is this level of sensation that most women simply surrender, and fear and tension give way to an awareness of their baby's form. This can be a spiritual and sexual experience of union, merging . . . what some women refer to as the orgasm of delivery.

Regardless of how sensitively a woman delivers her baby, the sudden sensation of emptiness immediately postpartum can come as both a relief and a shock. It is of greatest importance that the mother have access to her baby at once, so this shock does not deepen into numbness that will hinder her ability to bond. The practice of keeping the baby down on the mother's thigh until stable, or that of routine suctioning, cleaning, and cutting the cord before giving the baby to the mother, are unnatural methods which definitely disrupt the intimate needs of the emerging family. Make no exceptions to this; even the baby who is born "floppy" should be lifted onto the mother and stimulation begun with it resting against her skin. Her connection with the baby is integral to its survival and well-being.

It used to be my practice to place the baby directly into the mother's arms, but I have modified this for several reasons. First, I noticed that women who birthed upright, either squatting or with birthing stool, all seemed to need a bit of time before they were ready to touch or pick up their babies. Then I viewed Marshall Klaus' video, in which a newly born baby placed on its mother's abdomen crawled instinctively to her nipple! Ray DeVries, Ph.D., has speculated that our rush to put the baby in its mother's arms and get it nursing as soon as possible may come from our own unresolved birth traumas of separation. *Why not place the baby on the mother's belly and allow it to come to her, or let her embrace it when she is ready?*

THIRD STAGE

The key to a safe and easy third stage is **watchful observation**. Many a bonding period has been disintegrated by an overzealous midwife who insisted on using cord traction, or on having the mother squat for the placenta before the time was really ripe. Then again, many a prolonged wait for the placenta and/or excessive blood loss has been caused by a non-attentive attendant missing crucial signs of placental separation. Watchful observation means exactly that; the midwife's participation is indicated by specific signs and signals rather than by rote.

As soon as the baby is stable, carefully attend to the mother until third stage is completed. The umbilical cord should not be cut until it has stopped pulsing. Rest it between the fingers of one hand (don't use your thumb, as it has a pulse) and wait. When it is time, put one clamp close to the mother's outlet and the other about eight inches

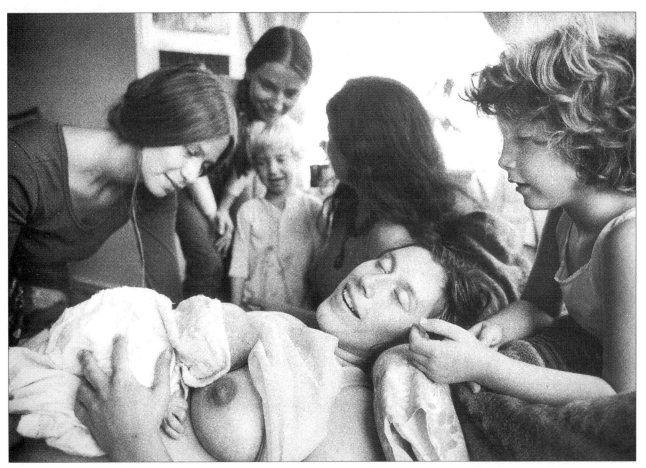

The ecstasy of delivery. One of the reasons for natural birth is this feeling akin to orgasm, of buildup and completion.

HERBS AND HOMEOPATHY DURING LABOR

by Shannon Anton

Most labors do not require the assistance or intervention of herbal or homeopathic allies. However, some labor circumstances can be aided by a skilled attendant utilizing these remedies appropriately. This support is offered primarily to preserve the precious energy of the laboring woman.

Early labor

If intense like transition, with contractions three minutes apart, and especially if the woman is shivering, try homeopathic **Cimicifuga** 200C. Labor may seem to decrease, but is actually finding a more effective pattern. This support greatly preserves the woman's vital forces.

If not yet regular, but unrelenting and not given to rest, promote regular contractions with homeopathic **Caulophyllum** 200C.

If on again, off again in nature, and especially if the woman is more whiny and clingy than usual, or needs a lot of validation that what she feels is emotionally normal, try homeopathic **Pulsitilla** 200C.

Active Labor

If one in which the woman appears to be scrambling away from herself and her contractions, try homeopathic **Sepia** 200C.

If the cervix is 100 percent effaced, about three cms. dilated, the os feels like a loop of thread, and labor appears very active or transitional, prepare for the birth as if it was imminent and give homeopathic **Gelsimium** 200C. Frequently, the cervix "pops" open to complete dilation. If the woman is not yet fully dilated but feels an urge to push, give **Arnica** 200C to prevent cervical swelling.

If there is a strong urge to push at only six to seven cms. dilation, or there is a cervical lip, try homeopathic **Sepia** 200C and **Arnica** 200C, followed by Sepia 200C every ten to fifteen minutes. I rely on these remedies absolutely, and find them to be among the best kept secrets of homeopathy for labor.

If dehydration or exhaustion occur, try homeopathic **China** or **Carbo Veg**, or **Ustilago** 200C. Additionally, an enema of warm water and **honey**, or a dose of **royal jelly** taken orally can greatly revive for the short term. Another good remedy is **Essence of Chicken**, found in Asian groceries and apothecaries.

Second Stage

If during second stage, contractions come less and less often, give homeopathic **Caulophyllum** 200C to keep labor going and to prevent postpartum hemorrhage. Each dose should have a noticeable effect. Repeat as necessary to establish a regular pattern of contractions.

Homeopathic Aconite is invaluable for helping women release fear or anxiety in labor. However, not all women benefit from crying or talking out their feelings; some are truly more internal in their process of release. Aconite 200C supports quietude and letting go.

Homeopathic Arnica is excellent when pain in labor seems out of proportion to the strength of contractions. Arnica can also render contractions more regular and effective. If the cervix is unyielding or swollen, Arnica 200C can alleviate irritation and reduce swelling. I give Arnica 200C to most mothers in my practice as soon as they feel bearing-down urges in second stage, dosing again as soon as possible after the baby is born. I rarely see swelling of the perineum postpartum, and almost never have to use ice. I suggest that my clients continue to take Arnica 30C for the first few days postpartum for soreness and body fatigue.

The Immediate Postpartum

I rely on two herbs during third stage: Angelica and Shepherd's Purse. I carry both in tincture form and keep them next to my pitocin. I find these herbs sufficient to handle most blood loss following birth. In case of sudden, torrential hemorrhage, I give pitocin IM as well as the appropriate herb. In some instances, I am sure it was the herb that stopped the bleeding, as the pitocin would not yet have had time to enter the mother's circulation. Nonetheless, with any dramatic blood loss, I give both.

Angelica tincture helps bring the placenta when the wait is prolonged. I give a dropperful under the tongue with a swig of water following. Remind yourself (and the mother) that Angelica brings the placenta "like an angel." Use also for partial separation of the placenta.

Shepherd's Purse tincture is best used after the placenta is out and you are certain it is complete. Because it promotes clotting so expertly, Shepherd's Purse can cause clots to form immediately as the placenta separates, which may lead to uterine distension and additional blood loss. If you are not sure the placenta is complete, use Angelica to bring on more contractions.

If you are confronted with a vaginal tear that has ruptured a small vessel, apply direct pressure to the tear and give a dropperful of **Trillium**, or Birthroot tincture. Trillium constricts small blood vessels and works perfectly in this application. You may find it unnecessary to tie off the vessel with suture.

Newborn Resuscitation: Homeopathic Remedies

While CPR and oxygen are essential, homeopathy is always appropriate and sometimes critical in newborn resuscitation. Most of these applications were taught me by Ifeoma Ikenze, pediatrician and homeopath. In my experience, their potency has been lifesaving. I keep these remedies near my drug box, with red labels to make them easily identifiable.

To give a remedy to a newborn, tuck one pellet in the cheek of the baby's mouth. A dose is assimilated by contact with the mucous membranes. In critical situations, repeat the dose in a minute or two. I have never heard of a baby aspirating a homeopathic remedy, even with use of an Ambu-bag.

Respiratory arrest

If there are minimal or no respiratory attempts, and the baby looks bluish or feels slightly cold, give **Carbo Veg** 1M.

Circulatory Collapse

If the baby is pale as a ghost, floppy, cold, weak, give **Camphora** 1M.

Weak Heartrate

If baby appears lifeless, pale, no respirations, give **Arsicum** 1M.

Mucous or wet lungs

If the baby is gray-blue, choking or gurgling, suction does not clear mucous, or lungs sound moist and sticky, give **Antimonium** 200C. Dose and repeat, along with percussion. Con[?] oxygen or steam from the shower.

Aconitum 1M is for a baby that is struggling and warm, perhaps crying inconsolably as if from a great fright, with rapid heart rate and respirations, and color red, not blue. This baby appears to be shocked by the suddenness of birth, and may have difficulty integrating all the stimuli. Another solution is **Rescue Remedy**, given orally or on the soles of the baby's feet.

Arnica 200C is a wonderful remedy for extreme molding or caput. If the mother chooses not to give vitamin K, homeopathic Arnica is appropriate.

Difficulty with Urination

A new mother may have difficulty urinating immediately after birth. It's important to make sure she is able to empty her bladder, as a distended bladder can interfere with her uterus staying contracted. Her bladder may also be injured if it becomes too distended. Homeopathic **Arnica** 200C can help reduce swelling of the urethra. Also try turning off the lights, dribbling water in the sink, having her put hands or feet in warm water, or putting a few drops of **Peppermint Oil** in the toilet before she tries to urinate. Give her privacy, but make sure she has support should she become faint.

Keep in mind that Peppermint oil will antidote any homeopathic remedies she has taken. This is usually fine, but if using homeopathic Arnica, dose again after she's settled back into bed.

Fainting In the Immediate Postpartum

Giving birth creates incredible changes in a woman's body. Getting to her feet, or even sitting upright, can cause dizziness and fainting. If so, place her in shock position and try this old, reliable but strange remedy: **burnt hair**. Take a lock of hair from her partner or closest relative present. Burn the hair to cinders, and place the crunchy bits under her tongue. Believe it or not, this will stabilize her dramatically. Some women benefit from a pinch of the **placenta** under their tongue. You may want to try a dose of **Rescue Remedy**. Or, using a soft bristled brush, stroke from her feet to her knees, then from her knees to her hips. Strong **black tea** will also help normalize her circulation.

away. Have the mother's partner or your assistant cut between them, several inches from the clamp nearest the baby.

Now, watch for **signs of placental separation**. Keep an eye on the clamp nearest the mother; it will move downward as the placenta detaches and descends, and the cord will appear to lengthen. Also watch the outlet for excessive bleeding. Usually, there is very little blood loss until the characteristic gush-flow of placental separation. Rarely, the placenta separates only in the center, with no blood evident at the outlet because margins remain attached. The uterus will increase in size and become boggy, and if the mother continues to bleed, she may go into shock. To rule this out, rest a hand on the fundus as soon as the baby is out, and keep it there until the placenta delivers. This maneuver is called **guarding the uterus**. But do not massage or prod the uterus, as this can cause uterine muscle spasm and result in partial separation and hemorrhage. No "fundus fiddling"; keep your hands still!

DELIVERING THE PLACENTA

Nine times out of ten, the placenta separates all at once. As you notice the cord lengthening, the mother says she feels like pushing. This is an opportune time for her to squat, as delivery of the placenta is best accomplished with the mother in an upright position.

If she is exhausted and doesn't feel like moving, you can assist her with expulsion. But first, make sure the placenta is fully separated. To do this, don a clean glove and gently follow the cord to the cervical os. If the placenta is either in the vagina or immediately behind the cervical opening, it is fully separated, and **controlled cord traction** may be used to remove it. But take care—if the placenta is not separated and you pull on the cord, you run the risk of **inverting the uterus**, i.e., turning it inside out, which could kill the mother.

To perform controlled cord traction, hold the uterus in place by pressing the edge of your hand in above the pubic bone and upwards towards the mother's head. As you apply traction to the cord, guide the placenta along the L-shaped curve of the birth canal—first down, then out. Do this when the uterus is contracted, and with the mother's pushing efforts.

What's the average time span for delivery of the placenta? About 20 to 30 minutes. Although separation may occur just moments after delivery, the membranes often remain adherent until the placenta drops to the cervix and its weight detaches them completely. It is therefore wise to catch and support the placenta as it delivers, for membranes may shred or tear if they are not yet separated and the placenta is allowed to fall any distance into the basin.

If the membranes do seem stuck, you can coax them out by holding the placenta with both hands and moving it with a give-and-take motion. Or twist the placenta around repeatedly so that the membranes form a rope, then coax outwards.

The placenta may deliver either fetal or maternal side first. If the fetal side presents, we call this **separation by the Shultz mechanism**, generally correlated to fundal implantation and separation beginning at the center of the placenta. If the maternal side presents, we call this **separation by the Duncan mechanism**, generally linked to low implantation and separation commencing at the edges. Students often remember these distinctions with slang terms: *shiny Shultz*, i.e., glossy membranes, and *dirty Duncan*, i.e., meaty maternal side.

Once expulsion is complete, check immediately to be certain the uterus is well contracted, and give it a few quick squeezes to expel any clots which may have formed behind the placenta. Then simply maintain watchful observation, keeping an eye out for any bleeding and feeling the uterus periodically for firmness. If the uterus feels soft or asymmetrical in shape, or you note excess bleeding at the outlet, rub up a good contraction and encourage the mother to nurse her baby, if she's not already doing so.

Slow trickle bleeding must be watched very carefully. Make sure the mother's bladder is not distended, as this can interfere with the uterus' ability to clamp down. Follow the recommendations above, and also give several droppersful of shepherd's purse and blue cohosh tinctures. Should blood begin to flow steadily or in spurts, it's time

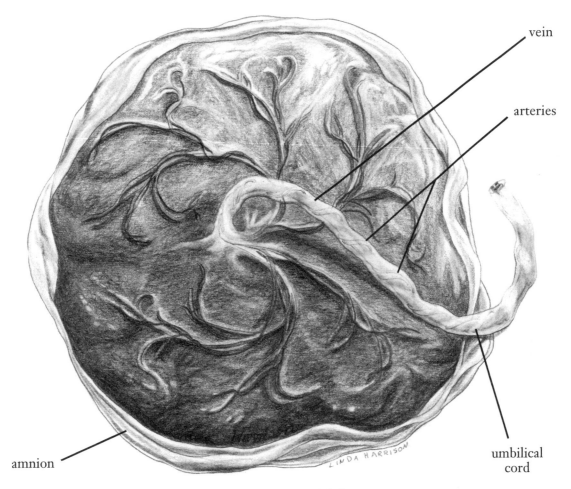

vein

arteries

umbilical
cord

amnion

Placenta: Fetal Side

to resort to emergency measures (see Hemorrhage, Chapter Five).

Also **examine the placenta thoroughly** to be sure it is complete. You can do this right at the bedside, as you keep watch on the mother. If she is bleeding and you are attending to that, have your assistant check the placenta, as retained fragments may be causing the problem. Anything retained in the uterus will prevent it from clamping down completely, and if such is the case, no amount of massage or pitocin will control blood loss for any length of time. The cardinal rule for managing postpartum hemorrhage is to **determine the cause of bleeding**, so you know how best to respond.

Examine the **maternal side** of the placenta first. Start by pulling away any clots, then hold the placenta in your hands so it opens convexly, exposing rents and separations clearly. Then cup it together, to see if the edges of the rents and spaces join evenly and match up. Check the edges of the

placenta to make sure they blend cleanly into membrane and nothing appears to have been torn away. If anything appears to be missing, hemorrhage may result.

Turn the placenta over to check the **fetal side**. Begin with the cord, noting how many vessels are present—there should be three tiny holes visible at the end, i.e., two arteries and a vein. If there are less, the baby may have anomalies not immediately apparent, and should be seen by a pediatrician. The white-blue material in which the vessels are suspended is called **Wharton's jelly**. This substance should be present at the juncture of cord and placenta—if the vessels are suspended in membrane alone, you've discovered a rare **velamentous cord insertion**. Next, determine where the cord joins the placenta—at the center, i.e., **central insertion**, or at the edge, i.e., **marginal insertion**.

Check too for any vessels running from the edge of the placenta off into the membranes. If any

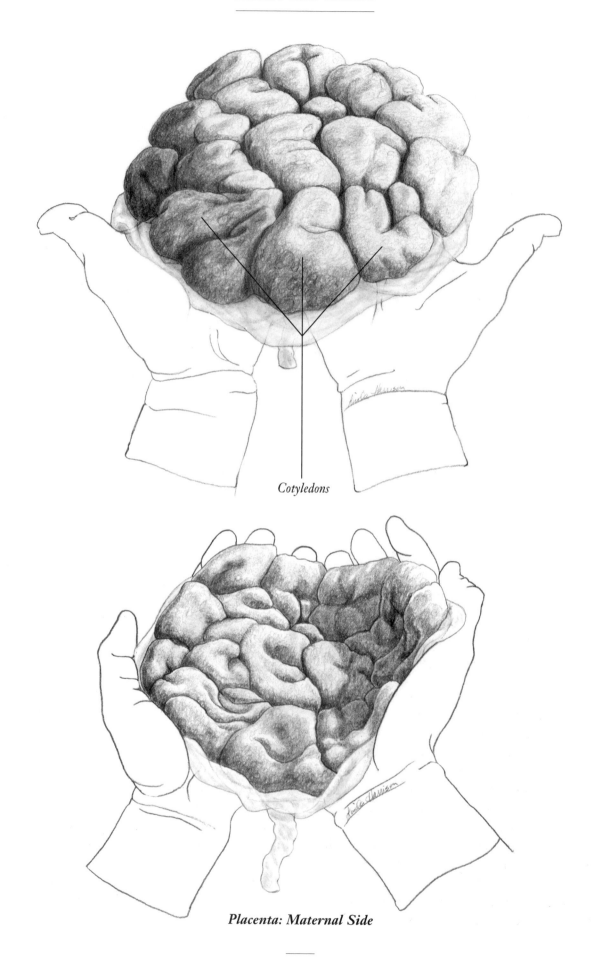

Cotyledons

Placenta: Maternal Side

of these vessels terminate abruptly with a hole in the membranes, it's probable that a **succenturiate lobe** (mini-placenta) is still retained in utero and will likely cause a postpartum hemorrhage. The lobe must be removed manually, either by you or by someone in the hospital (again, see Chapter Five).

Once the placenta has delivered, you have numerous minor tasks to attend to. Re-clamp and cut the baby's cord, get both baby and mother warm, cozy, and cleaned up, and facilitate breast-feeding. Your assistant can care for the baby while you see to the mother's comfort; this is very important. If she has slouched down in her pillows, help her into a comfortable sitting position, with enough support under each elbow to allow her to cradle the baby easily. Once she is relaxed and alert, she will nurse and bond more readily with the baby, which will help keep her uterus well contracted.

CHECKING FOR TEARS

Once the placenta is out and the mother is stable, she will want to know if she has torn, and you'll be anxious to resolve this question for yourself. Discard the bloodied underpads beneath her, and replace with several fresh ones. Wash the mother with warm water and Betadine. Arrange good lighting—a high-intensity lamp works well—then open some sterile gauze, put on sterile gloves, use gauze to part the labia, and see what you can see. (Sterile gloves must be used when checking for tears, since the cervix is still open and the uterus susceptible to infection.) Check for any abrasions, obvious tears around the urethra and perineum, or internal muscle splits at the floor of the vagina (see Chapter Five for further instructions).

If the mother needs no repair, her uterus is firm, her placenta is complete, and her baby has good color and responsiveness, you can afford to sit back for a moment and rest. As you do so, facilitate family integration with some heartfelt words of praise regarding the birth and the baby. This can help alleviate any self-conscious feelings the mother or her partner may have about their behavior during labor. As the new family relaxes and draws closer together, give them privacy and go out to the kitchen for a break of your own. Take

the placenta along for closer examination, and tell the mother to call if she feels herself bleeding, or feels at all weak or dizzy.

Check on her every ten minutes, and bring her juice and something to eat. As her band of supporters begins to disperse and she is ready to be up and around—perhaps to go to the bathroom—make sure someone goes with her. Then attend to cleaning up, changing the bed linens, straightening the room, etc.

NEWBORN EXAM

Because of HIV and hepatitis risks, wear gloves for newborn exam. Before you begin, make sure that the mother and her partner have had a chance to fondle and bond with the baby, and that it has nursed at least once. Do the exam on the bed so parents can watch. The room should be warm, as the warmer and more comfy the baby, the more cooperative it will be. If the room is cool, place a heating pad on low setting under a towel or several receiving blankets to create a cozy exam surface. Unwrap the baby gradually, exposing just the area being checked. Explain each step to the parents as you move along. Examine the baby from head to toe—first the front side, then the back. (Please refer to Newborn Exam, Appendix H.)

Begin by **checking the baby's heart beat.** Listen closely for arrhythmia or anything else unusual, then time it carefully and record. The heart rate often drops a bit after delivery; normal rate is about 110 to 150 BPM.

Next, note the **baby's general condition and activity level** with a brief description, e.g. "pink, vigorous, strong cry," or "good color and muscle tone, quiet, nursed at one and a half hours." Any general concerns regarding the birth or baby may be noted here, e.g trauma with delivery, need for resuscitation, etc.

Then **check the skin.** Note the color; a bright red tone is associated with prematurity and a condition known as **polycythemia** (excess red cells). This finding necessitates a hematocrit on the baby, or referral to the pediatrician. **Desquamation** (peeling skin) is common with postmaturity and in itself is no cause for alarm, but may alert you to more serious problems associated with this condition. Babies of African-American, Mediterranean, or Hispanic parentage may have **Mongolian spots**, dark splotches at the base of the spine which are normal and usually vanish in time (you may wait until you turn the baby over to check for these, and record then). Also note any birth marks, or hairy moles. If vernix is present, massage it into the baby's skin or it may cause inflammation, particularly in the skin folds.

It's important to **check the head carefully for excessive molding, bruising, or swelling**. All of these indicate some trauma during labor or delivery. Molding causes the head to assume an elongated, abnormal shape, but tends to diminish within a matter of hours. **Caput**, or generalized edema on top of the head, may result from extreme molding. **Cephalhematoma** is an abnormal, lump-like swelling confined to a particular area; it does not cross suture lines, and is associated with internal bleeding between the scalp and the skull. Cephalhematoma is a sign of significant trauma, necessitating administration of vitamin K to prevent further hemorrhage, and attention from a pediatrician. If cephalhematoma is combined with bruising and/or excessive molding, the baby should be seen as soon as possible.

Check the eyes for red spots, which are conjunctival hemorrhages from pressure in the birth canal. Instill medication; erythromycin ointment is standard, and is effective against both gonorrhea and chlamydia. The ENT abbreviation on the form means ear, nose, and throat. **Check the ears** by looking for skin tags and **noting ear placement**. The top of the ear should be level with the corner of the baby's eye; low-lying ears are often associated with kidney problems or other anomalies. If you discover this condition, have the baby seen immediately. Don a fresh glove to prevent any maternal secretions from entering the baby's mouth, and **check the lips and palate** to be sure they are normal. Feel carefully with your little finger all around the roof of the mouth and back to the throat, to make certain the palate is intact. In so doing, you will also note the sucking reflex—the baby should suck strongly on your finger as you check.

To **check the thorax for retractions**, observe how the chest and stomach move when the baby breathes. Ribs and belly should inflate smoothly together; if the skin pulls tight between the ribs, or the chest and the abdomen move in a seesaw fashion, the baby has retractions. This finding may indicate immature lungs, lung damage, or obstruction. A pediatrician should see the baby at once.

Next **check the abdomen**. Occasionally you will note **umbilical hernia**, which appears as a bulge at the base of the cord stump. This is not caused by any particular method of handling or tying the cord, but is a congenital defect which can be remedied by surgery when the child is around two years old. Also feel the belly for masses, lumps, swellings; all should feel smooth and even. (It's easier to do this if you flex the baby's knees toward the abdomen with one hand while checking with the other.)

Check femoral pulses by simultaneously placing fingertips (use the index fingers of both hands) in the left and right groin areas. You should feel pulsing on either side, and the pulses should be the same, i.e., symmetrical. If not, the baby may have a congenital heart problem; refer to the pediatrician immediately.

Femoral pulses can be difficult to assess. If you have trouble identifying them, try using less pressure with your examining fingers. The lighter your touch, the less chance of compressing the vessels so you can't feel the pulse.

Check genitals carefully to be sure that all essential parts and openings are present. Girl babies frequently have some vaginal mucus present. Boys should be checked to see that both testes are descended. This is not difficult; simply place your finger at the top of one side of the scrotum to close off the inguinal canal and feel carefully for the testicle, then repeat on the other side. This is especially important in breech births as trauma may cause torsion and swelling, and one testicle may be lost unless the problem is detected within several hours of delivery.

If the scrotum is very edematous and difficult to palpate, shine a flashlight against it. Illuminating the swollen scrotum will help you locate an evasive testicle.

Reflexes have usually been demonstrated by now, at least sucking (with palate check) and swallowing (by breastfeeding). To verify the grasping reflex, have the baby grab your little fingers, and see if you can lift its body slightly off the bed. Check the Moro, or startle, reflex by supporting the baby's body and tipping it back suddenly; the arms and hands should extend evenly. These reflexes are important, as their presence is a sign of neurological health and maturity.

Next, turn the baby over and **closely examine the spine**. This area can be easily overlooked. Check for incomplete fusion, and look for dimples or sinuses (openings), especially in the sacral area. Also note Mongolian spots and record with other findings regarding the skin. **Check the anus** by observation; it is not necessary to insert a thermometer to check for patency. Even if the baby has not passed meconium, it will often have a plug visible at the opening; this is also proof of patency.

Then **check the lungs**, listening through the baby's back. Position your stethoscope up near the shoulders, and then again at mid-back level on either side. The lungs should sound clear, air resonating as if in a hollow chamber with no rattling or scratchy noises. This is particularly important if there has been any meconium at delivery; if such is the case and the baby's lungs sound obstructed, try percussion and steam (see Chapter Six) or take the baby to the pediatrician right away.

Of greatest interest to parents and friends are the baby's **weight and measurements**. Measure the head circumference at the widest point, from occiput to frontal bone, and record in centimeters (average measurements are 34 to 37 cms.). Then measure the chest; the difference between head and chest should be no more than a few centimeters. If the head is much larger, there may be an abnormal amount of fluid in the cranium, which should be checked immediately by a pediatrician. If the chest measurement is the same or larger than that of the head, and the baby is over nine pounds, the mother may have had some degree of glucose intolerance and the baby should be checked for hypoglycemia. Measure length by setting the tape alongside the baby's body with top edge level with the tip of the head, then stretch the leg out and measure at the heel. Chart in both centimeters and inches. To weigh, use either a standard baby scale

or the more convenient hanging style, which has a hook from which the baby is temporarily suspended in a stork-style bundle. Whichever you use, don't forget to subtract the weight of the blankets. Chart in both pounds and grams. Also take the **axillary temperature,** and record.

Finish by **checking the extremities**. Save this for last, because when you check the hips the baby may cry, and this way, you can hand it directly to the mother. Begin by counting fingers and toes, checking for webbing. Note symmetry of muscle tone in the arms (largely accomplished already by checking the Moro reflex). This is crucial if there has been a tight squeeze with the shoulders, which could cause nerve damage known as **Erb's palsy** or injury to the clavicles. Check each clavicle by palpating from the sternum to the shoulder—if there is fracture, you will note an unmistakable crinkling sensation called **crepitus**.

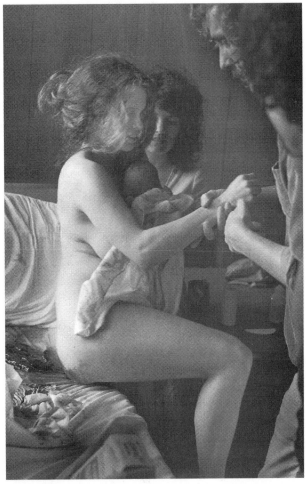

Triumphant and tender, the new mother gets up with her baby for the first time.

Finally check the hips by doing the "click test," rotating the legs firmly in their sockets as your fingers rest on the hip joints, and feeling for clicking that might indicate dislocation. Then flex the knees to the abdomen, and as you press them gently, feel once more for any clicking or unnatural movement of bone slipping out of the socket. If you find anything unusual, turn the baby over again and check hip creases from the backside. These should be symmetrical; if not, have the baby seen by a physician.

Wrap the baby in dry blankets. If it is content, this may be a good time for the mother's partner to hold it while she takes a shower or stretches her legs a bit.

POSTPARTUM WATCH

Your postpartum watch should last for at least two hours, longer if there has been repeated or recent bleeding, meconium at delivery, or any other concerns regarding the baby. The mother should have something to eat and drink, should urinate and nurse successfully before you go, and all her vital signs—blood pressure, temperature, and pulse—should be within normal range for at least an hour. Be sure to leave copies of the Birth Record and Newborn Exam for the parents to take to their pediatrician. Go over your postpartum instructions carefully (see Appendix K), making sure that parents understand everything. Encourage them to call you anytime, about anything, at any hour. And don't go until they seem to feel comfortable with you leaving.

You should also be sure that you are in stable condition before leaving. Particularly after a grueling labor or difficult delivery, you may be absolutely exhausted and should rest and relax with your assistant or midwifery partner before attempting to drive. A midwife from my area had the great misfortune of falling asleep at the wheel on her way back from a birth; her car hit a tree and she sustained major injuries. Those first few hours after the birth fly by; *make a habit of getting something to drink or eat immediately after the delivery* so you're ready to go when it's time.

GOLDEN TIPS FOR EXPECTANT PARTNERS

Here are some special ways to assist your partner during labor:

1. If labor begins at night and is mild, help her back to sleep with a massage.

2. If labor begins during the day, take her to a place you both love where you can get used to labor together.

3. Help her to eat as long as possible; prepare (or buy) her favorite foods.

4. Wear something she likes, and keep in close, relaxed physical contact with her.

5. As labor progresses, help her relax by encouraging her to let her body "go limp," and stroke her gently to reassure her.

6. Breathe with her if she starts to panic.

7. Don't be embarrassed to use common endearments with your midwives around; she needs to hear them from you!

8. In transition, speak tenderly to her between contractions, and maintain eye contact during contractions.

9. Once she is pushing, get your body close to her somehow so she feels your reinforcement.

10. Let her know when you can see the baby's head, and help her reach down and touch it.

11. Tell her you love her, especially after the baby comes out.

CHAPTER 5

Complications in Labor

Complications arising during labor are challenging to any midwife, no matter how experienced. Prenatal problems are not so crucial, as there is usually time to consider, consult, and re-evaluate from visit to visit. But labor is so condensed that decisions must be made both carefully and quickly. Close and vigilant attention is the key to detecting complications at their inception. Beyond that, sensitivity and objectivity must be combined to evaluate whether a particular course of treatment is proving effective. Labor is so intensive that feedback is fairly immediate, as long as you stay open to it.

When birth becomes complicated, one of the attributes of a good midwife is an ability to consider the total picture, while pinpointing the area on which to focus a remedy. In the midst of every difficult labor it is crucial to keep the overview, and to track any loose ends which may require attention later in labor or postpartum. And never should belief in the principle of non-intervention be used as an excuse for laziness or indifference! There is a delicate balance between the parents' right to give birth undisturbed, to proceed at their own pace and learn their lessons, and the midwife's responsibility to use her knowledge in such a way that stamina and safety are maintained to the end.

The effect of maternal emotions on labor should never be underestimated. There are definitely instances when emotional problems portend physical danger, yet there is still safe leeway for turning the tide and getting labor back on course again. Changes occurring with emotional breakthrough can be miraculous, and are as integral to positive outcome as are physical diagnosis and treatment.

Handling complications means *facilitating change*. This is part art, part logic. Take it step-by-step, like this:

1. Determine the possible cause or causes of the complication;
2. Test your diagnosis through further observation plus discussion with your partner and the parents;
3. Modify your diagnosis if need be, suggest a remedy, and implement it with the parents' agreement;
4. Follow up with close and careful checks on vital signs and progress to determine effectiveness/ results; and
5. Watch carefully for any side effects, and re-evaluate as indicated.

It helps tremendously if the entire birthing team is intent on working together. If you sense a non-committal attitude from the parents despite your best counsel and encouragement, it may be that the birth is not meant to happen at home. Waiting in limbo is dissipating, particularly when labor forces are struggling to move ahead. If the parents concur that transport is a good idea, the move to the hospital should be made as quickly as possible.

Sometimes parents request transport, not out of fear or desperation but because they sense that something is about to go wrong. Never try to dissuade parents from such a decision; always honor their instincts in this regard.

Transport is a complication and trauma in itself, especially if labor has been long and everyone is tired. Parents usually need help with preparations for leaving: getting dressed, packing a bag, making childcare arrangements, and calling a few relatives.

The woman's partner may be moved to tears out of sympathy for the mother, out of sadness for the loss of their homebirth dream, or out of sheer frustration and exhaustion. Some get angry and accusing. Meanwhile, you must contact the obstetrician and call the hospital to arrange for admission. Trying to be lucid and medically articulate while suffering from stress and/or sleep deprivation can be quite a challenge. It helps to have your chart in order, so questions from hospital personnel can be kept to a minimum when you do arrive (you can update in the car if necessary). A one-page transport summary sheet is also helpful.

Life-threatening emergencies seldom arise, but when they do, the focus is on survival (with little or no time for integration). But in the majority of transport situations, you have the opportunity to give reassurance, support, and hope to the parents on the way to the hospital—one of the greatest services a midwife can render.

PROLONGED FIRST STAGE AND MATERNAL EXHAUSTION

Prolonged first stage has many causes, some emotional and some physical. Often the two are interwoven, and it's up to you to sort through numerous factors to arrive at the primary problem. For example, say you are assisting a mother with a large, unengaged posterior baby; it's common to see an arrest of progress at around six centimeters due to lack of descent and insufficient cervical stimulation. She may become frustrated and impatient, but in this case, no amount of counseling or encouragement can override fetal malpresentation as the principal cause of arrest.

In itself, a long latent phase is no cause for concern as long as the mother is handling her contractions well and is able to eat, exercise, and rest in good measure. Latent labor should not interfere with normal life; encourage her to go for a walk, to a movie, or to visit friends. If she is only one or two centimeters dilated and is panting, groaning, and plugging away, she needs help winding down in order to conserve energy and keep her sense of humor for the hard work ahead.

Occasionally, you have the confusing case of a mother who seems to be in active labor, with contractions coming every five minutes, strong and lasting a minute or more, but no more than two or three centimeters dilation over a period of some hours. To call this a "long latent phase" would be a mistake. Going by the length and strength of contractions, this is actually an arrest of early, active labor.

There is a stereotype that tends to this problem—the woman with a strong athletic or intellectual component unable to let go and give up control. Uterine fatigue and inertia are likely to result; if so, a complete break for everyone is usually the best solution. Although the uterus has made a first attempt at active labor without success, never fear—it will start up again after a period of rest (and dilation may take place quite quickly!) Still, you may feel rather foolish for having coached and monitored so diligently, only to end up with two centimeters dilation and no more contractions. It's natural to wonder, "What was I doing here, anyway...maybe I just should have waited at home!" Strong contractions rightfully prompt assessment of mother and baby, but at this point it probably is best to go home for a meal and some rest, and suggest that parents have the same, with a glass of wine to help them relax before they get some sleep. The chance to be completely alone, with a taste of true labor behind them, will often set a couple to talking about any unresolved conflicts, or their more immediate needs for intimacy. This sets the stage for rapid progress in the next round.

I attended a birth classic in this pattern; for 12 hours (mostly at night) we had the mother walking, squatting, in and out of hot baths, drinking stimulating teas, etc. It felt rather ironic but liberating to be sitting around the following afternoon with labor halted, sharing a glass of champagne (we went ahead and opened it) and simply relaxing together. With no sign of maternal or fetal exhaustion, why worry? We went home, and after a six-hour break were called back to find the mother dilated to seven centimeters, handling her labor well and birthing shortly thereafter. When we asked what had happened she replied, "Well, after you left we got in bed and talked a lot, fell asleep, and then it just started up again really strong."

Fetal Asynclitism

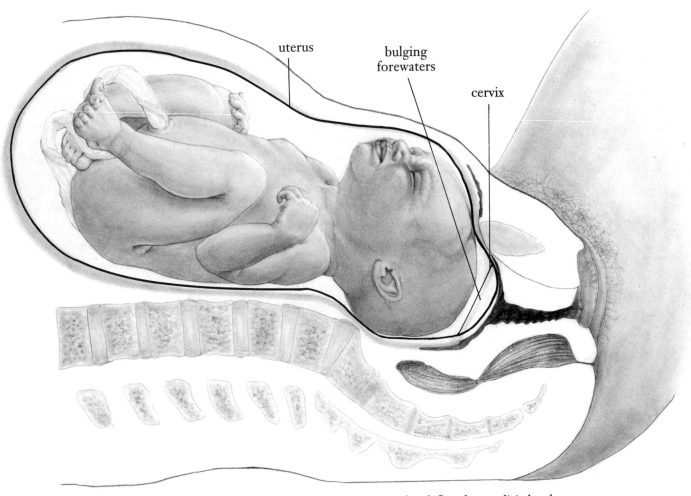

Relative CPD caused by a posterior position and a deflexed, asynclitic head.

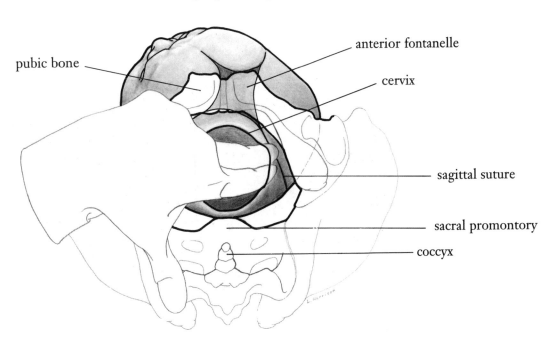

Correct asynclitism by centering the sagittal suture.

Once a woman has passed six centimeters, an arrest of progress is more serious because the uterus is now hard at work, and tends to persist regardless of maternal tension. This means that if the mother resists her sensations and works against her body, she may reach a state of **clinical exhaustion** long before her uterus takes a break. The symptoms of clinical exhaustion include ketones in the urine, with elevated pulse and temperature. This condition is also known as **ketoacidosis**, because the mother's blood pH becomes increasingly acidic. If the fetus in turn becomes acidotic, cardiac output goes down and the blood carries less oxygen. In other words, unless this condition is reversed, maternal exhaustion will lead to fetal distress.

In order to prevent this, the mother should be carefully monitored throughout any phase of arrest and if signs of ketoacidosis manifest, remedial measures should be initiated immediately (see page 93). The baby must also be monitored more closely for any signs of distress. It must be understood, however, that merely treating symptoms of arrest will not rectify the situation. You must do your utmost to *determine the cause*.

Begin by doing a thorough vaginal exam to ascertain any impediments to fetal descent. Check carefully the position of the head and how it's presenting. Posterior babies often present somewhat deflexed, which increases head circumference and may hinder descent. In this case, or if the baby is quite large, **asynclitism** may also be noted. Asynclitism occurs when the baby is having difficulty negotiating the pelvic inlet, and compensates by leading with one side of its head only; upon internal exam, the suture line is found either to be running high or low in the pelvis, rather than directly across the cervical opening (see illustration, page 119). Asynclitism may be a cause *or* a sign of **cephalopelvic disproportion (CPD)**, particularly if other factors, such as size of the baby, size of the mother's pelvis, and the condition of cervix tend to concur. Conditions of asynclitism, malpresentation, and CPD must be ruled out before considering other possibilities (please refer to forthcoming sections for more detail).

Another cause for delay may be **cervical edema**. If swelling occurs as early as five or six centimeters, and the cervix is not well applied to the head, rule out causative factors of malpresentation or CPD. If cervical edema occurs around eight centimeters and the mother has been favoring prone positions, chances are the cervix will thin out rapidly once she is upright. Prone positions often cause compression of vaginal tissues adjacent to the baby's head, which impairs venous return from the cervix and results in swelling. Having her change to a standing or squatting posture should increase pelvic space and circulation so dramatically that the problem quickly resolves itself.

On the other hand, if she has already been upright and her labor has been particularly painful or intense, cervical edema may be better alleviated by having her lie down on her side for a while, then switch to the other side. Even if the cervix is relieved of pressure one side at a time, edema will gradually resolve.

Sometimes a **cervical lip** is the last obstacle to complete dilation. This is swelling of the anterior portion of the cervix (the rest being fully retracted), due to pressure from the descending head against the bottom edge of the pubic bone. It is most common with persistent posterior presentations. Reposition the mother, as above. For a stubborn lip, one midwife recommends the application of ice, placed in the finger of a sterile glove and held against the cervix. Once the swelling is reduced, or if the lip is soft enough, try pushing it back. As the mother prepares to bear down, push the lip over the baby's head as it descends, and hold the lip up behind the pubic bone as the contraction recedes. If the lip is gone, you've succeeded; if not, try again. You may exert some pressure with this maneuver, but never force the cervix for risk of tearing it. This may be somewhat uncomfortable for the mother. It helps if she is in a squatting position.

Sometimes tense membranes retard descent and/or dilation. This is most common at approximately eight centimeters. You may wish to perform **artificial rupture of the membranes (AROM)**, but first make sure the head is low enough in the pelvis to prevent cord prolapse. As a rule, the head must be at 0 station, but it is common for a larger head (or one slightly deflexed and posterior) to fill the pelvic cavity snugly at -1 station. If the head is too high for AROM to be safe, the mother must walk, squat, relax, and wait until it descends. Be forewarned: this may take hours, so be sure the mother drinks plenty of water, takes tablespoons of honey, eats if possible, and keeps her bladder empty.

You may occasionally be tempted to intervene by artificially rupturing the membranes early in labor. I once made the mistake of doing so at four centimeters, hoping that descent would result and additional pressure on the cervix would stimulate progress. This decision was made after 38 hours of erratic contractions, and another twelve hours of regular, moderately strong ones. A tense bag of waters was forming, and the baby's head (which was small and engaged) was not well applied to the cervix. The mother had a generous pelvis with no abnormalities, so I reasoned the water bag was holding the baby up. Surprisingly enough, rupturing the membranes did not bring descent. The real problem was that the mother was still early enough in labor to have active control; she used her excellent abdominal and vaginal muscles to hold the baby up inside her so she'd feel less pressure on her back. The result of my intervention was to create a new complication—prolonged rupture of the membranes, which eventually necessitated pitocin induction as more time elapsed and infection became a concern.

To perform AROM, don a sterile glove, squirt a bit of sterile gel over your fingers, and splint an amnihook between them. As a contraction ends, insert your fingers, push the hook to the bag, then lift up and pull the tip towards you to snag the membranes. Remove your fingers slowly and carefully, keeping the hook fully guarded. It's best to do this with the mother fairly upright. Be sure to take heart tones immediately afterwards, and chart.

Once you've determined that there are no physical obstacles impeding progress, you have to consider both psychological and environmental dynamics. There are many different reasons why the mother or couple might resist the process of opening up. Usually, emotional problems revealed at prenatal visits will have given specific clues as to what might go awry, but here is a general list of possibilities:

1. Mother not feeling enough love, communication, or faith from her partner;

2. Partner unable or unwilling to let go and give, due to inhibitions with self, or fear of labor;

3. Worries for both about becoming parents; for the mother, loss of personal attention she enjoyed during pregnancy; for her partner, moving from limbo to new levels of responsibility;

4. Awareness of sexual dysfunction awakening with the physical-emotional intensity of labor, including unknown history of sexual abuse, or;

5. Disharmony in the environment—too many people, too many comings and goings, no sense of privacy, or a family friend or relative who is undermining or threatening the mother in some way.

With the possible exception of past sexual abuse, these problems are usually resolved by facilitating intimacy between the mother and her partner. As mentioned earlier, it may be tempting for the midwife to step in and take over, simply caring for the mother herself. But for the couple's sake, it is better that she stay neutral, exemplifying techniques for the expectant partner and subtly enlisting his/her participation. Demonstrate helpful ways to touch and massage the mother during contractions, and model an appropriately loving and tender tone of voice. Once the couple is working comfortably together, take any necessary vital assessments and leave them alone for a while.

As for the environment, the labor room can get rather stale after a while, so change the scene frequently. If the couple feels a veritable party impinging on their privacy, friends within earshot of their bedroom door, how free will they feel with intimate expression? Clear out well-wishers kindly, explaining that it may be many hours before the birth takes place and now is the best time for a break. In any event, get the mother up and walking in the backyard, or at a nearby park, beach, or wooded area. Being in touch with nature can work wonders for her morale. If you accompany her, have your partner (or other birth team member) straighten up the room, remake the bed, bring in fresh tea, water, flowers, etc. while you are out.

Emotionally-based arrests typically occur at four centimeters, seven to eight centimeters, and sometimes at nine centimeters. *The four centimeter threshold* is the reckoning point of labor, the time when a woman must humble herself to her need for assistance and support from her partner and/or friends. *Difficulty at seven to eight centimeters* is due to early transition sensations, strong surges of vaginal pressure which may cause the mother to fear she will split apart and lose the last remnants of her identity. If there is any history of sexual dysfunction, it may surface now. *An arrest at nine centimeters* may reflect conflicts about parenting, but these issues more commonly arise in second stage (see section on Prolonged Second Stage).

Keep in mind that emotional release is a major catalyst to progress. In the absence of physical impediments, the mother who fully surrenders all psychological resistance can dilate very rapidly. I've seen a number of women go from five centimeters to complete dilation in less than an hour—spilling out fear and anxiety one minute, easing into sensation the next, and suddenly feeling like pushing. *Never leave the mother alone, or take her outside for a walk, if you sense this kind of release is about to happen!*

In the event of emotionally-based arrest, be certain to keep on top of vital assessments. Check for signs of maternal exhaustion. A full bladder can hinder relaxation and descent, so make sure the mother urinates frequently. Take maternal blood pressure and fetal heart tones often, as emotional tension may impact both.

Emotionally-based arrests occurring when the mother is already physically depleted can rapidly deteriorate into pathology. You must guard the baby's welfare; sometimes, this means shaking sense into the parents by being frank about any immature behavior. If physical symptoms of emotional distress begin to manifest, discuss the possibility of transport. This may elicit determination or despair, but a decision must be made promptly. Give the mother and her partner a bit of time to consider their options, be encouraging but firm, and the appropriate course of action will soon become evident.

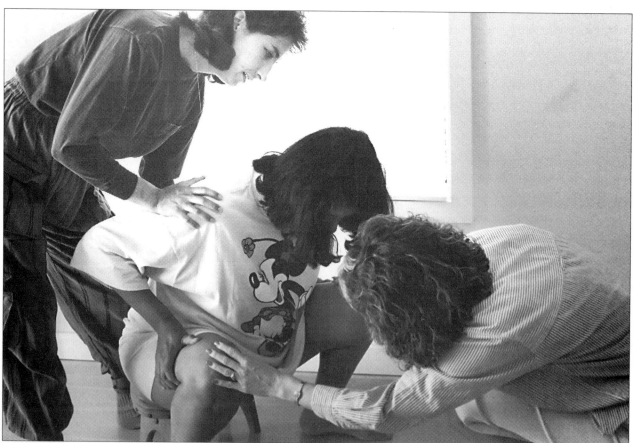

Obstructed labor is often more painful; the sooner you let go of easy birth fantasies and ask for help, the better your chances for progress.

CEPHALOPELVIC DISPROPORTION (CPD)

CPD is a condition in which the baby's head cannot engage or pass through the mother's pelvis. As *Myles Textbook for Midwives* states, disproportion can be pelvic or cephalic in origin, due to small pelvis, large baby, or a combination of the two. But it may also be due to malpresentation, e.g., if a posterior baby for which the mother has plenty of room presents an excessively large diameter of its head due to deflexion, disproportion may result. Other relevant factors include the degree to which the fetal skull is moldable, the amount of flexibility in the maternal pelvis, and the strength of uterine contractions. If the mother is upright and relaxed, her uterus working efficiently, even a moderate degree of CPD can be overcome. It's been said repeatedly that, "The best pelvimeter is the baby's head," which is absolutely true.

Thus CPD cannot really be diagnosed before labor, unless the head bulges over the pubic bone in a rare condition known as **fetal overlap**. If the head seems easier to palpate than usual in the final weeks of pregnancy, check for overlap by seeing whether the head can negotiate the pelvic inlet. To do this, grasp the head firmly just above the pubic bone and attempt to to press it against the mother's spine and down into her pelvis. If you sense "give" front to back with room for descent, there should be no problem. If space seems limited, plan to monitor labor very closely. Yet another option is to induce labor—see forthcoming pages for suggestions.

Failure to engage before labor cannot be considered diagnostic, as large babies frequently stay at - 2 or - 3 station until strong contractions bring them down. Mothers with very strong or tense abdominal muscles sometimes hold their babies high until active labor begins. Extremely poor abdominal tone may prevent the fetus from being properly aligned with the pelvis for descent, thus hindering engagement. Nevertheless, only 2 to 3 percent of all cases of CPD are due to a genuine discrepancy between the size of the baby and that of the mother's pelvis.

CPD can occur at any of the three prime pelvic dimensions: the inlet, the midpelvis, or the outlet.

Pelvimetry performed during pregnancy should have alerted you to any reduced dimension, helping both you and the mother prepare for labor. A pelvis which has a roomy inlet but a flat, heavy sacrum may render descent and engagement difficult. See that the head is well flexed in the last few weeks of pregnancy, and encourage the mother to walk and squat throughout the day, so as to stretch pelvic cartilage as much as possible. Or, if you find a pelvis to be basically gynecoid (roomy inlet, deep, rounded sacral curve, and ample pubic arch) but notice rather close-set, prominent spines, you can anticipate some delay due to midpelvic contraction. The pregnancy should not go much past term, as the baby's head must mold well to adapt. The mother should understand that it is sometimes necessary to push hard in second stage, for an extended period of time. She will need to be in top shape. Then again, if the pelvis is otherwise ample except for a narrow pubic arch and reduced outlet dimension, delay at the high point of fetal head compression may lead to fetal distress and necessitate episiotomy and/or cause a perineal tear. You must help the mother conserve her energy in labor, and work carefully during delivery to maintain flexion of the head. Squatting practice, vaginal awareness, and visualization are crucial to her preparation.

Be prepared, but don't be paranoid. It's quite miraculous sometimes to find borderline CPD suddenly overcome by fetal rotation, or by some subtle repositioning of the head. Even if progress does halt at home, pitocin augmentation may increase uterine powers just enough to avert a cesarean section. So even if you must transport, don't be pessimistic about the possibilities of vaginal delivery but give hope to the mother as honestly as you can.

How does one diagnose CPD during labor? First, it must seem a reasonable suspicion based on foreknowledge of the baby's size, gestational age, and the mother's dimensions. **Inlet disproportion** is signalled by lack of descent past - 3 or - 2 station, asynclitism, and cervix not well applied to the head. Particularly ominous is the cervix hanging "like an empty sleeve." Dilation commonly arrests at six cms.; without adequate pressure from the presenting part, the cervix can dilate no further. Another oddity in this case is the tendency of the cervix to reclose. I recall several cases in which the cervix, hanging loosely during a contraction, spastically closed up as the contraction ended. This is what happens if the cervix has nothing to hold it open, neither the head nor adequate strength in the lower uterine segment. The result is weakening, incoordinate contractions, with maternal symptoms of asymmetrical, isolated, spastic pain.

Midpelvic disproportion presents a bit differently. The head generally engages without trouble, dilation proceeds normally, but second stage is prolonged. Sometimes the baby gets stuck in **deep transverse arrest**, meaning that the head gets wedged behind the ischial spines and cannot rotate to the anteroposterior position.

Outlet disproportion is also correlated to prolonged second stage, but more commonly affects the perineal phase, after + 2 station. If the pubic arch is reduced, the head will press deeply into the pelvic floor and may tear the bulbocavernosus muscle or perineum. Or, if the ischial tuberosities are close-set, molding or caput formation may be extreme as delivery, particularly the crowning phase, tends to be prolonged.

Any tricks you can try for CPD? If inlet disproportion is due to malpresentation, i.e., deflexion or asynclitism, you can attempt to manually reposition the head. This works best with intact membranes, as they serve to cushion internal manipulations. Have the mother in knees-chest position to reverse the force of gravity. To **secure flexion**, follow the directions and diagrams under Posterior Arrest. To **correct asynclitism**, press the protruding side of the head firmly inward until the suture line is centered. If the head feels tightly wedged or is too high to reach, have the mother try **duck-walking**. To do this she must squat and "walk" by shifting her weight from one foot to the other. This helps open the pelvis, and at the same time encourages the baby to reposition itself.

For midpelvic disproportion and cases of deep transverse arrest, secure flexion (as above) and attempt to rotate the head to the anterior position. You may also wish to try the **pelvic press**,

popularized by Nan Koehler, author of *Artemis Speaks* and authority on VBAC. This must be performed with the mother in a squatting position, and will require a bit of physical strength. Kneeling behind her, place your hands firmly on the iliac crests (hip bones) and press them together as hard as possible, or until you feel some motion (see illustration, page 125). Pressure on the iliac crests flexes the symphysis and sacral-iliac joints, opening the midpelvis so the head can rotate and descend. Do this during a contraction. As you are trying to effect descent, have the mother bear down, even if she is not fully dilated. Check heart tones immediately afterwards, and repeat as necessary. Results are often quite remarkable.

The pelvic press is also useful for outlet disproportion, as it stretches the symphysis pubis open and increases the bi-tuberous diameter. To deepen pelvic relaxation, additional measures such as hot compresses and vaginal massage may help in borderline cases.

In terms of time, there are some limits. If one waits endlessly for descent to occur as the lower uterine segment thins away to nothing, there is danger of uterine rupture. However, maternal exhaustion and/or fetal distress will probably arise and necessitate transport long before this becomes a real possibility. Once CPD is confirmed and all reasonable efforts to correct it have failed, the mother should be taken to the hospital before she has frittered her energy away in hard but ineffective labor. Likely interventions of pitocin augmentation, delivery by forceps, suction, or cesarean section are all somewhat traumatic, and are best handled by a mother and baby still in good condition.

Pitocin administered with care can work wonders in borderline cases. After so many hours of difficult labor, pain relief may also be beneficial. Particularly in the presence of strong contractions, complete pelvic relaxation induced by epidural or other pain medication may allow the bones to give just enough to let the head pass through. This decision may be a real disappointment for the mother, both during labor and postpartum. But the midwife can help by reassuring her that the pain of obstructed labor—bone wedged against bone—is very real, and different from that of ordinary labor.

The Pelvic Press

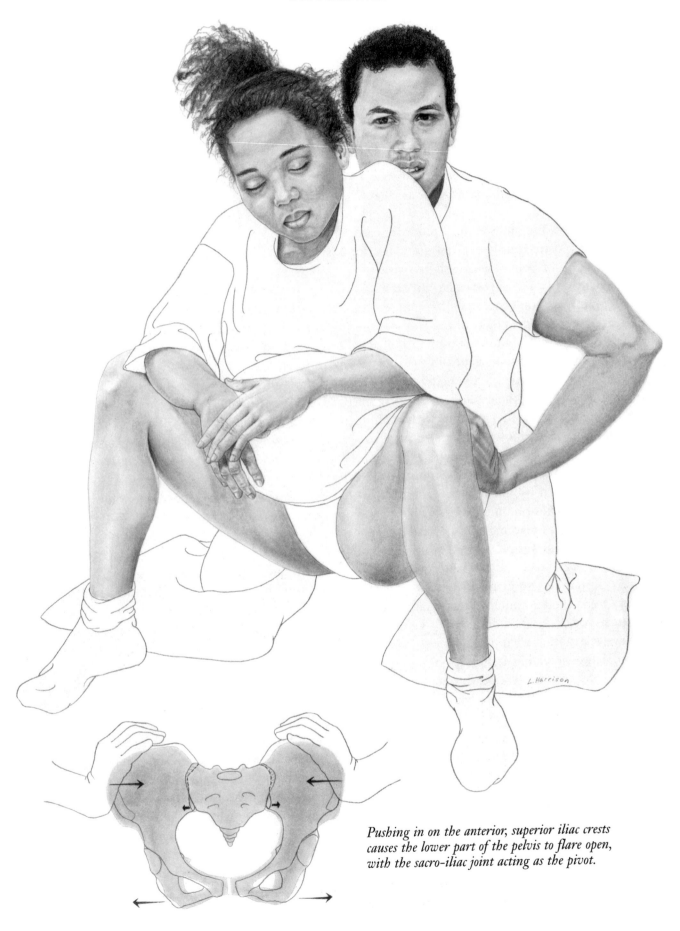

Pushing in on the anterior, superior iliac crests causes the lower part of the pelvis to flare open, with the sacro-iliac joint acting as the pivot.

Even if nothing seems to work, at least the mother may be content with the fact that she has tried everything, and has had a chance to work through feelings of hope, frustration, despair, and resignation. Seeing a woman through a rough labor that ends in cesarean birth is difficult at best. However, more and more hospitals routinely use local/epidural anesthesia and encourage the mother's partner to be present for the surgery, so the moments of birth and bonding can be shared as they should be.

Nevertheless, the mother will need extra care and support postpartum (see Resources list in Appendix). You or your assistant should visit the hospital daily, and do what you can to pave the way for the family's homecoming. Encourage the mother to nurse and get plenty of rest, see that she has healthy food brought to the hospital, and have her get up and walk as soon as possible (with staff clearance and support). This helps eliminate painful gas and speeds the healing process.

Years ago, I coached a woman with a nine-pound baby in breech position, arrested progress, and eventual need for cesarean section. Both the father and I were present in the operating room. She had been given a spinal but was unable to tolerate the sensation of numbness in her lungs; she felt as if she wasn't breathing. So she asked for general anesthesia and was put under.

Her mate got to hold the baby immediately, she was taken to recovery, and the baby went to the nursery to be checked out, where the father and I took turns rocking and holding it. During the next few days, the mother went through periods of very intense depression and paranoia; even though she had her baby with her, she felt incapacitated, vulnerable to hospital personnel, worried about her two-year-old son and husband at home, and extremely disappointed in her experience. One night, she was so upset that she called and asked me to come and stay with her at the hospital. We did a lot of talking in the weeks and months that followed; she repeatedly asked questions about the moments of birth, needing not just simple reassurance but my specific observations, fine nuances of the baby's behavior, and every little detail that I could give her. A year later I received a picture of myself holding her baby girl in the nursery, along with this letter:

Dear Elizabeth,
It is a year on the 11th. Thank you so much for all that you gave me. What words can I use to tell you that without you my birth experience would have been really cold, my hospital stay a nightmare, but most of all, I would not have had a true witness to the birth, and how beautifully and perfectly you filled these needs. How I counted on you!
I hope that I am able to give something so wonderful into the great supply of love in the Universe.

POSTERIOR ARREST

Posterior arrest occurs when the baby is stuck in either LOP or ROP position during active, first stage labor. When the head enters the pelvis posteriorly, the occiput may snag on the sacral promontory, forcing the sinciput to descend first. Deflexion of the head renders its circumference enlarged, which hinders descent and prevents a firm, smooth fit of the head against the cervix. Lack of pressure on the cervix causes contractions to become irregular, incoordinate, and weak. Posterior arrest occurs most commonly at about six centimeters dilation, with station of - 3 or - 2. Occasionally, cervical edema develops and serves to compound the problem.

Findings by internal exam are very similar to those with large baby and small inlet. But with continuity of care, you should know enough of the mother's dimensions and baby's size to set this possibility aside. Assuming there is adequate room and that malpresentation has caused some degree of CPD, it is obviously necessary to do something to reposition the head and effect rotation. What are your options?

In the past, the only solution I knew was hospital transport for pitocin augmentation, in hopes that stronger contractions might force descent and rotation. Of course we would try everything we possibly could at home—positioning the mother on hands and knees or having her squat, giving her cohosh tinctures or pulsatilla homeopathic remedy to stimulate stronger contractions, nipple stimulation, etc. It was frustrating to encounter this posterior pattern repeatedly, and to pretty well know in advance that all of our efforts would probably be for naught and we would end up in the hospital.

Then I discovered a technique of **manual rotation** advocated by the Australian obstetrician, Hamlin, in his out-of-print work, *Stepping Stones to Labour Ward Diagnosis*. He claims success with this technique in over a thousand attempts. With practice, I've modified his method somewhat, but the basic principles remain the same. It is definitely worth a try, but requires two skilled midwives to make it work (see diagrams, opposite).

You must first make certain of your posterior diagnosis. You may not be able to find the posterior fontanelle if the head is deflexed, but you should be able to feel the anterior fontanelle at the anterior edge of the cervical opening. Once you have found the anterior fontanelle, you can undertake maneuvers to flex the head. But you must first slightly disengage it, i.e., dislodge it from the point where it is wedged in the pelvis by exerting pressure on one of the parietal bones. With this, flexion and rotation may occur spontaneously.

If not, exert steady, even pressure on the bony edge of the anterior fontanelle, as if tucking the fontanelle back inside the mother's cervix. At the same time, attempt to rotate the fontanelle to a transverse position. As soon as you have the anterior fontanelle in a transverse position and almost out of range of feeling, reach for the posterior fontanelle and prepare to complete rotation to the anterior.

Keep your finger in place, and have the mother lie back, with ample room on either side to fling her leg over her body as she rolls to a right or left side position. Which way she will turn depends on which way you are rotating the baby—it will be one and the same. Your assistant should sit facing you, next to the baby's back. As you begin to rotate the baby internally, your assistant can help by attempting to grasp the baby's shoulder and backside, lifting and pushing the baby's body to the anterior position. As you and your assistant coordinate your efforts, the mother should roll over slowly. This makes it easier for your assistant to reach the baby's body, and further

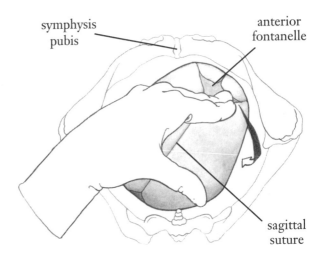

ROP to RPT

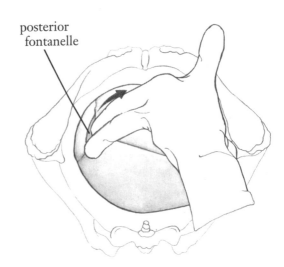

ROT to ROA

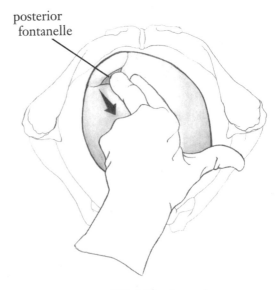

ROA Flexing

127

facilitates rotation. Once the mother has turned to her side, immediately check fetal heart tones. If all is well, have her sit fully upright to secure the baby in its new position.

How much force do you need to use? Hamlin uses the image of "dialing a telephone," but this is a bit misleading, as there is considerable effort involved in maintaining flexion during rotation maneuvers. If you feel strong resistance at any point, attempt no further.

If you are working without an assistant, you can use the suggested maneuvers alone, with the mother in knees-chest position. (As the mother's position is reversed, you must of course reverse your manipulations.) Knees-chest has advantages of increasing pelvic capacity and encouraging the baby to disengage, crucial if the membranes have ruptured and the uterus has closed tightly around the baby's body. *In fact, all internal maneuvers are much easier to accomplish with the membranes intact.* Amniotic fluid provides a much needed cushion for rotating the baby or otherwise adjusting its position.

The simplest but least effective technique of internal rotation involves placing two fingers on the sagittal suture line, then turning them to rotate the baby. In any case, if rotation to transverse or anterior positions proves impossible, the baby can instead be turned OP. This may dislodge it sufficiently to allow for rotation to the anterior position, but even if the baby stays OP, at least it can descend and birth that way.

If you do succeed in turning the baby, check the heart tones with every contraction for the next 20 minutes or so. And do another internal exam after a few contractions to be sure the baby is still in place. Sometimes the baby reverts to its original position, and it appears that your efforts have been for naught. But don't be discouraged; if rotation were to be accomplished easily, it probably would have occurred by itself. It may take another two or three attempts; with each, the baby is likely to flex and descend a bit more, and eventually stay in place.

Here is an interesting case history. This mother was two weeks past due; her baby was large and in ROP position. She had a long latent phase of about 12 hours, and took three more hours to dilate from four to six centimeters. By internal exam, the head was at - 2 station and sharply asynclitic, with the posterior parietal bone presenting. The cervix was not well applied to the head, and I couldn't even feel the sagittal suture line, which was way up behind the pubic bone. After a few more hours, cervical edema began to develop, but the head had come down a bit and the suture line was now within reach.

With the parents' agreement, my partner and I decided to make an attempt at rotation and managed to turn the baby to ROA. It promptly rotated back to ROP again, but gained a centimeter of descent. An hour later and with good contractions, we tried once more, and this time the baby settled at ROT, - 1 station. With yet another try, as we rotated the baby to ROA, it spontaneously flexed its head and came down to 0 station, at which point we artificially ruptured the membranes to secure engagement. Fetal heart tones were fine throughout, and the baby was soon born in good condition.

In retrospect, the mother said the procedure was definitely uncomfortable but given the choice between it and the hospital, there was no question in her mind. In terms of minimizing trauma, attempt rotation early when mother and baby still have the fortitude to handle it.

PROLONGED SECOND STAGE

After the cervix is fully dilated, delay may be caused by one or both of the following factors: 1) poor management of second stage; or 2) some degree of CPD.

How long is too long for second stage? It all depends on the nature of the obstacle; your fingers will tell you if there are bony or muscular impediments. One thing is certain, it is foolish to let the mother flounder with strong contractions, hoping she'll eventually get the knack of pushing. Instead, check and advise her frequently. Once the bearing-down urge is established, the first-time mother seldom takes more than an hour and a half to bring her baby down to the perineum, and multiparous women generally take less than 45 minutes to push their babies out.

If vaginal exam reveals plenty of room for descent but the baby remains high, maternal tension is probably at issue, so try to help the mother loosen up and relax. Massage her shoulders and back, and have her focus her energy downward. If she is willing, have her partner massage her inner thighs. Try hot perineal compresses, or have her sit on a heating pad, or perhaps push on the toilet. But if you note variable decelerations at this stage, cord entanglement may be hindering descent. Listen to the baby with every contraction; if bradycardia develops, you may need to transport or effect delivery immediately.

As stated earlier, prominent ischial spines or a narrow pubic arch can also lead to second stage delays. Midpelvic disproportion may cause caput to develop, which feels like fleshy enlargement of the baby's head. Caput indicates considerable head compression within a particular pelvic dimension, causing impaired venous return and swelling (it may reach a thickness of an inch or more). If you detect caput accompanied by lack of descent, especially in the presence of strong contractions, check for any unusual tension in the vaginal muscles, and

help the mother relax as much as possible. Even if the head is still high, you can start internal massage on tense areas if the mother agrees.

Squatting is a tremendous aid, shown to increase the pelvic outlet an average of 28 percent over the supine position. But is is tiring for the mother, so have her alternate squatting with periods of semi-reclining. This gives you a chance to auscultate fetal heart tones, which will tell you how well the baby is handling head compression. You can consider early decelerations normal as long as they go no lower than 80 BPM, and as long as recovery is complete as the contraction ends. Whatever the cause of midpelvic disproportion, the mother needs to focus and concentrate her efforts, and bear down fully with her urges. She should also breathe deeply between contractions, i.e., "breathe to the baby."

If second stage is prolonged in spite of the mother's best efforts, consider the pelvic press to effect descent (described previously in Cephalo-Pelvic Disproportion). You may wish to combine

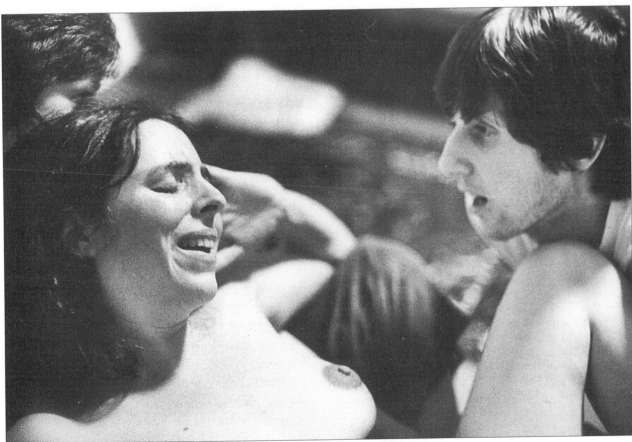

A look of anguish on the laboring woman's face can be frightening, but is often just a stress reaction to great exertion.

this maneuver with a bit of **fundal pressure** during a contraction, in conjunction with the mother's pushing efforts. This is not advisable if more than a minor degree of disproportion exists, if the head is not molding, or if mother and baby are in anything less than top condition. *Do not attempt to apply fundal pressure unless you've had enough experience to be sure of all these factors.* This procedure remains highly controversial, as it can lead to uterine rupture if used inappropriately. Monitor the FHT closely throughout, and desist immediately with any sign of distress.

Delay at the outlet is yet another problem, and is most commonly caused by strong, thick, or tense musculature. If such is the case and the baby is in distress, episiotomy and rapid delivery may be necessary; otherwise, employ the use of perineal massage and hot compresses. Delay due to outlet disproportion is another matter. A reduced pubic arch inadvertently forces the baby's head deep into vaginal and perineal tissues. It is unrealistic to expect a tear-free delivery, but do your best to protect the perineum and to prevent minor tears from extending. If for any reason you must do an episiotomy, carefully guard the apex of the wound as the head delivers.

There are also emotional issues that can cause late second stage arrest. Fear of becoming a parent can definitely cause perineal tension and deep decelerations. It's often enough to say, "You've got a strong, healthy baby, but it's time for it to come out now." Fear of sensory overload can be mediated by helping the mother feel safe enough to completely let go. Last minute fears of "splitting open" may be alleviated by having her feel the baby's head, or take a look in the mirror. One glance will remind her that she is still in her body, and that she is stretched no more than what she has seen in pictures. Objectifying herself this way can help her feel secure and aid her concentration.

FETAL DISTRESS

Fetal distress has been covered in many sections of this book; Chapter Four has numerous references to unusual FHT patterns and appropriate responses. In the event of transport for fetal distress, **internal monitoring** is likely. This requires

an electrode be attached to the baby's head, rendering a more accurate reading than external ultrasound devices. Internal monitoring may also be mandated by pitocin augmentation, particularly if the uterus does not seem to be responding. For this, an **internal pressure catheter** is inserted through the cervix to determine the precise strength of uterine contractions. Tracings from this device also show whether the uterus is returning fully to baseline as contractions end—if not, the baby may be compromised by lack of oxygen. In contrast, the ultrasound and pressure-sensing units used to determine uterine activity and fetal response in **external monitoring** are less precise, and may be readily replaced by periodic fetal auscultation.

Some hospitals utilize **fetal scalp sampling** to assess fetal well-being. This test involves taking a bit of blood from the baby's head, the pH of which is tested immediately to determine whether or not the baby is acidotic, i.e., truly hypoxic. Fetal scalp sampling more accurately identifies fetal distress than does fetal monitoring. Even in the presence of an ominous FHT pattern, an otherwise stressful labor may safely proceed if the scalp sample is within normal range. In other words, fetal scalp sampling can sometimes make the difference between cesarean section and vaginal delivery. Readings at or above 7.26 are considered normal.

Increasingly, obstetricians use **fetal scalp massage** in lieu of fetal scalp sampling. Massage should be performed for about ten seconds. A 15-point acceleration lasting 15 seconds is supposed to indicate a pH of at least 7.26.

CORD PROBLEMS

There are several types of cord problems which can affect blood flow to the baby and cause fetal distress. **Cord nipping** means the cord is being pinched between the head and pelvic bones, causing variable decelerations in the FHT. During first stage, repositioning the mother usually eases pressure on the cord and brings the FHT back to normal, but in second stage, nipping may easily progress to cord compression, depending on how low the cord is lying. One trick for remedying variable decels in second stage is to gently press on

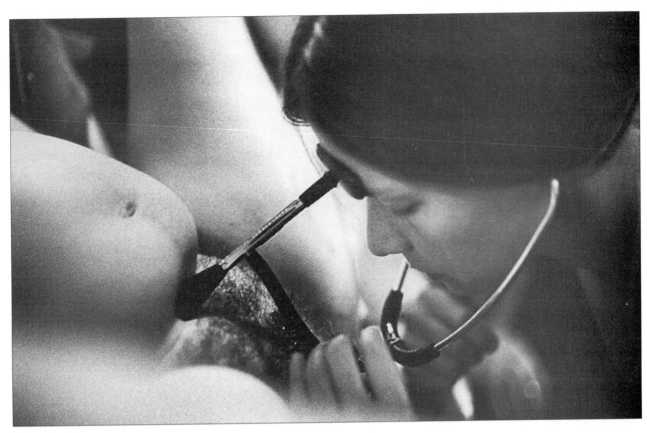

Using the Fetascope

the mother's abdomen where the baby's back is located—this frequently shifts the baby off the cord and improves FHTs.

Cord compression may be due to **occult prolapse**, meaning that the cord is low in the pelvis and is being compressed by the head as it descends with the force of contractions. If cord compression is severe, bradycardia is likely to develop. There is also a possibility that the FHT will return to normal if the head moves past the cord entirely. You need to listen assiduously, as persistent bradycardia constitutes a crisis with very little leeway. Try repositioning the mother, and give oxygen by mask at six litres per minute. Check the FHT with each contraction. If there is no improvement after four or five contractions, transport.

If it's a case of **cord entanglement**, i.e., the cord is wrapped repeatedly around the neck or about the limbs and body, descent will probably be inhibited and you may hear cord sounds over the FHT (cord sounds make a swishing noise like placental or maternal artery sounds, but at the baby's rhythm). A very tight cord around the neck may

also deflex the baby's head. The bottom line is persistent bradycardia, necessitating transport.

The obstetric disaster of **complete cord prolapse** tends to occur if the presenting part is high when the membranes rupture. It is also linked to conditions of polyhydramnios, multiple pregnancy, breech or compound presentation, or transverse lie. Complete cord prolapse can occasionally be diagnosed by internal exam in the last weeks of pregnancy with the discovery of pulsations at the cervix or through the lower uterine segment that are synchronous with the FHT. This finding necessitates immediate hospitalization and cesarean section to save the baby.

If the membranes rupture during labor and the cord prolapses, call the paramedics and place the mother in a knees-chest position with your fingers inside her cervix, holding the head up and away from the cord. Place the cord gently back inside the vagina if it is exposed. If there is not room, wrap it in gauze or a washcloth soaked in warm water with a pinch of salt, and cover with a plastic bag. Rough handling of the cord or exposure to air can cause spasm and constriction. If you must transport the mother yourself, lay a chair back-down on the floor and ease her on to it, then lift and tip her slightly backwards until her head is lower than her hips. Keep her in this position in the car, with fingers inside to alleviate pressure on the cord until the cesarean is performed.

Complete cord prolapse occurs very rarely, but if head is high in the pelvis near term and the mother reports labor's onset with rupture of the membranes, immediately go and check the FHT.

MATERNAL HYPERTENSION

Hypertension in labor is a danger to both mother and baby because it may progress to preeclampsia, even with no previous signs. Thus it is critical to watch the mother carefully. Urinalysis for proteinuria is somewhat unreliable in labor, as cells in the amniotic fluid may wash down and give a false positive reading. Check for clonus/hyperreflexia, and transport at the first sign. Hypertension in labor also increases the risk of placental abruption.

Herbal remedies may stabilize or lower blood pressure; the best is tincture of hops, one of the most effective sedative herbs known. Tincture form ensures potency (much stronger than tea) and quick assimilation (placed under the tongue, it absorbs directly into the blood stream, whereas tea or anything else by mouth digests very slowly in labor). Skullcap, passionflower, and hawthorne tinctures are also useful, as is bathing with Epsom salts (magnesium sulfate).

If hypertension has been a problem in late pregnancy, check blood pressure hourly in early labor. Labor is sometimes therapeutic for gestational hypertension. If blood pressure remains elevated as active labor begins, check every 20 minutes, and if it continues to rise, transport. On the other hand, if blood pressure has been normal during labor, do not be alarmed if it rises as high as 140/90 with second stage exertion.

If blood pressure does rise as labor becomes more intense, place the mother on her left side to maximize oxygen delivery to her and the baby. Also push fluids, as dehydration may exacerbate hypertension in labor.

In the event of transport, standard procedures for hypertension include intravenous magnesium sulfate for the mother, and continuous fetal monitoring of the baby. Magnesium sulfate may reduce blood pressure somewhat, but primarily serves to prevent changes in brain activity that could lead to convulsions. It may also slow labor, necessitating pitocin augmentation, and is associated with risks of pulmonary embolism and postpartum hemorrhage. Nevertheless, apart from the nuisance of IV and monitor hookups, the mother can still have a spontaneous, beautiful birthing if the hospital staff is amenable. The probable course of events should be discussed with parents as soon as the problem develops, so they will be adequately prepared.

Any woman with borderline hypertension prenatally or during labor is at risk for an even greater rise in blood pressure after delivery. There is a type of eclampsia which can develop in the immediate postpartum—be on the lookout for this.

PROLONGED RUPTURE OF THE MEMBRANES

Prolonged rupture of the membranes (PROM) is a potential complication of labor. Although it is quite normal for the water bag to break at the beginning of labor, there is concern that the time lapse between rupture and delivery may put the baby at risk for infection because the uterus is no longer closed to germs present in the vagina. Conventional procedure is to wait no more than 24 hours before inducing labor, and some physicians start even earlier to see that the baby delivers before 24 hours have elapsed.

The problem with this standard of care is that it does not incorporate factors of the mother's health, her personal cleanliness, or that of her environment as relevant to her risk of infection. Women planning home birth are usually in top condition, and it is a proven fact that risks of infection are much less at home than in the hospital, where patients are apt to be exposed to particularly virulent strains of microorganisms for which they have no resistance.

In 1996, a major study was completed at the University of Toronto, involving 5,041 women from Canada, Britain, Australia, Israel, Sweden, and Denmark with PROM who were randomly assigned either to have their labors induced, or to wait for up to four days for labor to start spontaneously. Results showed very little difference between the two groups—in both, about 3 percent of babies developed infection, and about 10 percent were delivered by cesarean section. Study authors concluded that physicians should present this research to patients, who should choose the option they prefer.

This study was, however, conducted in hospital. Risks of infection are undoubtedly less for the low-risk woman giving birth at home, with resistance to organisms commonly encountered in her own environment. Infection due to prolonged ruptured membranes is thus a theoretical complication. Who wants hospitalization and pitocin induction for a problem which may not exist? The issue is political; induction is the prevailing standard of care, which has yet to catch up with the research.

Yet another study published almost a decade ago in the *Journal of the American Medical Association* indicates that the risk for infection with ruptured membranes increases dramatically *24 hours after the first vaginal exam or other internal procedure*. This makes sense, for how can we expect to move fingers or speculum through an organism-rich vagina to the cervix—gateway to the sterile uterine environment—without exacerbating risks of infection? Thus it is crucial with PROM to avoid vaginal exams and cultures as long as possible. The only exception would be to visually inspect the cervix and vagina for herpes lesions, if the mother has any history.

In my experience, it's not unusual for mothers to go 24 hours after the waters break without even starting labor. But in order to minimize risks of infection, here are some commonsense guidelines and rules for the mother (also given in Chapter Four):

1. No tub baths until the mother is in advanced, active labor;
2. No hand-mouth-genital contact;
3. Use utmost care when using the toilet, wiping backwards, and washing hands both before and after;
4. No underwear, just clean loose clothing, and preferably no sanitary pad unless flow is considerable, in which case pad should be changed often;
5. Have plenty to drink, in order to replenish amniotic fluid and keep system flushed;
6. Increase dosages of vitamin C, up to two grams per 24 hours, or 250 mg. every three or four hours;
7. Eat good quality, unconstipating foods, to keep energy levels high; and
8. Take temperature readings every three or four hours, reporting any elevation at once.

Some physicians want daily blood work on the mother for white cell counts, checking primarily for elevated banded cells (generated in response to acute infection). It is possible for the mother's uterus to be barely infected, with the baby decidedly septic. If this is the case, fetal tachycardia will usually result. Once membranes have been ruptured for 24 hours, check fetal heart tones periodically to rule out infection.

Basic management of ruptured membranes includes close phone contact with the mother during the immediate post-rupture period to check her morale and make sure she is following basic guidelines for avoiding infection. Avoid exams and/or internal manipulations until the mother is in active labor; rely on observation and intuition as much as possible. If you must check, use antiseptic solution with a sterile glove, and avoid inserting your fingers into the os.

The Centers for Disease Control recommend that women whose membranes are ruptured for more than 18 hours be started on prophylactic antibiotics against group B strep (GBS). Midwives can inform women about GBS at 35 weeks, and let them decide if they wish prenatal screening. If the mother is GBS (-) and PROM occurs in labor, everyone can afford to relax and wait. If she's GBS (+), she could be started on large doses of antibiotics by mouth if she decides prophylaxis is important to her. If a woman is GSB (+) with PROM and declines antibiotics, her baby should be seen by a pediatrician as soon as possible for a blood draw and culture.

Whenever neonatal infection is a possibility, make certain that the mother understands normal newborn behavior. An experienced pediatrician colleague says the first sign of newborn infection is often failure to nurse. Any baby who acts listless or irritable should be checked at once by a pediatrician.

Now for some birthing tale examples:

This first labor was that of a woman with large baby in posterior position. Her labor began with ruptured membranes, a few sporadic contractions, and light meconium in the waters. I went to check on her immediately, but the baby sounded fine and the meconium was very light. The mother was well rested and wanted to get things going. She tried walking, cohosh tea, and nipple stimulation, but the baby was so high in the pelvis (- 3 station) that this did little good. She remained in prodromal labor throughout the night and was still in early labor at 24 hours.

In the morning she tried castor oil and an enema, and soon appeared to be in active labor. About six hours later, with meconium still light and baby still fine, we checked to find her at five centimeters. Although her pulse and temperature were normal, she had moderate ketoneuria so we gave her a snack and extra fluids with honey.

The original rupture was a hind-leak and at seven centimeters, the forewaters broke with a gush. Still light mec only. The baby descended, internal rotation occurred, and the mother was soon complete. She pushed for two hours, we did DeLee suction on the perineum, and she gave birth to a baby boy with 9/9 Apgars, no problems postpartum. Total time since rupture, 40 hours.

* * *

Another woman went into labor just under 37 weeks, but I palpated her baby to be over six pounds and near term by its recent, consistent growth pattern. Also, she had always felt intuitively that she would go early. At her last prenatal she was already 85 percent effaced, and one to two centimeters dilated. She had few contractions for about 16 hours, then took castor oil and was in active labor by 24 hours. All vitals were within normal range. Baby delivered at 40 hours after SROM,

7/10 Apgars, no postpartum problems. Gestational age by exam, 37 + weeks.

* * *

Last comes the most complex; a woman with reduced midpelvis, palpated at 38 weeks to have possible fetal head overlap. This woman had also frequently come to clinic in a state of physical and emotional disarray. Due to her numerous personal problems, we decided she would birth at the alternative birth room in hospital. When her water broke one morning we planned to meet her there, but the obstetrician said she could wait at home for a while if she kept track of her temperature and reported any rise. She was admitted to the hospital at 24 hours with no contractions and was given pitocin IV.

Her labor was so very difficult for her that all our energies were focused on emotional support. Eventually she requested an epidural. After many hours of labor and several of pushing, it was clear that CPD was preventing delivery. She had a cesarean with general anesthesia at 37 hours. The amniotic fluid was found to be both stained and infected so the baby was given a complete septic workup. In light of her condition prenatally, this woman was at risk in many ways so the outcome was no surprise. Anyway, the baby had to spend time in isolation, the mother's recovery was slow (her incision became infected), and she had many emotional problems postpartum.

* * *

This last example shows how prolonged ruptured membranes, if compounded by other factors, can become risky. But the other cases show how common sense measures of care are keys to good outcomes.

UNUSUAL PRESENTATIONS

Face Presentation: This is quite rare, occurring once in every 250 deliveries. You should notice a marked degree of deflexion (by palpation) some weeks before term. If you discover this before the head is down in the pelvis, make an attempt at securing flexion. This is a simple procedure (see Chapter Two, page 45) and works unless the baby is posterior, in which case the occiput is

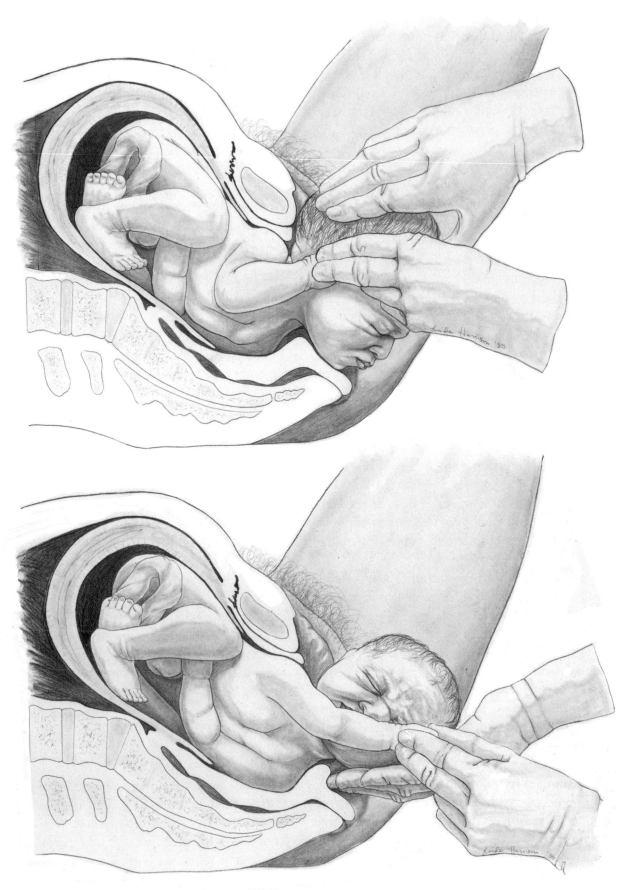

Extracting the Nuchal Arm

impossible to reach. Keep in mind that face presentation is sometimes caused by a tight cord around the neck deflexing the head as it descends, so if you attempt to flex the head, proceed slowly, and have your assistant continually assess the FHT.

Another cause of face presentation is inlet CPD. Be relatively sure at the onset of labor that this is not the case, lest you waste precious time and energy at home on a seriously obstructed labor.

The mechanics of delivering the face presentation are such that the baby must be born with its chin at the pubic bone, and body in a posterior position. Although labor may begin with the baby anterior, descent in this position is impossible because the crown of the head will impinge on the symphysis. As the baby delivers, the midwife must hold back the baby's brow by applying counter-pressure to the perineum until the chin escapes, which keeps the chin from getting caught behind the pubic bone. Obviously, the occiput will put extra pressure and strain on the perineum. Tearing is common with face presentation; you may not be able to prevent it. Suction is usually necessary because the baby is facing upwards and likely to get a nose full of fluids as the head delivers.

The baby probably will be born with considerable bruising and swelling, so be sure to administer vitamin K. Also watch for breathing difficulties due to tracheal edema.

Brow and Military Presentation: These deflexed positions of the head can be remedied prenatally during the last few weeks of care. If they are discovered in labor by internal exam (via location of the fontanelles) you may be able to flex the head by internal maneuvering. See the section on Posterior Arrest for instructions.

Compound Presentation: Most frequently this means a little hand and arm coming down alongside the head. Usually compound presentation is not discovered until the head is birthing; it all depends on how far down the hand is extending.

The biggest problem associated with "nuchal arm" is perineal lacerations, as the head and arm together create an unusually large circumference at crowning. You may be able to avoid this while the head is still high by gently pinching the baby's finger, which may cause it to retract its hand. If this

doesn't work, prepare to extract the arm so the shoulders can be born. The easiest way to do this is to grasp the hand, and manually restitute the head while bringing the arm across the chest and outward. This maneuvering comes naturally in times of crisis; it's mechanical logic that flows of necessity. Still, it's wise to think it through so the sense and feel of it are imprinted and ready at need.

Membranes Presenting at Delivery: This is not strictly a presentation problem, but an unusual quirk of delivery. When the membranes present and are bulging from the vagina, they will usually rupture as the head distends the perineum, but sometimes the break occurs farther up and away from the baby's head. This leads to a condition known as **delivery in the caul**, in which membranes envelop the baby's face as it is born and will obstruct breathing unless removed.

Some midwives routinely break a presenting water bag so the baby can be born through the rent, with membranes pushed aside and out of the way. But some mothers resent this interference, especially due to superstition that birth in the caul brings good luck. Once thing is for certain, the sensation of pushing a full water bag plus a baby is quite intense! If the mother shows signs of overwhelming discomfort or asks you to break the waters, just be sure to warn her immediately before performing AROM, as the release of pressure can come as a shock.

If the bag is left intact and the baby is born in the caul, you must immediately hook a fingernail into the membrane below the chin and peel it back over the face so the baby can breathe. My daughter was born in the caul, and my midwife used a sterile receiving blanket to catch and lift the membrane edge. Whatever you do, be sure and quick.

SHOULDER DYSTOCIA

Shoulder dystocia is a serious delivery complication, which becomes fully evident once the head has birthed and the shoulders fail to appear. Shoulder dystocia occurs when the baby's anterior shoulder is impacted behind the mother's pubic bone: the shoulder girdle is simply too broad to pass through the anteroposterior dimension of the pelvis. There is also considerable chest compression for the baby because it is squeezed so tightly in the birth canal, which can impair venous return from the head and lead to intercranial bleeding, brain damage, and death if not handled swiftly and competently.

It is easy to panic with this complication, but less likely if the problem has been anticipated beforehand. The mother with a baby large for her pelvic dimensions is a prime candidate for shoulder dystocia. Nevertheless, it's important to remember that if the head can pass through so can the shoulders, although you may need to do a bit of fancy maneuvering to make this happen.

Here is the usual course of events. An unusually large head passes over the perineum, then pulls back or retracts against it—this is known as the **turtle sign**. Restitution may take place slowly, haltingly, or not at all. Both these occurrences are due to shoulders too high in the pelvis to allow the head normal freedom of movement. Checking for cord is difficult, no shoulder presents, and the baby's color rapidly deepens to dark purple. Despite the mother's pushing efforts and reasonable downward traction on the head, nothing changes, and a diagnosis is made.

Immediately have the mother roll over to the hands-and-knees posture. Rolling will often rotate the baby out of the anteroposterior diameter to the oblique, making delivery of the shoulder easier. Hands-and-knees promotes full pelvic relaxation, and enhances your ability to maneuver. If the shoulder does not deliver spontaneously with this, use the **screw maneuver**. Reach inside the perineum to the posterior shoulder, and place two fingers in front of it, against the juncture of chest and armpit. Just take care not to hook your fingers in the armpit, which can cause nerve damage. Rotate backwards, pulling the baby outwards at the same time (with a screw-like motion). This should dislodge the anterior shoulder, collapse the shoulder girdle and bring the baby out. A 180° turn is usually enough to free the baby, though occasionally you may need to reverse this process for the other shoulder.

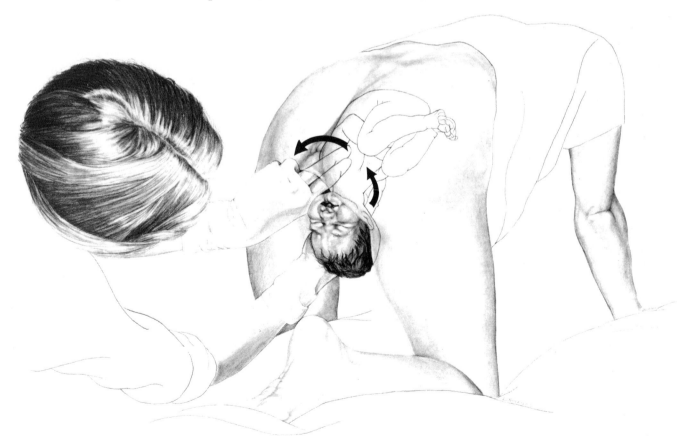

Managing Shoulder Dystocia

An alternative is to use the McRoberts position in which the mother is fully supine with her knees hyperflexed. This posture lifts the pelvis off the bed, increasing flexibility of the joints and available room to maneuver. Have an assistant gently lift the baby's head up towards the mother's pubic bone, or do so yourself as you hook two fingers behind the posterior shoulder and move it to an oblique position. Often just rotating the bottom shoulder will birth the baby, but extracting the arm will further reduce the diameter if necessary. To do this safely, you must splint the arm with two fingers and sweep it across the chest, so you can grasp the hand and complete the maneuver.

It sometimes helps to have your assistant give **suprapubic pressure** to help dislodge the anterior shoulder. Suprapubic pressure should be applied at an angle, from behind the baby's shoulder and towards its face, rather than straight down. Don't confuse this with fundal pressure, which will only impact the shoulder further unless it is given in conjunction with firm suprapubic pressure. This may be necessary if the posterior shoulder cannot be reached.

Which of these positions is best? Experienced midwives agree that change of position is more crucial than choice of position, as any movement on the mother's part serves to loosen the pelvis. Some midwives swear by having the mother in a standing squat.

The worst case of shoulder dystocia I ever encountered was forewarned by another midwife. She visited me a few days prior to this experience, and told me of a shoulder dystocia she recently handled where nothing, not even the screw maneuver, had worked. "Well, what did you do?" I asked, and she said, "We pushed, pulled, and prayed I guess until finally the baby came out." This sounded like a panic scene I'd just as soon avoid, but sure enough, a few days later . . .

This mother was of small stature. She had been artificially inseminated, and knew nothing about the father. At her last prenatal, fundal height was 40 cms. After a long labor, the head delivered smoothly and without a tear, but I had to push the perineum back over the chin and there was no restitution. As the face rapidly turned purple, we had her move to hands-and-knees.

My senior apprentice was assisting—this was to be her first catch. She tried the screw maneuver, but couldn't reach enough shoulder to get traction. Then she called for suprapubic pressure and tried again, but no change. So I stepped in and tried the screw maneuver myself, and had my apprentices apply both fundal and suprapubic pressure. At last, blessings be, I could reach the shoulder sufficiently to complete the maneuver. The baby was quite depressed at birth and needed resuscitation, but was fine shortly thereafter (Apgars were 2 and 8). But the mother tore all the way through her rectum; I had done an episiotomy to create more room and it extended badly.

My junior apprentice said she had seen the "Angel of Death," and it certainly felt to me for a time like we might lose the baby. But I gave in to my fear, and as adrenaline shot through me, I used it to help me complete the maneuvers. And yes, I guess I prayed, or at least offered up my total concentration.

On another occasion, I was co-managing a planned hospital birth with one of my favorite backup obstetricians. This mother had experienced a difficult posterior arrest and transport with her first birth, and chose hospital birth this time in case she wanted pain relief. She started out in the alternative birth room and progressed to about six centimeters, then opted for an epidural and was transferred to labor and delivery. She dilated rapidly to complete, but slowed dramatically in second stage. The physician was concerned, but offered to leave the room because he noticed she did much better when he was away. She was hooked to the monitor, but I had her squat on the floor by the bed and the baby crowned immediately.

I called for assistance as the head delivered, and it soon became apparent that the shoulders were stuck. Both the physician and I were quite disoriented. He was used to having epidural patients in lithotomy position, and I was used to having women roll over to hands-and-knees, which the tangle of monitor tubes and wires prevented. As I was hands-on, he told me to "pull down, down, down" on the head, until fearing I'd damage the neck, I said, "No, you do it, you know what you're doing." Apparently he did not, because he began twisting the head this way and that, and I realized he was panicking. Suddenly, my mind cleared. I pushed his hands aside, applied suprapubic pressure, and directed him to go for the posterior shoulder, at which point the baby promptly delivered.

Later, as he was filling out the chart, he pointedly asked me, "What would you call that delivery position?" The mother had actually been sitting on the lap of my partner who had been kneeling, so I suggested the term "supported squat."

"Hmm," he responded, "Sounds good…and that was suprapubic pressure with rotation to the oblique, was it not?" A nice gesture of acknowledgement, to top off a most challenging co-management experience.

On rare occasions, you may find you can reach the posterior shoulder, but cannot rotate the baby in either direction. As the situation becomes critical, you may have to resort to the extreme of **breaking the baby's clavicle** in order to collapse the shoulder girdle and effect delivery. Yes, this is a horrifying prospect, but it is certainly preferable to fetal brain damage or death! To break the clavicle, position two fingers against the anterior surface of the collar bone, open your fingers slightly, then place your thumb behind the bone and push between your fingers. One midwife forced to resort to this procedure relayed that the clavicle "snapped like a matchstick." As long as you break the bone outward, you avoid the risk of puncturing the baby's lungs. The baby should be seen by a pediatrician immediately, but don't worry—clavicles heal very readily.

Check every baby who has had shoulder dystocia carefully for bruising, injuries to the clavicle bone, or possible Erb's paralysis due to nerve trauma. Severe dystocia is an automatic indication for vitamin K. Consult a pediatrician at once if anything is abnormal.

SURPRISE BREECH

Even if you have decided not to handle breech births at home, it is wise to practice an emergency delivery routine until it is memorized and flowing automatically. How does surprise breech occur if the midwife has palpated assiduously? If the baby is extremely posterior, the sides of the head may feel remarkably like the iliac crests of the hips. Firm maternal abdominal muscle, excess fat, or extra amniotic fluid may also confuse your evaluation of fetal position. Whenever in doubt, vaginal exam may clear things up, as the feeling of hard round head in the vagina is quite distinct from that of the soft, irregular butt. Sonogram is another option.

But even if you clearly determine the baby to be head down in pregnancy, it may still change position at the last minute, especially if high in the pelvis at term. Suddenly you have a surprise breech on your hands. Be ready for it.

Assisting Breech Birth

1. *The mother must not push until she is completely dilated, and the breech is down to the perineum.* If the baby descends too rapidly, the cervix may not be dilated enough for the head to pass through. Once the body and cord are exposed to air, the baby will attempt to breathe, thus it is crucial that the head be free to deliver at this point. It may be stressful for the mother to hold back during pushing urges, but she must pant-blow through most of her labor.

2. *If the breech is frank or complete and delivery of the body is delayed, it may be necessary to "break down the breech" by extracting the legs.* This problem becomes obvious if the baby's body is exposed to the cord stump and then begins arching up towards the mother's pubic bone. If the legs do not birth spontaneously, splint them one at a time, then bring them across the body and down.

3. *Once the baby has birthed to the umbilicus and the legs are out, pull down a loop of cord to create some slack for delivery.* This is to prevent undue traction on the cord stump as the body delivers.

4. *Wrap the baby's body in a towel or two blankets to keep it warm and to prevent stimulation of respiratory efforts.*

5. *Grasp the baby at the hip bones and gently rotate the body to the anteroposterior position (shoulders vertical), then assist delivery of the shoulders one at a time.* It is important to hold the baby only at the hip bones, as undue pressure on internal organs could cause serious damage.

6. *Rotate the body again so the baby is face down, and reach a finger inside the vagina to create an airway.* This is in case the baby attempts to breathe before it is delivered. Once you have created an airway, use your forearm to support the baby's body. Lower your arm, and the occiput will clear the mother's outlet first, which helps prevent perineal lacerations.

7. *Once the occiput has cleared (hairline visible), have an assistant apply suprapubic pressure as you lift the baby up and over the perineum.* This is much safer than hooking your finger inside the baby's mouth to maintain flexion of the head; to do so might damage the mouth or jaw.

8. *Bring the baby all the way out, place it on the mom's belly, and then assess the need for suction, stimulation, etc.*

9. Remember that babies born breech are much more frequently in need of extra stimulation and/or blow-by oxygen to help them get started.

HEMORRHAGE

Hemorrhage is a complication we would all just as soon avoid. That is why it is crucial to take an exhaustive medical history and do thorough prenatal screening, including appropriate lab tests, so women likely to hemorrhage may be identified and either treated or risked-out in advance of labor. All women should have a complete blood count early in pregnancy or following the initial visit, with a repeat at the onset of the last trimester. An adequate HCT/HGB reading is crucial to ensure maternal well-being during pregnancy, and maximum resilience if bleeding does occur with delivery.

History of previous postpartum hemorrhage doesn't necessarily contraindicate home birth; it depends on the cause of bleeding. If the mother reports, "I was fine right after the birth, but then the doctor pulled hard on the cord...it really hurt, and I really started to bleed a lot," you can assume third stage mismanagement was probably at fault. Additional information about subsequent measures required to stabilize the mother, such as medications or transfusion, will give you a more accurate picture of the woman's tendency to hemorrhage and her recuperative abilities. Nevertheless, any history of postpartum hemorrhage or excessive bleeding following injury, surgery, or dental work should be investigated via lab tests for clotting factors. These tests are numerous and complex to interpret, so seek medical consultation on this.

Yet another possible cause of, or precursor to, postpartum hemorrhage is close-set child spacing, i.e., the mother has given birth to several children in quick succession. Childbearing and breastfeeding can take their toll on a woman's body; if abdominal muscle tone is not adequately restored postpartum, the uterus may not be able to contract effectively during labor or after delivery. Take a good look at the woman; observe her energy level, vitality, appearance. On this basis, recommend exercise to strengthen her abdominal muscles, and/or brisk walking or swimming to stimulate her circulation. You may also wish to suggest appropriate herbal or homeopathic remedies. Cayenne pepper (three to six capsules daily) serves to revitalize the system. She might also take alfalfa tablets regularly during her last weeks, as alfalfa is rich in vitamin K (which facilitates the clotting process).

Intrapartum Bleeding: There are two principal causes of bleeding during labor, placenta praevia and placental abruption.

Placenta praevia has already been defined in Chapter Three. For review, this term refers to implantation of the placenta low in the uterus, either over the cervix or at its edge, so that separation and bleeding occur automatically with effacement and dilatation. It is commonly diagnosed in the last trimester of pregnancy by painless spotting or bleeding, and appropriate management is determined at that time.

Placental abruption, also discussed in Chapter Three, is premature separation of the placenta, i.e., separation before birth occurs. This poses grave dangers to both mother and baby; the more the mother bleeds, the more the baby's oxygen supply is reduced. The only way to control blood loss is by immediate cesarean section, unless the abruption is marginal or the mother is in second stage and about to give birth. Here are the symptoms:

1. *severe, persistent abdominal pain,* different from the ebb and flow sensation of contractions;

2. *abdominal tenderness*, abdomen rock hard to the touch;

3. *fetal distress*, with FHT pattern indicating hypoxia; and

4. *blood appearing at the outlet*. However, this will not occur in the event of concealed abruption, as blood loss in this case is trapped behind the placenta.

Any woman with sudden, severe and persistent abdominal pain must be transported at once, and should be given oxygen en route to the hospital. Treat for shock, being certain her head is down and that she is covered and warm.

If a woman complains of sharp but sporadic pain, apply heat to the affected area of the uterus and keep a close check on the FHT. The pain may be due to incoordinate uterine action, but transport immediately if it becomes persistent or acute.

Vasa praevia is an exceedingly rare complication in which vessels running from the placenta through the membranes present over the cervical opening. They may be running to an accessory, or **succenturiate lobe** of placental tissue. If the membranes rupture where vessels run, the mother will hemorrhage and the baby may die. Occasionally this complication is detected in the last few weeks of pregnancy by internal exam—a pulse may be palpated, the membranes may feel irregular, and unusual changes in fetal heart rate may be noted immediately afterwards. If not discovered in pregnancy, vasa praevia is often identified in early labor. Otherwise, rupture of the membranes may be combined with intrapartum hemorrhage. If so, give the mother oxygen and rush to the hospital.

Third Stage Hemorrhage: Third stage hemorrhage refers to an excess of two cups, or 500 ccs. blood loss after the birth of the baby, but before delivery of the placenta. Estimating blood loss is not easy for beginners; try pouring a measured amount of liquid on an underpad (some midwifery instructors use a mix of liquid starch and red food color) to get some idea of what a loss of one or two cups looks like. Don't forget that clots must be added into the measurement.

There are three major causes of third stage hemorrhage; 1) partial placental separation; 2) cervical lacerations; and 3) vaginal tears. **Partial separation of the placenta** is the most life-threatening of these, as blood loss is usually greater than with lacerations and more difficult to control. Why is this so? As long as portions of the placenta remain attached, the uterus will be distended and blood will continue to flow from vessels exposed at areas where the placenta has already separated. The only solution for this problem is delivery of the placenta, as this permits uterine muscle fibers to contract fully and close off bleeding vessels.

Nevertheless, whenever she is confronted with postpartum hemorrhage, the midwife must quickly **determine the cause of bleeding** before initiating treatment. For blood loss in third stage, quickly rule out other possible factors of cervical or vaginal lacerations. **Cervical laceration** is highly unlikely unless pitocin, forceps, or vacuum extraction have been used to force labor. **Vaginal lacerations** are more common with compound or face presentation, persistent posterior position, or with large and/or deflexed heads. With these, vaginal tears may be deep enough to involve small arterioles, which tend to bleed in gushes and spurts not unlike blood loss from partial separation. Check the vaginal floor and vault swiftly but thoroughly, dabbing with sterile gauze at any torn areas. If it appears that a vessel or arteriole has been torn, clamp an artery forceps wherever the blood flow is most concentrated and use tie-off suturing to control bleeding (see Suturing, this chapter).

Partial separation of the placenta has several causes. One is incoordinate uterine action, generally caused by "fundus fiddling" attendants. In the vast majority of cases, the uterus will clamp down uniformly and release the placenta completely if left to itself. But if the uterus is poked and prodded, it may contract only in certain areas and release only certain portions of the placenta. Other causes of incoordinate uterine action include prolonged labor and precipitous labor; with the former, the uterus is too tired to separate the placenta in a single effort; with the latter, the uterus more or less grinds to a halt following its highly concentrated and rigorous efforts. Rarely, portions of the placenta are morbidly adherent and resist the retracting of uterine muscle, no matter how strong and coordinate contractions may be. This is due to a condition known as **placenta accreta**, which results from a defective decidua basalis and is characterized by the attachment and growth of the chorionic villi directly into the myometrium. This may involve little or all placental tissue (see Retained Placenta, this chapter).

Partial separation is signaled by bleeding with no apparent lengthening of the umbilical cord, and no desire on the mother's part to expel the placenta. To make a certain diagnosis, put on a fresh sterile glove and follow the cord up to the cervix. If the placenta is at the os, it is indeed separated and can be expelled by the mother's efforts, or you may use controlled cord traction to remove it. But if your fingers trail through the os and up into the uterus, you have diagnosed partial separation and should: 1) immediately give the mother tincture of angelica; 2) begin vigorous nipple stimulation (if the baby is not ready to nurse); and 3) administer 10 to 20 units of pitocin by intramuscular injection (or by intravenous drip if you are able). These measures all serve to contract the uterus, hopefully enough to expel the placenta in a matter of minutes. (And do not worry that pitocin will close the cervix. It contracts the longitudinal fibers of the uterus only, not the circular ones at the cervical os.)

How you proceed from this point depends on the amount of blood loss. If bleeding continues in small gushes and spurts, you can assume that only a small portion of the placenta is separated. If you attempt to remove it manually, you might encounter large sections morbidly adherent and impossible to detach, and cause significant blood loss by distending the uterus with your hand. Give pitocin if you've not done so already, or repeat at five minutes after your initial dose. Some midwives inject a mix of 10 cc. normal saline solution and 10 cc. pitocin directly into the cord (providing it has been cut), which sometimes helps complete separation.

Again, follow the cord to the cervix to see if the placenta is present. If not, and bleeding persists, transport. Remember that anything over two cups blood loss is considered a hemorrhage—some women will go into shock at the loss of four cups. You must figure transport time, so make a conservative decision. And be certain to physically attend the mother during transport, treating her for shock (she should be reclining, feet elevated, warmed with blankets, oxygen by mask) as you continue to assess blood loss and watch for signs of separation. You may also repeat pitocin injections at eight minute intervals, 10 units IM. This will usually control the bleeding and stabilize the mother's condition somewhat. But if she starts bleeding heavily, your only option is to manually remove the placenta then and there.

The same is true at home, if blood loss is heavy from the start. Fortunately, heavy blood loss indicates that a considerable portion of the placenta is already separated (lots of uterine blood vessels exposed) so manual removal should not be too difficult. Sometimes the placenta is fully separated but has lodged just inside the cervix, in which case it is easily grasped and removed. But if it is still attached, you must remove it.

Manual removal of the placenta may be painful for the mother, and may lead to postpartum infection. Thus it should only be performed in dire necessity. The procedure is fairly simple. Don fresh, elbow-length sterile gloves, pour some antiseptic over your gloved hand and insert through the os, using your other hand at the fundus to prevent the uterus from being forced upwards. Slip your hand between the separated portion of the placenta and the uterus, then pry the rest of the placenta away, using your hand like a spatula and working your way across the entire surface. Once you have the placenta removed, quickly go over the uterine wall to remove any fragments, then grasp the placenta and bring it down and through the os. Your assistant should give methergine and/or pitocin as soon as the placenta is out, and vigorous uterine massage should be started at once. Assess the mother's blood loss and vital signs. If her blood pressure is low, she looks pale, feels cold and clammy, or her pulse is thready or erratic, give oxygen and transport at once, treating for shock. If she is stable, push fluids, keep her warm and quiet, and continue to assess vital signs. The placenta itself should be examined carefully to be sure it is complete. If there is any question, take the mother to the hospital immediately for a consultation (she may need a D & C). Bring the placenta in case evaluation by a pathologist is suggested.

If sections of the placenta cannot be removed manually and the mother continues to bleed, methergine can be given as a last resort. This will cause very strong contractions and may close the cervix, but your priority is to save the mother's life by minimizing blood loss during transport, particularly if she has lost more than three cups of blood and transport time is more than twenty minutes.

I once had an uncanny experience with partial separation. After the mother called to tell me her labor had started, I lay down to clear my mind and focus my energies on my upcoming tasks when my inner voice said clearly, "There's going to be a partial separation."

"Well," I thought, "that's reasonable, she had bleeding in the first trimester. No problem, I'll just go up inside the cervix like I've done before and grab it."

"No," the voice insisted, "this time it's different, this time you'll have to go all the way up and really pry it off."

Now I was frightened! But I put it out of my mind, dismissed it as a logical fear based on the mother's history, and went on to the birth.

But it paid to be prepared. The baby delivered beautifully, then torrential bleeding began. I followed the cord up and felt it meet the placenta just inside the cervix and thought, "Oh good, it's right here," but as I attempted to grasp it, I realized the cord was inserted at the placenta's edge and upper margins were still attached. Before I knew it, I was doing a complete manual separation. I had my assistant give 20 units of pitocin IM (which I'd drawn up in advance) as the blood poured down my arm. But the process was quickly completed—I felt like I was on "automatic pilot." The uterus firmed up right away, and the mother was stable with an estimated blood loss (EBL) of 800 ccs.

Another cardinal rule of dealing with a woman who is hemorrhaging is to keep her attention focused on the here and now. This means commanding her to stay with you, to look you or her partner in the eyes, or to touch and speak to her baby. In truth, you must call on her to rally her life essence or vital force, particularly if she is drifting or fading out. This is one reason why prenatal communication has to be authentic: you must have channels open and ready to be activated in case of emergency.

To illustrate: a former midwifery partner told this story of her second birth. She lived way out in the country, up a rough road, and her husband had gone to get the midwives when she delivered precipitously and unattended. After she birthed the placenta, she began bleeding heavily and somehow managed to pull out a syringe, load it, and inject herself with pitocin.

She later told me, "You know, Liz, I really got how women can just slip away when they bleed like that. I was already so high from the birth, and it would have been really easy just to check out completely. It was the coziest, warmest, most delicious feeling—it just felt so good." I never forgot this, as only then did I appreciate how firmly and passionately the midwife must tell the hemorrhaging mother to stay present.

Fourth Stage Hemorrhage: Fourth stage hemorrhage refers to blood loss in excess of two cups or 500 ccs. after the placenta has delivered, but within a 24 hour period following the birth.

Eighty to 90 percent of fourth stage hemorrhage is due to a condition known as **uterine atony** (atony means lack of tone). Nevertheless, it is essential to eliminate other possible causes of bleeding before proceeding with a remedy, unless blood loss is torrential (covered later in this section).

Begin by ruling out cervical or vaginal lacerations. Also check to see if the mother needs to urinate, as a full bladder can cause postpartum hemorrhage by interfering with the ability of the uterus to descend into the pelvis and fully contract. Ask the mother if she needs to go to the bathroom, or palpate the bladder to see if it is enlarged.

Retained placental fragments can also cause fourth stage hemorrhage. Check the placenta thoroughly, as described in Chapter Four. If missed, retained fragments may lead to delayed bleeding in the first two weeks postpartum, particularly if their presence has been masked by the use of oxytocics after delivery.

Another possible cause is **sequestered clots**, which form if the uterus does not clamp down firmly after the placenta delivers. As blood clots form and distend the uterus, more bleeding and more clotting occur, on and on in a vicious cycle. The best way to deal with sequestered clots is to prevent them. Massage the uterus firmly after the placenta delivers, or better still, have the mother birth the placenta in an upright position so her internal organs automatically compress the uterus and squeeze blood out, preventing clots from forming. Suspect sequestered clots if the uterus feels slightly enlarged or somewhat soft, or if a slow trickle bleed begins after placental delivery and gradually increases. Check for clots by doing a gentle, sterile exploration at the cervical os, and remove clots from the uterus if need be.

Apart from lacerations, the above are mechanical factors which interfere with the ability of the uterus to contact. Oxytocic herbs, homeopathic remedies, or drugs will do little good if the bladder is distended, placental fragments are retained, or the uterus is full of sequestered clots.

But oxytocics are crucial for treating uterine atony, which can result in considerable blood loss. There are several causes: one is a long, drawn-out labor rendering the uterus too exhausted to clamp down efficiently; another is precipitous labor, with contractions so rigorous that the uterus is unable to downshift and make the sudden adjustment to its reduced volume. A uterus overdistended by polyhydramnios, a large baby, or multiple fetuses may also have difficulty contracting effectively after delivery. These cases can usually be managed with fundal massage and oxytocic drugs or herbs unless there is a pathological condition of the blood which inhibits coagulation.

If you are faced with a seemingly uncontrollable bleed following delivery of the placenta, and uterine massage and medications don't work, you must immediately call for help while giving the mother oxygen and **bimanual compression**. In addition to the method pictured in the illustration on page 145, you can also perform this maneuver externally by grasping and lifting the uterus firmly with both hands, then pressing them together as hard as possible. Treat the mother for shock and give fluids (by mouth or intravenously). Help her summon her vital forces and stay present.

I had an interesting experience with a young Venezuelan mother who had just given birth precipitously. During pregnancy, she and her adoring partner told me repeatedly, "If there is anything wrong, just tell us and we will fix it." I thought them a bit naive, but admired their dedication and devotion to one another. Shortly after giving birth and delivering the placenta, she began to bleed quite heavily. My partner and I massaged her uterus, felt her bladder, but could find no obvious cause, at which point we encouraged her to nurse and began to prepare the pitocin. Her partner turned to look at us and asked, "What is wrong?"

"She's bleeding too much," we said, "and we'll have to give her an injection."

"Wait a minute," they said. And as though it were scripted, they joined hands, looked into each other's eyes and began to chant, "No mas sangre, no mas sangre" (sangre means blood in Spanish). In a matter of minutes, the mother stopped bleeding as abruptly and completely as if someone had turned off the faucet. And that was that!

Sometimes you have a case of **slow trickle bleeding**, a lazy, sporadic flow, which, barring other factors, may reflect the mother's emotional state. Particularly if the birth has been difficult, or if for some reason the mother isn't glad to see her baby, she may become passively withdrawn (emotionally shocky). Take a strong stance—ask her firmly to stop bleeding and pull herself together. Have her touch and talk to her baby, kiss her partner, stay involved with her support team. Give her something sweet to drink, with plenty of praise and encouragement. Tinctures of angelica and shepherd's purse may help; give a large dose, a dropperful of each under the tongue.

Watch the slow trickle bleed very carefully. It may start and stop repeatedly, so blood loss must continually be reassessed. If it exceeds 750 ccs. (3 cups) you must transport, even though the situation may not appear critical. Sometimes it is necessary to give pitocin or methergine as much as 45 minutes after delivery if blood loss has accumulated

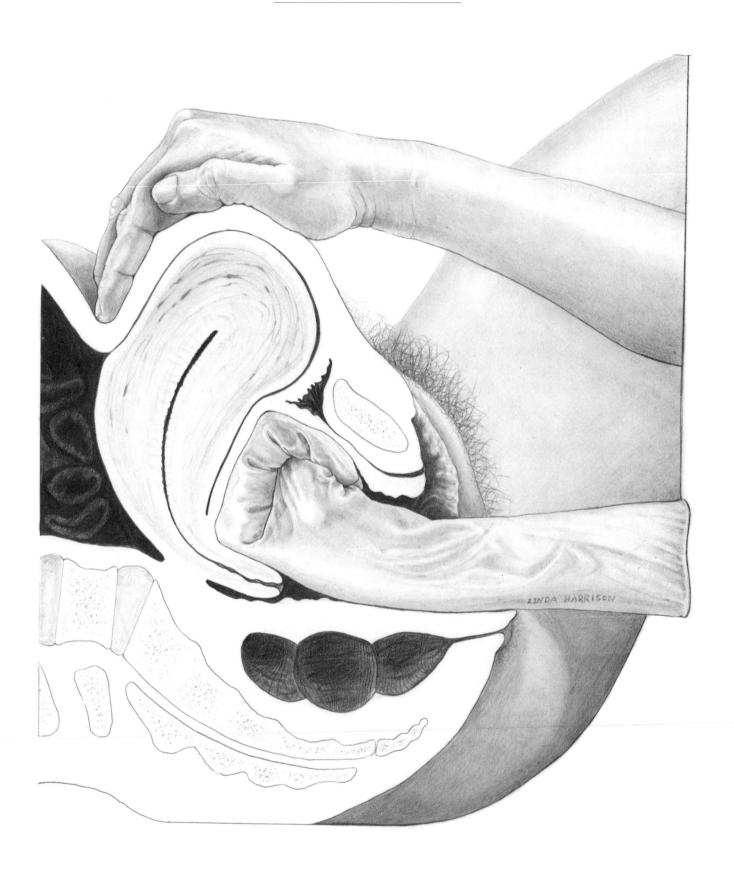

Bimanual Compression

to a critical level and the mother shows no signs of stabilizing. Experts on the subject repeatedly advise, "It's rarely the torrential hemorrhage, but the slow trickle bleed, that kills." Stay alert, and do not leave the mother until blood loss has been fully controlled for at least an hour—longer if it has exceeded 600 ccs.

RETAINED PLACENTA

The placenta usually comes away from the uterine wall with the first strong contractions following delivery. This may take 10, 20, or 30 minutes, as the uterus must recover its strength and reduce in size sufficiently to shear the placenta away. Absence of the characteristic "separation gush" is a definite sign to wait and see.

Nevertheless, bring the mother's attention to her sensations as soon as you notice that uterine contractions have resumed. She may not feel much at first, but may suddenly become distracted from her baby, or throw you a questioning look. If physical signs concur, advise her that it's time to birth the placenta, and assist her into a squatting position. If you stick to this routine, you'll find the placenta usually delivers within the first half hour postpartum.

Certain circumstances may interfere with this. One is prolonged labor, which may leave the uterus so exhausted that it can't quite finish its job. If the mother is tired and baby not yet nursing, try nipple stimulation, or tinctures of cohosh and angelica. Another solution is to administer pitocin IM or by intravenous dilution. If none of these work, there may be a problem of abnormal implantation.

The rare condition of placenta accreta (see previous section) argues against cord traction under any circumstance. An unforgettable picture in *Williams Obstetrics* shows a fatal case of inverted uterus pulled completely out of the vagina, with placenta still attached. Upon transport, D & C may be sufficient to remove the placenta depending on the amount of tissue affected, or hysterotomy (opening the uterus for surgical removal of the placenta) may be required. Rarely, placenta accreta necessitates hysterectomy if there is no other way for the placenta to be removed.

GIVING AN INJECTION

1. Take a moment to steady yourself.
2. Flick the ampule to get all the medication into the base and break the tip off and away from you, being careful not to touch the edges.
3. Remove the syringe from the package.
4. Remove needle cover, place needle into ampule and pull back plunger to draw up solution. See that the tip of the needle is all the way into the ampule, to avoid drawing up any air.
5. Pointing syringe upward, tap sides to bring air bubbles up, and press plunger to remove air and bring medication to needle level.
6. Locate the outer, upper quadrant of one hip.
7. Use left hand to cleanse injection site with alcohol by starting in center and circling outward, then hold area firmly, skin spread flat.
8. Plunge needle in about three-quarters of the way in one quick movement.
9. Draw back on the plunger to see if a vein has been entered. If blood comes up, push needle in a bit more and check again.
10. If clear, inject slowly, pushing plunger all the way down to the base.
11. Draw needle out quickly in one smooth movement, and put pressure on site with alcohol pad until bleeding stops. You may cover area with a spot bandage.
12. Dispose of needles and syringes properly, i.e., in the sharps box provided by your lab.

More commonly, it's a matter of maternal inertia which stalls delivery of the placenta. I recall one birthing which went quite quickly; when we arrived, the mother was already nine centimeters dilated. She and her partner had established their own coping routine, and regardless of our closeness to them prenatally, we felt a bit like intruders. She birthed with very little assistance, then we began to wait for the placenta. Two hours later, after having nursed her baby and taken tinctures repeatedly, she went into the bathroom to pee and delivered the placenta herself, in private. She came out and handed it to us, saying good naturedly, "Here's what you wanted!"

Occasionally a woman resists letting go of the placenta because it represents the last remnant of pregnancy, the final barrier to full-fledged motherhood. Focusing her on the beauty of her baby or on the pleasure of nursing will often bring the placenta. Sometimes a bit of encouragement, "Let's just get the placenta out now and you'll feel so relieved," will provide the necessary prompt to let go.

How long is it safe to wait? You might try an injection of pitocin at 45 minutes. As long as there is no bleeding, the uterus remains firm, and fundal height is stable, you can afford to wait another hour or so. Beyond that, extended watch may cause anxiety and fatigue for both the mother and her attendants. Also, the cervix begins to close after several hours, presenting an obstacle to placental delivery. Infection is another potential danger, as germs may migrate up the cord to the uterus. After two hours, talk about going to the hospital, and after another twenty minutes or so, go ahead and transport.

ASSESSMENT AND REPAIR OF LACERATIONS/EPISIOTOMY

One of the most interesting facets of my apprenticeship was observing the unique ways in which various midwives did their suturing. Also interesting were decisions regarding when, and when not to repair. After observing healing time and relative discomfort caused by various techniques, I developed a personal preference. This method is presented in the following section, along with many other critical elements of technique, by my friend and mentor, John Walsh.

Always remember that episiotomy is rarely justified, except in cases of fetal distress necessitating emergency delivery. An episiotomy may be easier to suture than a laceration but one is obliged to cut through muscle, whereas lacerations are often more superficial. Episiotomy weakens the musculature unless perfectly repaired, and causes much greater discomfort and slower recovery for the new mother.

With most deliveries, the mother's perineum is intact. Otherwise, she may have but a few minor abrasions (my midwife friend Tina calls them "skid marks"), none of which require stitches. These are most likely to occur on the labia, and look rather like chicken breast with skin torn, but flesh smooth and intact underneath. Suturing these is contraindicated, because stitches will not hold unless imbedded in the flesh.

Sometimes, a minor internal muscle split of the bulbocavernosus muscle occurs, even though the perineum remains intact. If bleeding from this internal tear can be controlled with a bit of pressure (using sterile gauze), I usually do no suturing at all. Internal tear edges will usually meet and join together as long as the split is no more than halfway through the muscle. Superficial, first degree perineal tears will also heal by themselves if the woman takes good care of them.

But be sure to make a thorough and honest assessment of each and every laceration. Unfortunately, there is a strange status quest among midwives regarding the ability to do tear-free deliveries; do not let this prevent you from suturing when it is clearly necessary. Sometimes the mother will be more comfortable if sutured, especially if tear edges do not approximate, i.e., fit together by themselves.

IN CASE OF TRANSPORT

1. *For the mother: don't panic!* It is easy to feel despair, and to lose control upon arriving at the hospital. But you have a better chance for a good outcome if you stay relaxed.

2. *For partner or father: if your partner is exhausted or nearly so, don't expect her to make complex decisions about hospital routine or physician recommendations.* Here is where all your study and investigation during pregnancy really pays off. The better you know your stuff, the easier it is to respond to suggested procedures with either agreement or alternative solutions.

3. *For both of you: ask for what you want, or enlist your midwives' assistance in doing so.* You have only one birth of this baby; don't hold back! The hospital can be an intimidating place, but just because the routine runs a certain way doesn't mean it can't be altered. For example, you can definitely refuse: 1) to wear a hospital gown; 2) people running in and out of your room continually; 3) attendants talking during contractions; 4) bright lights in the labor or delivery room; 5) routine IV; 6) routine episiotomy; 7) stirrups for delivery, or; 8) baby not given to you immediately (barring emergency complications).

4. *In the event the baby is temporarily stable but requires care in the nursery, keep the baby with you as long as possible.* Partner or father should go with the baby to the nursery until the mother can join them. Once in the nursery, maintain physical and verbal contact with the baby (the isolettes have holes you can put your hand through).

5. *If you are unsure about any recommended test for your newborn, ask your midwives or pediatrician.* Don't be railroaded into a package treatment; let staff convince you that each test is truly necessary for the baby's welfare—not just for liability reasons.

6. *If you must stay in the hospital, activate your postpartum support system immediately.* Don't think you can wait until you get home—you need it now! Have fresh fruit, vegetables, bread, cheese, water, etc. brought in daily, as hospital fare is inadequate in quality and quantity for a breast-feeding mother.

7. *Don't hesitate to ask for privacy, or to be left alone for a while.* Routine checks on mother and baby occur on a regular schedule, but unless they are truly necessary because of some specific concern, refuse this constant monitoring or you will never get any rest! You may also find that as shifts change and new nurses appear, each will have some suggestion about wrapping, feeding, or caring for the baby. Cheerfully thank them, but explain that you'd rather figure things out yourself. If they press you, reassure them that you are fine, and they needn't worry. Otherwise, you'll go crazy with input and could lose confidence in your natural mothering abilities.

8. *If you've been in the hospital for a few days due to some complication, be prepared to be absolutely exhausted when you get home.* You don't get much sleep in the hospital anyway, but combine this with the stress of transport and adjustments to the newborn, and you can imagine how tired you'll be. Arrange it so no one is there when you first get home, except other children and their caretaker.

9. *Take it easy on the processing; it may take some time before the whys and the wherefores of transport become evident.* If you start to feel emotionally overwhelmed, call on your midwives.

SUTURING TECHNIQUE
by John Walsh, PA/Midwife

Unlike most obstetricians who prefer to make an episiotomy for a variety of rationalizations, midwives take great pride in maintaining an intact perineum. This is the hallmark of a real midwife and is genuine proof of her patience and loving touch. Nevertheless, tears occur commonly and sometimes surprisingly. A nine-pounder slides out without a nick, while a five-pounder creates a second degree laceration unexpectedly. Often the head is guided out exquisitely, only to have the shoulders do damage because of some urgency. And what does it gain a woman to have a wonderful birth at home only to have to pack up, drive to the hospital, and be sutured by strangers who may receive her with rudeness or even pointed hostility?

After the first 15 or 20 deliveries, every midwife has had to reckon with a few serious tears. They are simply going to happen, no matter how ideal things are. In fact, she may even decide to do an episiotomy on rare occasions, and this requires a repair job.

Every midwife should learn to suture and do it without recoiling. It is one of those skills with a great aura of mystery about it. This is probably because suturing is usually considered part of the province of surgery, with firsthand experience not easy to come by. Although it is a skill best acquired by actual practice, it requires understanding and rehearsal in advance.

It is essential to set up properly for the procedure, or you won't be able to do a good job. The mother should be made comfortable on the bed's edge. She should have a clean, dry underpad beneath her. You must have excellent lighting; carry your own tensor lamp and extension cord, or forehead mounted system to eliminate this worry. Also, you must find a comfortable position in which to begin—your back will definitely begin to ache, and sweat will pour down your nose. This is really hard work.

The first step in repair is careful examination. Wear sterile gloves for this. It is helpful to place several gauze sponges in the vagina to aid exposure and to sop up the oozing which obscures your

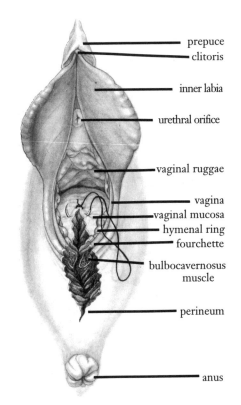

Anatomical Landmarks

prepuce
clitoris
inner labia
urethral orifice
vaginal ruggae
vagina
vaginal mucosa
hymenal ring
fourchette
bulbocavernosus muscle
perineum
anus

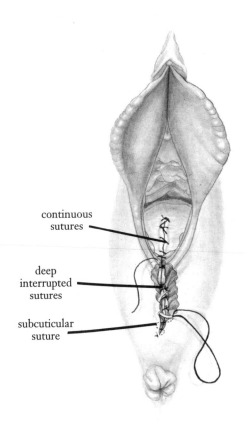

continuous sutures
deep interrupted sutures
subcuticular suture

Repair Technique

landmarks. Roll up the gauze and insert like a tampon. Just don't forget to remove it when you are done—it will be practically invisible because it will be bloodsoaked.

Take your time to be sure you see the full extent of any tears or bleeding sites. Don't assume that everything is OK. You must look. If the mother is uncomfortable during the exam, it may be best to give local anesthetic (1 or 2 percent lidocaine) now, and continue the exam as it takes effect. It will help if she is arranged comfortably and is holding her new baby, not paying much attention to what you are doing. However, it is important to warn her gently whenever you begin something painful like injecting.

Lidocaine does not completely anesthetize tissue. Usually women can feel moderate pressure or pulling sensations, although these shouldn't be painful. This worries some women, as they are afraid your next movement will hurt a lot. Don't do anything suddenly, and the mother will begin to relax and stop anticipating pain.

The basic suture kit needs to contain:

1. **A needle holder.** The five-inch Baumgartner is probably the best. The tips are small and serrated to hold the needle tightly without slipping. A hemostat should not be substituted, because the balance and the grip as the needle is driven through tissue makes a subtle but important difference in doing a good job;

2. **A tissue forceps.** These look somewhat like tweezers but are called forceps. A very delicate kind called Semkin-Taylor or Addsons are a good choice. They have tiny, interlocking "rats teeth" at their tips and with them you can hold and lift tissue very nicely without pinching or destroying membranes. Thumb forceps or dressing forceps are not suitable for handling skin, and the usual tissue forceps found in medical supply houses are too large and clumsy to do precise and careful work;

3. **Two or three mosquito hemostats.** As their name implies, these are hemostats with small tips used for clamping small "bleeders." They should never be used for anything else;

4. **Scissors.** A pair with sharp tips is used for trimming tissue and cutting suture material precisely. This should not be the same pair of scissors used during delivery or for cutting the cord;

5. **4 x 4 sterile gauze pads or sponges;**

6. **Betadine solution;**

7. **Suture material.** Generally, 3-0 chromic gut on a round half-circle needle is the most useful. A 4-0, 3/8 circle with cutting edge is best for labial tears; it pops through skin easily but can bend if used for deep muscle sewing. The half-circle needle is sturdier and penetrates deeper. By the way, "cat-gut" really comes from the submucous connective tissue of sheep intestine. It dissolves in five to seven days, unless it is impregnated with chromic oxide which prevents it from decomposing so readily. A new suture material, vicryl, is increasingly preferred to catgut as it is less likely to cause tissue irritation. The designation 3-0 refers to the diameter and tensile strength of the suture. 5-0 is smaller, weaker; 1-0 is thicker and stronger. 3-0 has a pulling strength of approximately two and a half pounds. 4-0 has about one and a half pound knot-pull tensile strength. Sooner or later, you will break a suture just as you tie an important knot. It is exasperating, but you will learn a finer touch. The needle itself is swaged onto the suture material so there is no "eye" or bump of thread to pull through tissue.

The repair instruments should be kept wrapped up and sterile until the local anesthetic has been given. Suturing must be done by **sterile technique**. This may seem complicated and difficult to organize at first, but practice makes perfect. It is essential to have an assistant, and you both must know exactly what to do. For the purpose of making the following explanation clear, the one doing the suturing will be called "A" and the assistant will be called "B."

1. *A opens her pair of sterile gloves and puts them on, then places the sterile inner wrapper down to serve as the sterile field.*

2. *B opens outer suture wrapper and drops sterile suture packet on sterile field, then does the same with*

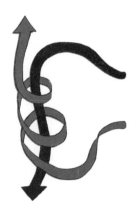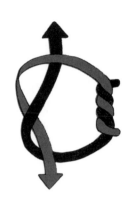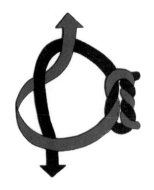

Triple-tie Knot

the sterile gauze pads and the syringe (this should be 10 ccs., 23 gauge, 3/4-in. needle).

3. A takes the sterile instruments (needle holder, scissors, mosquito hemostats, and tissue forceps) and places them on the sterile field.

4. B wipes the lidocaine top with an alcohol pad.

5. A picks up the syringe, and draws up an amount of air equivalent to the amount of lidocaine she wishes to inject—5-10 ccs. B holds up the bottle, A injects the air through the rubber stopper and then draws up the lidocaine. A and B must be careful not to touch each other's hands or tools; this requires a delicate choreography between them.

6. A now begins injecting lidocaine around the edges of the wound and prepares to suture.

7. B puts on a pair of sterile gloves, and assists by holding the labia open while A does the suturing. She can also reach for gauze and dab while A is stitching.

A word now about injections. Always rule out an allergy to lidocaine by reviewing the mother's medical history. And read the package literature that comes with lidocaine—especially the part about side effects. If the mother says she feels peculiar after you have injected, stop everything and assess the situation carefully. Every now and then, a woman may have a reaction which is simply one of distaste for shots and needles. Make sure that's all it is. If she is feeling faint, suddenly says she feels hot and shaky, or has a metallic taste in her mouth, watch for signs of shock. Take blood pressure and pulse, monitor skin color, check the uterus for

firmness, etc. True drug reactions are rare but emotional reactions common.

It will be easiest to inject if you start at the top of the tear and work downward. Inject directly into the sides of the laceration, parallel to the skin. It takes a surprising amount of force to squirt medication into tissue. Be patient; if you inject too quickly it will sting the mother. As you inject, you will notice that you change and distort the tissue as it distends with anesthetic. Try not to plunge the needle all the way to the hilt, as that is its weakest point. Inject no more than one cc. at once, pulling back the plunger each time to make sure that a vein hasn't been entered.

Now you are ready to begin suturing. The repair of a second degree midline laceration goes something like this (there are many variations). After the anesthesia has taken effect, use tissue forceps to examine the edges of the internal vaginal tear. Continuous sutures are begun at the apex of the tear. The tissue forceps grasp the edge of one side, the needleholder directs the needle in a curving motion, and a "bite" of tissue is taken. The needle pops through the other side to be clamped by the holder again, and is reinserted about three-eighths to half an inch below the first stitch. By pulling slightly on the strand as it is placed, the edges to be closed next will come into view easily. It is also a good idea to re-approximate edges (hold them together) every stitch or two, to make sure they are matching up correctly. The continuous suturing is continued until the hymenal ring is reached. Cut the suture string to leave a dangling end of about four inches (you will tie this to the strand used to repair the perineum).

The next step is to join the deeper perineal muscle tissue with a series of two or three interrupted sutures. These will bring the edges of the skin closer together, evenly distributing tension and eliminating dead space. Start at the top and work your way down. The first of these, where the tear is the deepest, should be done in two parts, one bite on each side (like halves of a circle). Be sure to keep your needle holder vertical to avoid entering rectal tissue. Your final stitch should be triple knotted like the others, but do not cut both ends—leave the suture string attached.

Now close the superficial layer of outer perineal skin with subcuticular stitches. Make your first stitch immediately beneath and parallel to the skin, running from your last internal stitch down to the bottom of the perineal split. Run a second stitch upward, on the opposite side (again, like halves of a circle). *Now reverse your needle position in your needle holder.* The point of the needle should face opposite of how it has faced thus far—instead of pointing left, it should point to the right, or vice versa. This allows you to aim your next stitch up the other side of the perineum. Keep switching your needle position back and forth, as you zig-zag towards the hymenal ring. Your final stitch should end slightly inside the hymenal ring back in the vaginal mucosa, opposite your loose end. Pull each end separately until snug, then triple tie together. Here are some basic principles to keep in mind for any type of suture job:

1. *Close lacerations (no matter where they are) in layers-muscle, fascia, skin.* The basic idea is to eliminate tension in any one spot. Always make sure your deep stitches are placed horizontally and run level from side to side, so the pull on deep layers is distributed evenly. This is especially important in mediolateral lacerations (those starting at the fourchette and going off to one side) or they will heal in a distorted manner. Things may look alright on the surface, but if deep layers are not joined symmetrically, there will be puckering.

2. *Eliminate dead spaces between layers.* If you don't,

oozing can occur and a small (or large) hematoma can form. These are terribly painful swellings which can lead to infection, and may cause the entire repair to fail.

3. *Don't suture too tightly or you will impair the circulation.* Anticipate slight tissue swelling after you complete the repair, and compensate by sewing loosely. Don't use too many stitches either, as each will interfere with circulation to some extent. Use just enough sutures to bring tissues together and reapproximate edges. Vaginal tissue is highly vascular, and good at healing itself. In fact, the fewer stitches, the better.

4. *Check your landmarks carefully and repeatedly.* If you have waited several hours to do a repair, significant edema may confuse the picture. Double check what goes with what. Go slowly. It is sometimes helpful to tack the middle of a laceration together, instead of working from both ends only to find that things don't quite match up. The bulbocavernosus muscle at the mouth of the vagina is an important landmark; it should be united very meticulously. A deep interrupted stitch should be used to join both sides so that the skin will meet exactly. Take care not to pull too tightly. Also, when a second-degree tear is deep, you must be certain that the levator ani muscle encircling the anus has not been torn either partially or completely. Repair of a third-degree laceration is strictly a job for the experienced! Don't attempt it if you don't know how, and more importantly, don't neglect it, thinking, "it's only a little tear." Anal incontinence is very difficult to remedy later on.

5. *Sutures should be placed so that the depth is greater than the width.* This is the best way to produce a closure where the edges meet correctly. This is a fundamental principle of suturing and it is important to figure out why this is so.

6. *The curved needle is best grasped at about two-thirds of its length.* If it is held at the end, it frequently bends or worse, breaks. The needleholder itself should be grasped firmly, piercing tissues by using the entire hand and wrist in a twisting motion. It is sometimes very difficult to pop the needle through the skin; use the tissue forceps to hold the area steady with your other hand.

7. *Every suture should have three alternating knots.* The first should be a friction knot (put end through loop twice before pulling snug), and the other two should be alternating slip knots. This triple-knot process creates a very strong, true square knot. Be careful never to clamp the suture with the needleholder, as it will tend to break at this site. Suturing is easier if you wet the suture with Betadine before beginning, and again as needed. This keeps the string from sticking to itself (and to your gloves).

8. *Your assistant can be very helpful by cutting sutures as they are placed.* This saves you the movements of laying down the needleholder and forceps to pick up the scissors. You should hold both strands up rather tautly as your assistant prepares to cut. She takes the scissors and then, with the index finger pointing down the blades, opens the scissor tops just slightly, places them slowly on the strands at just the right spot, and quickly snips. The tails on interrupted sutures should be a half centimeter in length—if they are too short they may slip, whereas long ends may cause irritation by poking adjacent tissue.

If there is swelling after the repair, apply an ice pack (crushed ice in a sterile glove works fine). Make sure to tell the mother to rinse off with warm water with a squirt of Betadine added, each time she uses the toilet. After the first 24 hours, it is perfectly OK for the mother to soak in the bathtub. It will not dissolve the sutures. It is also a good idea to expose the perineum to a lightbulb or sunlight to dry it. The mother should avoid applying vitamin E or other oils to the wound as these retard the healing process. If you have done a good job, the majority of the healing will take place in a few days.

* * *

INFANT RESUSCITATION

Here is a topic you need to discuss with parents before the birth. In order to explain your procedures for resuscitation, you must cite the main causes of severe neonatal depression. It's important parents realize that some occurrences, such as cord accidents (prolapse, true knot) or placental problems (abruption, vasa praevia) can lead to fetal demise regardless of your best efforts, and that the presence of resuscitation equipment is no guarantee of absolute safety or security. Beyond that, neonatal resuscitation procedures should be described so if they become necessary, parents will have a sense of what is taking place and can support your efforts.

Much has been said already about monitoring fetal well-being so that fetal distress is not allowed to persist and deepen into depression. The most common cause of last-minute distress is severe head compression, which seldom presents a problem if the baby is born promptly. However, the baby's ability to tolerate more or less hypoxia is based on many factors, including maternal and fetal well-being in pregnancy, intrapartum complications of prolonged labor or fetal distress, even a minor degree of outlet disproportion. Remember that the baby of a clinically exhausted mother can react suddenly and severely to head compression in the final stages of labor. As stated earlier, bradycardia or early decelerations to 60 BPM or less are definite indications for effecting immediate delivery.

Whenever a baby is born in compromised condition, your top priorities are to clear the airway and provide warmth. Regarding the latter, it is crucial to appreciate the folly of trying to bring a baby around if it is chilled. Naked and dripping wet, the newborn loses body heat rapidly unless placed on the mother's belly and covered, from head to toe, with two or three flannel blankets (preferably oven-warmed). Suction the baby as indicated, but be careful not to stimulate the gag reflex by placing the bulb syringe too far back in the throat. The American Heart Association and the American Academy of Pediatrics have jointly developed a course on neonatal advanced life support (NALS). This includes intubation techniques and is more comprehensive than the basic CPR course. Call (800) 242-8721 for information, or contact the nearest branch of the American Heart Association.

Unless at risk due to stressful labor, postmaturity, prematurity, or intrauterine growth retardation, a baby with a hypoxic phase of less than ten minutes will usually come around quickly if given sensitive stimulation and kept warm. Minor last-minute depression causes no major change in blood pH (acidosis) that could hinder spontaneous recovery. Remember that the baby will continue to receive oxygen from the mother as long as the cord is left pulsing—this allows time for complex internal changes that establish respiration to be completed. This transition takes some babies a bit of time; it is not abnormal for 20 seconds to elapse before significant respiratory efforts are made.

In contrast, true neonatal depression, or **apnea**, literally means "without breath." There are two categories: primary and secondary. A baby who has not been hypoxic for long but has attempted to compensate by making respiratory efforts/gasping attempts in utero is in a state of **primary apnea**. This baby will generally respond well to stimulation and blow-by oxygen, or a few breaths mouth-to-mouth. But the baby who has suffered a greater degree of hypoxia and has made a second round of gasping respiratory attempts is in **secondary apnea**. It will not attempt to breathe on its own again, so waste no time with stimulation. This baby needs oxygen, via mouth-to-mouth or bag-mask resuscitation, sufficient to reverse the acidosis caused by severe hypoxia.

Determine appropriate resuscitation techniques by taking your cues from the baby's skin color, muscle tone, and general in-the-body quality. A baby who delivers with an APGAR of 6— blue, a bit floppy, minimal respiratory efforts but definitely present—needs stimulation via immediate, firm but gentle massage at the base of the spine and up the back. Do this with love—let positive energy pour from your hands. Keep the baby against the mother's skin for warmth and contact—you can reach under the blankets to massage. Gentle words of encouragement, e.g., "Come on, baby," help the parents stay connected and focused on the baby's well-being.

And get the mother to talk to her baby! Neonatal intensive care nurses have observed that babies' oxygen levels surge upon hearing the sound of their mother's voice. With all these modes of stimulation, response should occur within 10 or 15 seconds; if not, try using a see-saw motion of rocking the baby head to toe. This alters diaphragmatic pressure and can stimulate respiration. Remember to keep the baby warm, too—change dampened blankets promptly.

Prolonged labor may cause a minor type of depression in which the tired baby makes a rather slow transition. Sometimes the parents are likewise so exhausted that they cannot muster welcome and attention for the baby. I have seen several babies deliver in fine condition, then proceed to go pale and flaccid due to a lukewarm reception from the parents. Perhaps the baby is of undesired or unexpected gender. Come from the heart in moments like these: "What a gorgeous girl (or boy) you have!" Or to the sibling standing by, "You have a sister (or brother)!" Love kindles life— it's just that simple—and it's the midwife's job to bring this to bear.

Standard hospital management of the slightly depressed or tentative baby is quite different.

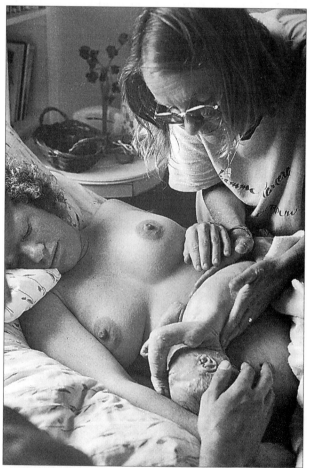

The midwife stimulates a baby making a slow transition, keeping the baby warm against the mother.

Duties are sharply divided between obstetrician and neonatologist, as per their respective liability. It is not within the obstetrician's scope of practice to stimulate or resuscitate the newborn. When confronted with an unstable baby, his/her immediate priority is to pass it on to the neonatal team. This necessitates premature cord clamping, placing the tentative baby in an even more compromised condition. The neonatologist responds by placing the baby in the resuscitation unit, applying mechanical suction to its nose/throat and then, more often than not, bag-masking the baby even though it is already breathing. Time and again, I've watched babies deteriorate rapidly with this treatment. It is noteworthy that in all this, stimulation is usually overlooked—no one touches the baby. Sometimes I simply do it myself, while encouraging the mother to talk to the baby from across the room.

The baby born in secondary apnea, easily recognizable by its shocking white and completely limp appearance, is another story (APGAR of 2 or less). As soon as suction is complete, this baby needs immediate mouth-to-mouth, or bag-mask resuscitation with oxygen. An assistant should get a heart rate, as pulse below 60 indicates the need for cardiac massage. A friend or the father should call for the ambulance at once.

Mouth-to-mouth resuscitation is usually sufficient for all but the most severe cases. Although we no longer administer the "kiss of life" directly, we can begin resuscitation immediately with a pocket mask while the oxygen system is readied. There is a special relationship between breathing to the baby and feeling the baby's response through your hands, which gives a clear and accurate sense of its revival. Often the baby will open its eyes and look straight into yours before it begins to breathe, which greatly boosts your intent and concentration.

Sometimes babies make gurgling noises as you resuscitate them. Depending on degree, you may need to suction again (use a DeLee for best results). Rarely, globs of thick mucus lodge in the throat, and must be quickly removed with a fingertip. But don't fuss too much with this—getting oxygen to the baby is your top priority.

I once had an experience with resuscitation that bears repeating. The baby was born after an hour-long second stage and trouble-free labor. Heart tones were good throughout crowning, the scalp tone was pink. No meconium in the waters, but there was tight cord around the neck which I clamped and cut at once. The shoulders then birthed without delay, so there was no reason to expect what happened next.

The baby failed to make any respiratory efforts, and lost what little muscle tone it had at delivery. APGAR at one minute was about 4. Stimulation helped somewhat, and the baby began to pink up a bit with DeLee suction (it actually sucked the tubing). I thought the baby had made it then, but instead it proceeded to go pale and flaccid. I tried more stimulation, gentle suction, and a few breaths mouth-to-mouth to which the baby responded mildly (although it had never really stopped breathing). It seemed to need more stimulation, but the moment I stopped, it began to fade away again.

Minutes had gone by, so I decided that I would take the baby and give it all the attention and energy I could muster (I also had my apprentice call the ambulance). As I started to do the diaphragmatic seesaw, someone in the room observed that the baby had not yet opened its eyes. At that, it winked its lids and I began to swing its body slowly from side to side, hoping to stimulate it to take a peek. Not much of anything, and I was getting desperate. Then I remembered that its strongest response had been sucking on the DeLee, so I put my little finger tip in its mouth. I felt a wave of tenderness sweep through me as I began to speak, "Come on in baby, it's not so bad here, come on, please come in." At that, it started sucking, opened its eyes and looked right at me, and turned nice and pink. The paramedics arrived, but soon realized that nothing but observation was needed and so left shortly thereafter.

How to explain the baby's in-and-out behavior? Likely causes, such as prematurity, infection, or maternal drug use did not apply. There were, however, extreme psychological tensions between the parents regarding each other and the baby. The father had been unfaithful to the mother repeatedly during pregnancy, and had made no adjustment whatsoever to his new responsibilities. Just moments after the birth, he got up and moved to the far side of the room, and the mother froze up completely. I think the baby felt unwanted. The father would not connect with it at all, the mother would not speak to it when I prompted her. No wonder it was tentative! This was why, when I gave it my finger to suck, I instinctively said, "It's not so bad here...come on in."

The part of this experience that overwhelmed me was the realization that the baby's life was entirely in my hands—that I alone would make the difference in its decision to live. I had never played this role before, and I still recall the confusion of trying to find the baby's soul, hoping to give enough of myself and my love that it would want to stay. I certainly learned the importance of clearing up chaotic personal issues between parents in advance! As it turned out, the parents separated shortly after the birth, and the woman moved out of the area. But she kept in touch, and proved to be a loving and devoted mother.

In any marginal situation like this, be sure to maintain an extra-long postpartum watch. Check the baby very carefully and repeatedly (especially the reflexes). You shouldn't leave until the parents are warmly attentive and the baby is glowing. And have them see their pediatrician as soon as possible.

FETAL ANOMALIES

Fetal anomalies may be caused by genetics or by certain viruses. Increasingly, drugs or chemicals found in the environment or workplace are implicated in fetal anomalies. Use a current issue of the *Physician's Desk Reference* to identify teratogenic effects of over-the-counter and prescription medications. Consult *Holistic Midwifery* (Frye) or *Will it Hurt the Baby?* (Abrams) for precise information on links between fetal anomalies and certain environmental or occupational exposures. Regional phone numbers for teratogen information, and referrals to various parent support organizations can be obtained toll free from the March of Dimes Birth Defects Foundation at (888) 663-4637.

Severe abnormalities are sometimes correlated to polyhydramnios or oligohydramnios. Careful

PRINCIPLES OF INFANT RESUSCITATION

If the baby is born limp and floppy, with white body:

1. *Provide warmth:* wrap the baby with blankets and cover the head.

2. *Clear the airway:* suction mouth with bulb syringe or DeLee if necessary.

3. *Position the baby so head is not overextended:* otherwise, the airway will be occluded.

4. *Begin mouth-to-mouth:* place mask unit over baby's nose and mouth, puff your cheeks full of air, and give four short puffs to the baby. Do not use your lungs! If this does not initiate breathing, continue at the rate of 30 breaths per minute. Switch to your ambu-bag as soon as possible, hooked to your oxygen tank. Watch the baby's chest—it should rise and fall as you work. If not, make sure you have a good seal over nose and throat with the mask, and that the head is level with the back.

5. *Have your assistant take heart tones:* if pulse rate is below 60, begin cardiac massage. Apply pressure on the sternum bone midway between the nipples, pressing with two fingers about 1/2 inch into chest. Continue at the rate of 80 to 100 times per minute.

6. *If performing cardiac massage, blow air into the baby every fifth beat as you release pressure, without interrupting the rhythm of your fingers:* this is full CPR.

7. *After a full minute, briefly stop and recheck pulse:* if absent or still below 60, carefully reposition your fingers and continue CPR.

8. *Periodically re-check pulse, but never stop for more than a minute:* continue as necessary.

palpation may disclose **hydrocephaly** (enlarged cranium) or **anencephaly** (little or no cranial vault, with extremely large, long limbs). Minor defects like cleft palate or club foot are undetectable until birth, whereas more serious ones like **spina bifida** (exposed spinal meninges) may be detected by early pregnancy testing (see Chapter Two) or by the use of ultrasound.

The most important thing to remember when a baby is born with anomalies is that parents need to see, touch, feel, and bond. Most mothers will readily embrace their babies regardless of defects, often emphasizing the beauty of other features. Just be sure to stay in close proximity to the parents until you are certain they have noticed the defects. Avoid pointing these out, unless parents are clearly in denial. Then do so simply and gently, and without lengthy discourses on causes, treatment, outcome, etc. All of this information will surely be requested later; let the parents set the pace for this.

Some midwives feel an odd sense of shame when first assisting delivery of a baby with anomalies. This is probably a carry-over from the medieval days, when midwives were accused of practicing witchcraft and causing fetal deformity. But it is also possible to feel all the joy and wonder of assisting a normal baby—maybe more so. As one midwife colleague reports:

I was always afraid of assisting a baby with deformities, but when it finally happened, I felt thrilled by his beautiful spirit, and very welcoming. He had lots of anomalies, but his body was secondary. I was shocked at how open I was to him, almost as if his imperfections made him more perfect in some way. This touched my heart profoundly.

It is also normal to feel concern, disappointment or sadness, but again, your most crucial task is to open your heart to the parents. You will have plenty of time to find your own support, and identify community resources for parents as they make their adjustment.

Most anomalies require no immediate treatment, except for spina bifida. Exposed meninges or open areas along the spine should be covered with sterile gauze soaked in warm sterile saline solution. However, babies with anomalies should be seen by

a sympathetic pediatrician as soon as possible, as there may be additional internal defects not readily detected by cursory examination.

If anomalies are so severe that it appears the parents will have little time with the baby, you must take your cues from them. They may or may not want to transport; you are obligated by professional ethics to respect their wishes. You must also give life support to the best of your ability, unless they outright refuse treatment for the baby.

I once heard a story of a couple whose baby was born with Down's Syndrome. Their obstetrician was a personal friend who could not bear to tell them. His way of resolving this problem was to drop a book on Down's Syndrome in their mail slot, ring the doorbell, and then slip away. By lack of communication, his kind intent clearly became an act of violence. But most medical personnel today are knowledgeable about the emotional issues surrounding fetal anomalies, and will offer support and information in a respectful, sensitive manner.

STILLBIRTH AND NEONATAL DEATH

Often death is caused by severe deformity, and it's clear at delivery that there are only moments of time for greeting, acknowledgement, and letting go. It's a blessing that birth generally renders everyone so refreshed and exhilarated that if death occurs, it is within a positive, open framework. If you sense that parents are in denial and you know the baby is departing, you should tell them simply that their baby has such serious problems that it is going to die. Seldom is this necessary, though—when death is part of birth, we all know it.

Many women considering the practice of midwifery pause at the thought of losing a baby. Is it the ambiguity of emotion, fear of accusation, or confrontation with death itself that is so terrifying? It helps to remember that birth and death are similar high-energy, transitional states, and guidelines for moving through both are virtually identical. Sure it's tragic and incomprehensible to lose a baby, but it's easier if everyone stays present, open, and connected.

It's different when a baby is unexpectedly stillborn: perfect, beautiful, and lifeless. Then there is

157

genuine shock plus loss, a reality warp in which the mind struggles to grasp, explain, control. If confronted with a stillbirth, try to set aside your thoughts and surrender to your feelings. Hold this possibility for other members of the birth team. Help the mother touch and claim her baby, encourage both parents to look and caress. Bear witness to this rite of passage. Don't give consolation or suggestion; there will be time for that later on.

The coroner must be notified of any stillborn infant weighing 500 grams or more. Autopsy is at the discretion of the coroner. But if it can be established that the baby has been dead in utero for some time, autopsy is optional. The coroner releases the body to a funeral home of the parents' choosing. With hospital stillbirth, the physician signs the death certificate; out of hospital, this is the coroner's task.

Some believe that naming the baby is important, and I agree. Parents may also want to save a lock of hair, or take a photograph. After assisting her first stillbirth, a midwife friend of mine was both surprised and honored that at the baby's memorial, each guest made a point of stopping and speaking not only to the parents and the reverend, but to her as well.

It is very difficult for the mother in the first few days postpartum. Her hormones fluctuate dramatically, and her milk begins to flow. Lactation can be suppressed with sage tea, or by binding the breasts. But the grief is something else. Plan to spend time with the parents daily for the first few weeks. Friends and family will stop by, and will look to you for reassurance and support (and they will have lots of questions). Take care of yourself and get plenty of rest, even as you see to the mother's recovery by guarding her privacy, if need be. Just being there as a witness and friend, ready to listen if she or anyone else needs to talk, is your most important task right now.

At some point, encourage parents to write a chronicle of the event, or make a scrapbook. And expect to be in touch with them for many months. Make a point of calling regularly, meeting them for

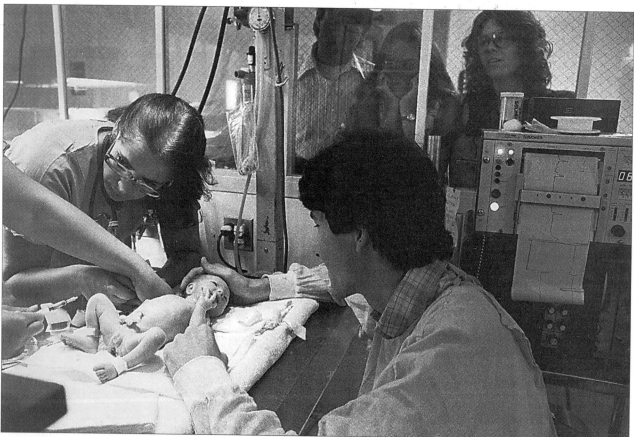

The machinery is intimidating, but your baby desperately needs your touch, the sound of your voice and your reassuring presence.

lunch, etc. Contrary to popular belief, grieving is often a lengthy, drawn-out process. It does not commence in an orderly, predictable fashion, but is comprised of rounds—some more vivid and painful than others—which may continue for a lifetime. Know the basic phases of grieving—shock, denial, anger, resolution—and be ready to share this knowledge with the mother and her intimates as appropriate.

And be sure to have referrals to support groups readily available, as well as written materials on how to talk to children/siblings about death. (See Appendix B for support organizations.)

LIAM ANDREW

by Shannon Anton

We watched the moon rise slowly from inside the jeep. The moon rose slowly, and slowly I watched every detail of her round, white fullness so pronounced. The speed of my life, every movement and interaction, has been altered to reflect the slow pace of grief. Next to the moon I can see a few people leaving the church. I wonder why they don't notice the moon right there, only then I realize she is behind them— concealed yet right there on the horizon, suspended silently in front of me, looking me right in the eye. I am familiar with this feeling in my heart. It is what I feel for an old, old friend that I have loved well but have not thought of for too long. Nostalgic and strange, because someone else now has died, that sadness is again permeating my days, slowing them until I can see the beauty in everything. Sometimes I must be slowed so very much before I can see it clearly; then there it is and the moment can pass to the next.

A few days ago I walked in the park, and crossed the landbridge between the ponds. On the sand were the usual folks, plus ducks and turtles, who always skitter into the water as I approach with my dogs by my side. A single turtle stayed on the sand, making no move toward the water. I was quite close before I realized she was still there, looking at me, unwavering. Her eyes held me in their gaze. I stopped. It was a long moment of slow stillness. The scent of the pond, the sand, the lush green on the banks became like a fog around me and mixed with the heat of hiking. I took a step forward to steady myself in her gaze. Once there I continued on, walking fast away from her because, I told myself, the dogs would bother her. Uh huh. And now I think of her stare and know that today I could meet her gaze completely.

What I remember most from Susan's pregnancy is her smiling face above her growing belly. We laughed easily during our visits. Her baby moved in response to our feeling his knees, his back, kicking us while we listened to his heartbeat. We guessed sometimes he was a boy, sometimes a girl. The Blessingway brought Jane and I into the circle of loving closeness that surrounds Susan and Mark.

Susan called me at 6 A.M. On the phone she was nervous and giggly; contractions woke her around 4 A.M. after not much sleep. We talked, and I planned to come when she called me back, or if I hadn't heard from her by 10 A.M., I would come by and check in. When I arrived at their house around 11 A.M., Susan was in early labor. She was kneeling on the floor with her elbows on the bed, beginning to be uncomfortable during her contractions. I worked to help her stay relaxed during them, to breathe deeply and loosely. She moved into the ease of that without struggle, and as she did, the contractions became longer. I took her blood pressure and we agreed to listen to the baby's heartbeat after the next contraction.

Susan leaned back on the bed and I pressed the fetascope to her belly. I heard nothing, and seeing from the shape of her belly that the baby was still posterior, continued to listen in other places, guessing how the sound of the heartbeat might travel around folded arms and legs. I sat back to stretch, and saw with some surprise that the bottom half of her belly was covered in the small ring-shaped indentations left by my fetascope. I had still heard nothing.

I grabbed my Doppler from my bag and explained that I wanted to use it to try and hear the baby; Susan agreed. I listened. I heard nothing. I asked Susan if she'd been feeling the baby move and she said she thought so, though as the contractions became stronger it may have been the start of each contraction that she had thought was movement. I jiggled her belly, rubbing the baby's knees, hoping for a kick to let me know all was well. Nothing. I put my Doppler on the charger, thinking maybe it wasn't working properly, and sent Susan downstairs for a glass of juice to try to wake the baby up.

A few minutes later we tried to find the heartbeat again, this time downstairs on the couch where we had always done prenatals together. I told myself that she hadn't been flat enough upstairs to hear easily. With the fetascope I again heard nothing, covering her lower belly once more with round indentations.

I went upstairs to get my Doppler again, and while I was in the bedroom I felt that same unsteadiness I'd felt with the turtle. I told myself I'd been on my knees too long and now I'd run up the stairs, no wonder. But once downstairs again with the Doppler, still I could hear nothing of the baby's heartbeat. Out of frustration both with the technology in my hands, and the feeling that at this point, I might not know the heartbeat if it bit me, I held the Doppler to my own heart and heard it clearly: boom... boom...boom.

Satisfied the Doppler was working, I held it again to Susan's belly. The words "silent uterus" rose up from somewhere deep in my mind. I thought how strangely accurate they were: I could hear no sound at all. Susan had felt nothing of movement yet, and was beginning to believe she might not have felt the baby move since the night before; she and Mark had spent time together, feeling the baby kick.

We went back upstairs so I could do an internal exam. I thought if I could stimulate the baby's head, he might give us a kick. We worked between contractions, Susan lying back while I reached with my fingers to find her cervix opened three centimeters and a bulging bag of water in front of her baby's head. The baby's head itself was slightly overlapping at the sagittal suture, and I thought the edge of the suture line had a jagged, shard-like quality to it. The baby's head was still high in her pelvis, high enough it seemed odd that there would be molding now, already. When I pressed against the head, I could feel a wrinkly, loose scalp over the crown. Thinking back now, things seem obvious, but then it seemed that nothing made sense.

I tried one more time to hear the baby's heartbeat and when I could not, I said to Susan and Mark, "This has never happened to me before, it's just never taken me this long to hear heart tones. We haven't felt the baby move and I don't know what else to try. I think we need to go to the hospital and try to get the baby on the monitor."

Susan and Mark agreed. I added, "We'll probably get there and find the heartbeat right away and I'll feel like an idiot, but I don't care. I'll go call now while you get things together."

I went downstairs and phoned labor and delivery. The voice on the other end was familiar, and when I identified myself, she said, "Shannon, it's Jan Randall. How are you?"

In a moment's passing my mind flashed through my experiences with Jan; she'd apprenticed with me for a short time. I recalled the sense of her at my shoulder as a young, single mom pushed her baby out after a few short hours of labor; the mom's laboring sounds and then the baby's cries echoing off the high ceiling of her Victorian apartment, grayish morning light filtering through tall windows. I also remembered her very pregnant body just a few months ago: she'd given birth at home herself, to a healthy baby boy.

Realizing time was doing that amorphous thing it does around birth (and death), I came back to the present, to Jan, and in the same breath I laid out everything that had happened so far. When I came to not having any other ideas except coming in, she agreed. She said it was a slow day there and she could take care of us herself; she wanted to keep things low-key for Susan and Mark.

I called my apprentice and gave her a brief version of what was happening. She would meet us at the hospital.

We drove on the freeway. I followed Mark and as we drove, I thought to myself how good it was that we were staying in the exit lane, since we were going so slow. I glanced at my speedometer and was surprised to find it at 60 mph. I looked around—even knowing this I would have guessed our speed at around 30 mph. I backed off Mark's bumper to a reasonable distance, vaguely aware that something was definitely up. I was in an altered state now and felt a sense of something important to come.

On arrival, we made our way to labor and delivery. The ward was quiet. No one was willing to meet my eye *directly, and after one nurse handed us a clipboard with admission forms on it, she turned abruptly on her heel and retreated behind the desk. I felt as if everyone there had heard of our concern and no one was quite sure how to respond to us in this limbo time of not knowing. So to be respectful, no one engaged with us. I stayed by Susan and Mark while they wrote down the few lines of information needed.*

Jane arrived. Then Jan came over to us and greeted us warmly, showing us all into a room. She made explanation of the technology at hand, reminding Susan that it takes a while sometimes to find the heartbeat with the monitor. Jan swept slowly across Susan's lower belly. She paused at intervals, waiting, looking at the monitor, listening for the familiar and reassuring blip of heartbeat. Nothing. She told Susan and Mark that she liked to have a second person try before being convinced that we couldn't get anything on the monitor. Jan looked at me and asked if I'd like to give it a try. I took the sensor in hand and repeated the search. My sense of the baby was obscure, not like usual when I have an idea where to try and hear heart tones. I knew I was in the right area but it still felt off, like I only thought I knew where to listen.

After searching across her belly again, I asked Jan, "What's next?" She recommended a sonogram; Susan and Mark agreed. Jan went to get a doctor, and we waited. The room was quiet. I didn't know what to say to fill the space, so I said nothing. We waited together quietly. Inside myself I was feeling a dread certainty; I hoped I was wrong and I hoped I wasn't too transparent.

The door squeaked open and Jan returned with a doctor following. The doctor came directly to look Susan in the eye and introduce herself. "I'm Dr. Frazier. I've brought a sonogram machine with me so we can have a better look at your baby. Is that all right with you?" Her voice had the kind steadiness that I knew from other transports when we'd worked together. I felt relieved to see her on duty, a friendly and familiar face. I felt like we were being buffered by a soundness of community that surprised and comforted me.

As Dr. Frazier moved the sono probe across Susan's belly, I held my breath. She was quiet, looking hard all around. Then she swept over the baby's ribcage and I could see clearly the brightly lit ribs in silhouette around the heart. There was only stillness. No movement, no heartbeat.

In a tone of voice that was kind but left no room for possibility, Dr. Frazier said, "I'm looking right now at your baby's lungs and heart and I don't see any movement. The baby's heart is not beating. Your baby has died."

Susan and Mark were stunned; my eyes were already tearing and I felt no breath in my own body.

After a brief pause, Dr. Frazier asked Susan, "Have you been laboring a long time?"

Susan's reply was like a reflex, "No! It's just really started."

"When did you last feel the baby move?"

"Well, I thought I was feeling movement with every contraction, but as the contractions got a little stronger, I think I was feeling the beginning of them, maybe not movement. But the baby was moving a lot last night, we both felt it." Susan looked at Mark and they held hands a little tighter.

"This is intense news I'm giving you, and I have to tell you I've been up all night. So before I say for certain, I'd like another doctor to have a look, just to be sure. Is that all right with you?" I knew that Dr. Frazier was willing, hoping to be wrong. But I also knew what I saw on the sono screen, what I sensed as time went on. I could appreciate her wanting to be wrong. Knowing but not wanting to believe. But still, knowing.

For the next hour we hung in a limbo that felt like days. Susan couldn't really let labor go on, she couldn't quite begin grieving, she couldn't feel all was well. The sono machine sat blindly against the wall, waiting with us. At one point Susan said, "Second opinions are good. We'll wait."

At long last, three doctors entered the room together. Dr. Frazier introduced Drs. Jones and Irwin. It was Dr. Irwin who repeated the sonogram and at 3 P.M., confirmed the baby was dead. There was a long moment of shocked silence, then we all began to cry. The doctors excused themselves, saying softly that we could have all the time we needed and to come get them when we were ready to talk about a plan.

The door swung shut and Susan and Mark, holding each other, began to wail. I felt the wall against my back, cool and solid. I slid down to sit at its base, the floor rising up to meet me. I could not look at Jane for a long time. My face was wet but I wasn't sure if I was crying. Jane caught my eye and crawled over to put her arms around me. We both sobbed.

I remember thinking how empty I could still feel with someone's arms around me like that. It wasn't Jane's embrace that was empty, it was the emptiness of loss that couldn't feel any better no matter who held me. That is the forlorn truth about grief. It's just in you until it's not anymore. It seemed tragic to have it fill me again, to know the hard path of its eventual leaving, that path stretching out long and lonely before us all, especially before Susan and Mark.

We mourned hard for the first hour after the news of their baby's death. At the end of that time, Susan's labor was beginning to pick up; she was getting practical. She looked at me squarely and not asking for confirmation, said, "I still have to birth this baby, right?"

I was standing close to her and Mark. I forced my voice out of my body, "Yes."

Susan looked first at Mark and then at me again and nodded, "OK."

"Should I go and get Dr. Frazier now?"

"Yes."

I moved through the door and down the hall. The lights were too bright, the skin on my cheeks and around my eyes was strangely tender; coming to the nurses' station I felt my eyes squint. Dr. Frazier was reading my chart on Susan. I sat down next to her and waited for her attention to turn to me. Another of those long moments passed.

"Hi, how're you doing?" she asked. I could only inhale and nod my head a little. She spoke directly, this time to me, "You gave her good care. There isn't anything you should have done that you didn't."

At this I had tears on my face, "Well, something like this happens, I have to wonder..."

Dr. Frazier took my hand and said, "She received excellent care from you. I'll tell her the same thing. If she'd been our patient she wouldn't even be here yet. She's 41 weeks, but that isn't enough for our postdates protocol to set in. You did a good job." She paused and added, "And we're not gonna do anything about this." I realized she was referring to having me investigated or arrested, and I couldn't believe how far that was from my mind. The thought of having to protect myself right now was too much. I just could do what I was doing. I felt so still inside, like movement or speech required incredible intention.

I sniffed and thanked her, "It's really nice of you to say that."

She nodded, "One of the docs here had a daughter getting top OB care at Stanford; at 39 weeks her baby died. They don't know why. We may not find out either." She turned back to the chart and asked, "Is she ready to talk?"

"Yes, I came to get you."

We walked into Susan's room and all attention turned toward the doctor. She spoke in soft tones and laid a hand on Susan's arm. The contractions were getting stronger. Dr. Frazier and Susan briefly discussed the options: staying here to have her baby or having her baby back at home. Then I heard Dr. Frazier tell Susan that there wasn't anything she should have done that she didn't do, that she had gotten excellent care with her midwives. Then she left us to the decision making.

The door closed and Susan asked me if I would still help her have her baby at home. I said, "Of course. We'll be wherever you are. If you stay here, we'll stay. Whatever you want to do is really OK." She asked if she could have her friends come to the hospital. Her contractions continued to get stronger. It seemed too difficult to return home at that point. I went to call Peg and Jackie.

For the next 24 hours, the labor of birthing and grieving coexisted. Alternately each would fill the room—laughter, tears. Friends and family came to call, more like after a death than in preparation for a birth. None of it felt wrong.

Susan worked with her contractions, breathing, moaning, sighing, until the last bit of cervix was dissolved around her baby's head. She felt pressure enough to make her want to push, and as she bore down she felt the need to be more upright. She pushed well that first time, very vertical using the squatting bar and coming a bit onto her feet at the end of the bed. After that contraction, I felt inside to check on the baby's descent and position.

Another contraction came quickly, and as I was removing my fingers from Susan's vagina, I could feel the bones of the baby's head shifting suddenly and sharply beneath the scalp. The molding was extreme and the scalp loose over it. The edges of bone felt sharp and shard-like, as I remembered from before.

I thought of a squirrel I'd skinned after a roadkill and how the skull was fractured into a hundred tiny sharp pieces. The sound those pieces made when I shifted the squirrel in my hands: it traveled not through the air to my ears but instead vibrated through my fingers and up my arms. Like broken glass but denser, like stoneware, but hydrated and suffused with the stuff of life. It was a sensation of sound in my body. The baby's head bones made a similar clicking and grinding.

For one frightening moment I could imagine the baby's head coming apart, the bones tearing through the scalp and compressing together flatly. I motioned to Jane to help me position Susan in a more reclining posture, allowing more space toward her sacrum for the baby's head to descend, removing direct pressure from the pubic bone.

She pushed again in this new reclining position, and I felt the need to check once more to assure myself that the worst was not happening. The baby's head then felt normal, still sharpish around the edges but molding in a reasonable way.

Susan pushed a bit more. Suddenly we could see the baby's head through her labia! I brought Mark down on the floor with me; on our knees we watched as more of the head gradually appeared. This baby had a good amount of dark hair, wavy and wet.

I felt inside again to see how the head was molding, how it was moving the bands of muscle out of the way toward crowning. I was afraid again of what might happen to the baby's head if I wasn't careful. I began pressing evenly on the muscle bands at Susan's vaginal opening. All I could think was, "I don't want the baby's head to come apart." I thought then, "Wow, I wonder if all bottoms feel this tight before the baby's really pressing more toward crowning? I never ever do this. Why am I doing this?" I stood up and stepped back, thinking, "Geez, girl, get a grip!" I looked around and saw Anne, our nurse, standing nearby. I whispered in her ear, "Have you been to a stillbirth before?" She nodded yes.

"How careful of the head do I have to be?"

"Oh, not very."

I looked at her with my heart and so completely trusted her that I just moved back to the floor, beside Mark, and knew I'd be all right, the baby would be born without damage, and Susan could see and hold her baby without ugliness or horror. I felt a huge worry leave my body. I was warm and relaxed all at once. The world around me slowed again.

I looked at Mark and said, "We'll do this together so neither one of us will be alone." He nodded and smiled a little.

Susan continued to push. Each time, the baby moved a little bit. I was glad to see the gradual movement, her bottom was stretching perfectly with the gentle pressure of the baby's head. Even though the head had begun to come around the pubic bone with her pushes, between contractions it would slip back up again. Susan could feel this and felt at first like she was losing ground. I assured her that with the next contraction, the baby would move right back down again. A bit of a running start. Sharon laughed at my joke and I realized what joy and expectation filled the room.

When the baby stayed in view between pushes, I kept pressure on the occiput of the baby's head to help keep it flexed, and to protect Sharon's urethra and inner labia. There was a lot of give in her perineum—she was stretching around the baby's head beautifully. She reached down around my hands and felt the bulge of the baby's head and smiled like when you just can't believe something so wonderful is happening.

Susan slowly crowned her baby's head. Little by little, the baby was born to his forehead. Mark's forehead, the baby had Mark's forehead! A long pause for the next contraction, and then the baby's nose and finally mouth and chin were born. Dark fluid drained from the baby's nose and mouth. I said to Mark, "The airway is getting squeezed clear now, this is really normal." Mark, not taking his eyes off the baby, nodded.

I felt along the baby's neck and found the cord, loosely there. I pulled an easy loop but it wasn't enough to go over the head. I reached for the first cord clamp and said, "The cord's around the neck and we need to cut it. Mark, do you want to cut it?"

"No, no, go ahead," he said. A little more time went by as I reached for the second clamp and then the scissors and said, "OK, Mark, you wanna cut it?"

"Oh....sure, why not."

I held the cord by the clamps and he slid the scissors under, along the baby's neck. My fingers protected Susan and the baby. Mark cut the cord and helped me unwrap it from the baby's neck.

The next contraction and push didn't change anything. I carefully reached inside along the baby's back to find the shoulders completely unflexed. The usual sweep that brings unflexed shoulders together only moved loose bones in their joints; the baby had no real form. Utter lack of muscle tone allowed movement away from my hands rather than my hands shaping the baby's movement. With two hands I gently rotated the shoulders, and ever so slowly the baby restituted to face the right.

I heard Dr. Irwin ask me if I wanted suprapubic pressure, and heard my reply, no, the shoulder was right here. Concentration consumed me. I had to support every bit of the baby's birthed body or it would fall loosely to the bed. Susan continued to push and slowly, slowly the baby's body was born completely.

Mark helped me hand the baby up to Susan's belly. We all stood around the edges of the bed, around Susan and the baby. I don't know what we expected; no one was prepared for such a beautiful baby. We all just stared with awe for a moment before tears began to fall. We cried hard in those first minutes. Mark lifted the baby's leg to see, boy or girl? He was a boy, Susan and Mark said his name right away: Liam Andrew. He was named. He was their son.

I looked down as I cried, and tears splashed on my left breast. I'd been in the same dress for two days; the weight of the cotton had the neckline plunging, my bosom quite exposed. The sensation of Liam's birth was so much on the surface of my body, the sensation of the tears on my breast filled and startled me. It somehow echoed on my skin, the sadness in my heart. I was transfixed with the moment: I could see birth and death, the cycle of life before me. I was filled with a deep and abiding trust in life. It was a moment when everything came together vividly to make sense, to make a whole; it was also a moment of blinding grief. Susan was glowing, triumphant in her birth, ravaged and grieving in her son's death. So much all at once. It was a sacred and perfect time. I hope never to experience it again; I pray never to forget its influence.

We stayed together for five hours after Liam's birth. We held him, prayed for him, bathed and dressed him. We took photographs. We even laughed.

After having seen Susan and Mark the next day, I stopped on my way home to to get food for my dog. When I returned to my car, it wouldn't start. It was a hot day and everything remained in slow, vivid motion. Moment by moment passed as I stared at the brightness in the air around me. The last thing I wanted to do was deal with a towing company. I just wanted not to talk to anyone. I left my car and began the two-mile walk home. I headed for Golden Gate Park, for home on the other side.

Walking felt heavy but good. Everything was blindingly bright. I think I walked with my eyes closed, the heat searing through my eyelids in a swirling red density. I'm sure I was not alone.

I strayed from the present just as I crossed the polo field. By the time I skirted the ponds and was overcome with the moist smell of the mud, the tall grasses and their whispering shuffle, I was back in Iowa, following another dirt path, and headed for the short track. I recalled that bright day well. Skeeter wore no helmet, he rounded a corner on his cycle and met Roger head on. Literally. Skeeter collided with Roger's bike and then his helmet and landed finally in the soft grass of the field. It was my first true loss. Grief held my hand as I crested the sandy bank of the pond. Today the turtles won't meet my eye, they skitter into the water and are gone. That rich muddy smell, all heady and ripe: I recognize the scent of decay, of loss and turning under. I am relieved to name it. I am comforted by the familiarity of it. I give a nod of greeting to my old dead friends and see Liam among them. All those nice boys together.

As I broke through the line of grass and found my feet on asphalt I was at once confused. I spun around, reeling, really, and the foreground popped back into focus. It is 1995. I am a midwife. I have a place on my left breast that is ablaze. That is where the grief leaks out, where it exactly meets the light of day. Darkness to light, inside to out. It is a small opening, like for a pinhole camera, and the view is incredibly sharp.

A few days later, in the chair with Natasha leaning over me, needle buzzing in hand, I read the sign on the wall that says "Yes, it hurts," and I think, "But not that bad." She asks me something and I don't know how to reply; it was a simple question I can't recall now, but what I did say was, "I'm a midwife and I had a stillbirth in my practice. Liam Andrew Brooks O'Donnel." She paused and looked at me closely. She didn't look away, but she went back to my breast, back to her work. It's a beautiful tattoo. Tending it was both painful and validating. Something physical hurt, but I could put salve on it and it felt better. At least on the surface.

CHAPTER 6

Postpartum Care

he postpartum period is the last frontier for midwives and those associated with maternal well-being. For too long, this phase of childbearing has been utterly ignored, with mother and baby virtually abandoned after a day or two of the most rudimentary care. Midwives now refer to the first three months following birth as the fourth trimester, with the understanding that pregnancy and birth are transformative experiences culminating in this crucial phase of reintegration. As more research is applied to the physical and psychological challenges of this period, important new information is emerging.

Preparation for this fourth trimester should begin prenatally. There is nothing more important you can do than connect pregnant women with one another, or better still, with others who have recently given birth. Exercise classes or support groups can serve to accomplish this. Once the baby is born and helpers have resumed their normal lives, independent women otherwise content to spend most of their time alone may be overwhelmed by the pressure and intensity of the routine mothering, with nothing to break the monotony. For those used to choosing their friends carefully and insisting on intellectual common ground, suggest a more pragmatic approach for the time being. Mothering in the early months is made up of many mundane questions and concerns, and contacts with others in the same phase, even if not the most profound intimacies, will serve a great purpose.

Sometimes pregnant women do not want to face the prospect of caring for a baby, in which case you should tune them in to what's impending by suggesting books on breastfeeding, mothering, etc. Give out a resource list, including contacts for local chapters of La Leche League. Part of the reason for doing this is simple practicality; you just can't continue to give your attention to every new mother with problems or you'd have no time for your current clients. Besides, a new mother enters a new stage of her life, and plays a changed social role (even if she has already had other children). Better for her to launch herself with a sense of self-reliance than dependency. Remember that midwifery is an art of facilitating passage! The midwife plays the guiding role for a while, but after the baby is born, the mother needs her own mechanisms of support.

A former client once approached me with a vision of postpartum outreach that might serve as a model for midwifery practices everywhere. Her idea was to connect the prospective mother with one who had already birthed and would be willing to help with baby care and light chores in the early weeks following delivery. The bonus of this arrangement is that it taps the veteran's natural interest in breastfeeding, infant sleep patterns, family life, and personal issues—and both mothers benefit from having time to talk, relax, and observe their babies together. This also frees the midwife to concentrate on physical caregiving postpartum, rather than trying to address the myriad emotional and physical concerns so common at this stage.

Postpartum care should include home visits on a minimum of days one, three, and seven, with phone calls in between. The final checkup should be given at four to six weeks postpartum.

DAY-ONE VISIT

When you come back the day after the birth, begin by appraising the environment for order and cleanliness. If laundry or dishes have piled up, or the refrigerator is bare, lend a hand as necessary. Also see what the mother has been eating and drinking thus far. Make sure there is a jug of water at her bedside. She may not have even had a chance to shower yet, so help her with this if need be. Ask how she has been feeling in general: any dizzy spells, extreme fatigue or emotional upsets? Much of this depends on what her labor was like, and on what kind of help she is receiving from her partner or friends.

It is extremely important that you stress her need for a *full ten days of absolute rest*. Tell her to follow her body's signals for sleep and nourishment just as she did while pregnant. Explain that during this time, high levels of oxytocin prompt **uterine involution**, i.e., the return of the uterus to its prepregnant size. On the other hand, if she is overactive or stressed, adrenaline will inhibit recovery of muscle tone in the uterus and upper vaginal vault. In other words, the more she rests and lets her body recover, the sooner she will look and feel her best. This message bears repeating, as it is critical to her recuperation.

The main purpose of the day-one check is to see that she's off to a good start: relaxed, happy, comfy with her baby, and well cared for. Always wash your hands thoroughly before examining the mother, use aseptic technique when handling the baby, and universal precautions when in contact with any secretions. Things to check include:

1. *The nipple, for soreness or cracking.* If soreness is just developing, immediately look to the manner in which the mother is breastfeeding. The vast majority of breastfeeding difficulties are caused by improper positioning of the baby at the breast. Be sure the mother is lifting the baby to the breast, that it is not hanging from the nipple and is taking in the areola uniformly. Even though you may have demonstrated this to the

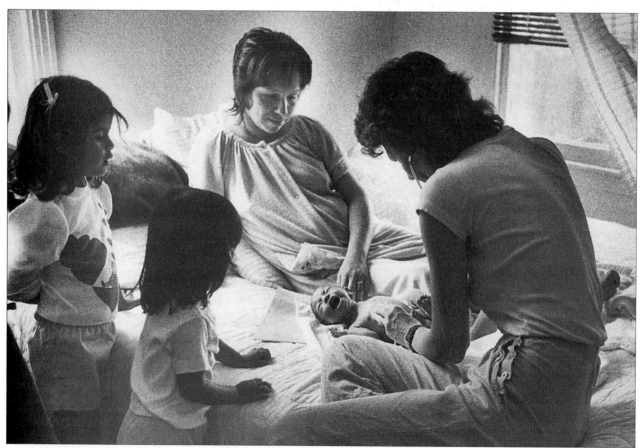

The midwife gives care to the entire family during the postpartum period.

mother immediately after the birth, she may have forgotten, or may have received conflicting advice from friends or relatives. Reassure her that she needn't limit how long the baby sucks, but must always remember to check that it is taking the nipple correctly. If the nipples are cracked, suggest she apply a bit of vitamin E oil between nursings. *Stress how important it is that she continue to breastfeed.* Have her begin with the least tender breast, then switch to the sorer side once she has a let-down.

2. *The uterus, for normal involution.* It should be just below the mother's umbilicus, and should feel firm, not tender. Massage it briefly to expel any clots, and have the woman sit up for a few minutes before checking her flow.

3. *The lochia, for color, amount, and odor.* Lochia is postpartum shedding of excess endometrium. On day one, expect **lochia rubra**, or red-brown flow in amounts like a heavy menstrual period. The odor should be fleshy, like menstrual blood.

4. *The perineum, especially if there has been swelling, tearing, or suturing.* All swelling should be gone; if not, suggest more ice, but also make certain the mother is rinsing her perineum twice a day with warm water and a bit of soap or Betadine. If swelling has increased and she complains of pain, check for a hematoma (see page 179).

   Also check the stitches to be sure they've held; the flesh should be pulling together, with wound edges dry and clean. Signs of infection include inflammation, pain and discharge; consult a physician if these are noted. If the mother complains of tenderness but the area looks healthy, recommend sitz baths three or four times daily. Fresh ginger simmered in water relieves burning and itching, and stimulates circulation. Even plain hot water speeds healing.

   Also check to see if she's had any pain with urination. If so, remind her to pour warm water over her vaginal area as she urinates. And check to see if she has had a bowel movement. Often, women are afraid their stitches will come out when bearing down. For comfort's sake, suggest a bit of counterpressure with a folded tissue.

5. *The mother's temperature record.* If the mother's temperature is elevated, she may be dehydrated or may have a uterine infection (see page 179).

6. *The mother's pulse.* If it is elevated, see above.

7. *The mother's blood pressure.* This is particularly important if it rose during or immediately after labor.

8. *The baby's cord stump.* It should look clean around the base, not red or swollen. Be sure that parents are folding diapers back so urine won't irritate it, and are swabbing the cord regularly with alcohol or hydrogen peroxide. Remove the cord clamp only if the stump is completely dry.

9. *The baby's skin color, inspecting for jaundice.* Depress the flesh on the baby's chest and extremities, checking for yellow undertone. Jaundice is unusual on day one, and should therefore be referred to a pediatrician. Depending on degree, the baby may need a bilirubin count (see page 175).

10. *The baby's skin consistency, for dehydration.* If the baby's wrists and ankles look cracked and wrinkly, it needs to nurse more often. Also note the temperature of the room—is it too warm, or is the baby overdressed? Dehydration can also develop in very hot weather. It's more apt to be a problem with postmature or SGA babies, as they tend to have very little subcutaneous fat.

11. *The baby's elimination pattern.* It should have passed meconium by now, and should be urinating frequently. If it has not had a bowel movement or urinated by 24 hours, consult a pediatrician;

12. *The baby's nursing pattern and behavior.* Sleepiness (especially after a long labor) is normal for the first day. Lethargy (characterized by drowsiness, apathy, disinterest in nursing, and lack of muscle tone) is of concern. The lethargic baby should be checked by a pediatrician, particularly if the mother's temperature is elevated or if neonatal jaundice is noted.

    Also ask parents about the baby's cry. If they report a high-pitched, cat-like wail, hypoglycemia (forthcoming section) may be at fault. Evaluate the cry yourself, and if questionable, refer to a pediatrician.

13. *Anything unusual in the Newborn Exam.* Reevaluate if parents have not yet seen a pediatrician.

Usually parents are in a state of bliss and happiness at this point; if they look frazzled or unhappy, you must try to find out why. It's quite common for the mother's partner to be totally exhausted, in delayed reaction to the energy demands of labor support and loss of sleep. If such is the case, suggest they send out for dinner, spend time in bed together with the baby, and take the phone off the hook until they feel a bit more stable. Many midwives also suggest a note be posted on the front door, to the effect of, "We had the baby, it's a____, we're fine but tired, please call in a few days so we can plan to have you over."

The parents may also wish to talk about the birth, particularly if it has been difficult. Make yourself fully available for this discussion (although parents typically want basic reassurance at this point more than detailed review).

If anything unusual is noted on day one, visit again on day two to follow up. It is better not to attempt reassessment by phone, as even minor physical concerns can exacerbate emotional breakdown in this fragile period. Specific indications for prompt reexamination at 48 hours include any problem with perineal repair, elevated maternal pulse or temperature, excessive blood loss, difficulties with breastfeeding, or signs of neonatal jaundice or dehydration. If everything was normal on day one, a follow up phone call on day two is sufficient.

DAY-THREE VISIT

By day three, the difficulties of integrating newborn care with daily life have become evident, and emotional outbursts are common. This coincides with hormone surges that initiate lactation; it is both common and appropriate for the mother's tears to flow just as her milk begins to come in. And since the baby must also make an adjustment to taking breastmilk, he/she may experience some fussiness or crying spells. This usually evokes emotional distress in the parents, which is exaggerated by fatigue. If the mother's partner has been frantically trying to handle everything—house, shopping, laundry, food preparation—he/she may be at the point of collapse. This may leave the mother somewhat stranded; if so, see that her postpartum support system is fully activated.

Discussions of the birth may either begin or resume, but tend to be more emotionally involved than on day one. To best facilitate the parents' honest disclosure regarding your care during labor, pose the question, "Is there anything you wish I had done differently?" Of course, you must be entirely relaxed and receptive if you expect them to be fully honest with you. Don't press, though—there will be plenty of time later on to talk things through.

Be sure to check:

1. *The breasts.* Check for engorgement by feeling for lumps along the sides of the breasts and under the arms, and looking for reddened areas. If engorgement is a problem, have the mother soak her breasts or her whole body in warm water, as this will stimulate the release of any backed-up milk. Then show her how to express milk.

   Many women find this easiest if they oil the entire breast, and using long strokes toward the nipple, work down from the collar bone with one hand and up from the base of the breast with the other. If specific lumps are noted, have her work from behind these areas. This may hurt a bit at first and she may need to work slowly, but make sure she applies enough firmness to bring the milk out. Up to ten sweeps may be necessary before milk appears at the nipple. Also demonstrate the proper way to grasp the areola, and how to squeeze it to get the flow started.

   Check the nipples carefully for cracks, and ask her how it feels to nurse (if the nipples are cracked, it won't feel good). Make sure she is positioning the baby properly at the breast, and recommend vitamin E oil on the nipples between nursings, if need be. Cold cabbage leaves tucked against the nipples also provide a lot of relief. And for lingering engorgement, hot ginger compresses under the arms or in the upper, outer quadrants of the breasts do a lot of good.

2. *The uterus, the lochia, the perineum, etc.* Recheck the perineum thoroughly, using guidelines from day one. Ask the mother if her flow has been consistent—any clots, heavy bleeding, dark red blood? By day three, her flow should be a bit lighter than before, beginning to change from rubra to **lochia serosa** (more pink than red). Palpate the uterus for enlargement, and note

any tenderness that might indicate infection. And check the odor on her pad to be sure it is normal. Ask how she feels when she's out of bed—any vaginal pressure, or dragging sensation? It is never too early to begin vaginal toning exercises, as long as they are started slowly.

3. *The mother's temperature.* Elevation to 101° is normal at the time the milk comes in. Nevertheless, rule out uterine infection by checking for symptoms (see page 179).

4. *The cord stump.* You can definitely remove the cord clamp by now.

5. *The baby, for jaundice.* A bit of a yellow tinge is normal in the face and down to the nipple line, but unusual in the extremities. Generally, excess bilirubin in the bloodstream is diluted and flushed from the system by breastmilk. If the baby is very yellow, speak to the pediatrician, and certainly check again the following day (see section on Jaundice later in chapter).

6. *The baby, for dehydration.* This is particularly important if noted earlier.

7. *Baby's behavior, nursing pattern, crying pattern, etc.*

8. *Mom's relationship to nursing.* This is crucial. Make sure she is not trying to impose a schedule on the baby, or limit the amount of time it nurses. In other words, replace any archaic, puritanical notions of structuring the baby's need for food with a sensual, loving approach based on trusting its instincts. The sensation of let-down varies from mild tingling to a sexual sort of release, and some women occasionally experience orgasm while nursing. Try to promote a positive feeling around letting go.

9. *Sleeping arrangements.* Check to see what has evolved. If the baby is in bed with the couple, how does the partner feel about this? If the baby is in a basket or crib, how does the mother feel about getting up to nurse? Is she getting enough sleep? Is her partner willing to get up and bring the baby to her?

There are often phone call ramifications of this visit, especially regarding the last three points. This is the time when concerns about discipline arise, and conflicts may develop between partners. Amazing as it seems, fear of spoiling the baby may actually become an issue this early! Men particularly tend to worry that the baby will be spoiled by too much attention, too much contact, too much love. Some respond by setting limits on how much time the mother spends with the baby, or by insisting that the baby be left to "cry it out" when it is fussy, which only exacerbates the problem. Whether due to cultural conditioning or simple jealousy, this reactionary approach should be set aside as soon as possible. Explain to parents that the baby has literally been enveloped by the mother for nine months, its every need immediately met. It has no experience of waiting to be fed or held, and cannot know when it is upset that its mother or father is close by in the next room. Babies need all the security they can get. *There is no such thing as too much love for a newborn.* If parents can surrender to the sensitivity and vulnerability engendered by love, they will be stronger and wiser in the end, and their baby will grow to be a loving, secure child. Encourage them to relax and get to know the baby through touch, play, and gentle massage. (Infant massage is also an important antidote for colic.)

Check in on parents for the next few days on the basis of findings at this visit. As with the day-one checkup, anything unusual is best followed up by a house call, rather than by phone. Otherwise, if everything is normal, a phone chat each day is sufficient.

DAY-SEVEN VISIT

By day seven, the mother's partner may be back at work, and friends and relatives may again be busy with their own concerns. No wonder the new mother may feel suddenly depressed and forgotten—her energy level is not nearly back to normal, and her emotions remain volatile. If she has additionally been entertaining well-wishers and trying to do more around the house than she should, she may be quite exhausted. A definite sign that she has been over-active is increased lochia flow, or change from serosa back to rubra. This is an optimal time for a close friend or relative to come help with major cleaning, laundry, shopping, or running errands, or the parents may want to hire someone to assist them.

Again, she may wish to discuss her birth. This is even more likely if it was traumatic, or the outcome was disappointing for her personally. Accept whatever feelings of resentment, frustration, or sadness she expresses. Try to supply any factual information she needs *without being defensive*. Pay tribute to her strengths, and downplay her shortcomings, if any.

And listen carefully to the scope of any current difficulties. Most women have no idea until they become mothers how hard they will work, let alone how much loss they will likely experience. Yes, loss—loss of friends who don't have children, loss of income for time off work, loss of sexual intimacy, loss of personal privacy, loss of sleep, loss of career-based identity, even the loss of pregnancy! Any two or three of these losses could precipitate a crisis in the most emotionally stable woman; taken together, and combined with hormonal upheavals and practical concerns of running a household, it is hardly surprising that many new mothers suffer some degree of **postpartum blues**. It is important to differentiate this condition from that of postpartum depression, though. The blues tend to diminish as adjustments are made to this new phase of life, but depression typically increases as the weeks or months go by, and is marked by persistent withdrawal and inability to cope. It is important that the midwife be able to distinguish these states, and acknowledge that there are times when professional intervention is indicated.

Physical symptoms of recuperation should be tapering off by day seven. If the mother had perineal repair, the skin should be drawn together by now. Breastfeeding should be fairly well established. Lochia flow should be decreasing. This visit is primarily for emotional support. Do your best to help the mother with any problems she is experiencing, because you probably won't see her again for several weeks.

You may also want to bring up the topic of sex. Advise every woman at day seven to wait on intercourse until her lochia flow has stopped completely. And of course, suggest she wait to see you before resuming intercourse. This is particularly important if she has had stitches.

Over the next few weeks, if the mother reports extreme fatigue or exhaustion, continued bleeding, or sensations of pressure/dragging in her vagina when she is up and about, see her at once. All of these symptoms indicate less than optimal healing, which must be addressed promptly if she is to recover.

FOUR TO SIX WEEKS CHECKUP

The timing of this visit depends on the mother's rate of recuperation. If her flow ceased at least a week prior to contacting you, you can assume her uterus is well involuted, her cervix firmed up, and that she is ready for her final checkup.

But if she had stitches, scheduling this checkup also depends on the condition of her perineum. If she is willing, ask her to wash her hands, and gently insert her fingers to see if the area is still sensitive to pressure; if so, she probably is not ready for sex or barrier method contraceptive fittings.

Nevertheless, wait no longer than six weeks to see her, for if adequate healing has not taken place by this time, you must determine the reason. Perhaps the mother had deep second-degree tears. These can take a while to heal, but if her lochia flow has stopped and she is feeling fine, you have no worries.

Sometimes emotional conditions precipitate scheduling this visit sooner than later. For example, if a woman calls at four weeks to report feeling severely depressed or emotionally incapacitated, see her at once, even though her physical recovery may still be weeks away.

One important reason for this checkup is to give the mother the OK for sex, along with suggestions on how to make the first occasion as pleasurable as possible. Recommend that she use plenty of lubrication, as breastfeeding will cause dryness and fragility of her tissues no matter how intense her desire. You must also raise the issue of birth control for heterosexual women. Although rare, ovulation can occur as early as six weeks after a woman has given birth. I have known a few nursing mothers (giving no formula or anything else to the baby) who conceived in the first two months postpartum.

Things to check at the final exam include:

1. *The uterus.* It should be out of range of palpation, except by bimanual exam. If it is enlarged, she is probably still bleeding, and her cervix will feel very soft by internal exam. All of these are signs of poor recovery. Pale discharge, or **lochia alba**, is all that should be present at this time. Prescribe rest, long relaxed nursing sessions to allow oxytocin to do its work, optimal nutrition, supplements as indicated, and involuting tea or tincture of black haw and shepherd's purse.

2. *The cervix.* It should feel firm, closed, and situated high in the vaginal vault as with initial pelvic assessment. However, some women do not regain their prepregnant cervical tone until they either stop or cut back significantly on breastfeeding, e.g. when solid foods are introduced to the baby.

3. *Internal muscle tone.* This should almost be back to normal by now if the woman has been doing vaginal exercises. If not, explain the importance of using the pelvic floor muscles for maintaining the uterus in its proper position, as well as revitalizing sexual desire and sensitivity. Check for tone high in the vaginal vault and just inside the vaginal opening. Often a woman has good tone in one area, but little in the other. Review vaginal exercise techniques (see Chapter Two).

4. *Lacerations or episiotomy, for complete healing.* If the woman sustained labial skin splits, they may still be somewhat tender as newly formed skin takes time to toughen up. This may cause some discomfort with sex, but adequate lubrication and creative positioning can help.

   If the perineum feels rigid with scar tissue, encourage the woman to do perineal massage using evening primrose oil to soften the area, and to prepare for intercourse. This practice can be emotionally and physically reassuring for any woman nervous about having sex again.

5. *The abdominal muscle tone.* Have the woman lie down, then lift just her head and shoulders as you place fingertips along the juncture of abdominal muscles running from the umbilicus to the pubic bone. If you note any gaping, suggest simple abdominal exercises, starting with single leg lifts progressing slowly to full sit-ups (with knees bent). Most women have about half an inch separation in their abdominals, while others have very little. You might also refer the mother to postpartum exercise groups or yoga classes, if such are available, or suggest she meet informally with several other new mothers for exercise interspersed with baby massage and conversation.

6. *The breasts, for tenderness or lumps.* It is said that the hormones of pregnancy tend to accelerate abnormal cell growth if any is preexisting. Even if the mother has seen a physician since the birth she may not have had a thorough breast exam, so do it yourself. This is also a good time to review self–breast exam with her.

7. *The cervix, by Pap smear.* For reasons stated above, do a repeat Pap even if the mother was screened in early pregnancy.

8. *The hemoglobin or hematocrit.* This is especially crucial if the mother appears weak or exhausted, or if she has history of hemorrhage either with delivery or during the postpartum period.

9. *The diet.* It's common for a new mother to forget her own needs once pregnancy is over and she becomes completely focused on the baby. Often, she finds she has no time to cook, and hardly time to eat. This may prompt her partner to take over food preparation, though perhaps not methodically enough to meet the breastfeeding mother's nutritional requirements. If she complains of chronic fatigue, nervous irritability, or upper respiratory infection, prescribe more protein, more calories, good sources of vitamins B and C, and trace mineral supplements. If her hematocrit is less than 37 or hemoglobin below 12 (nonpregnant standards), treat her for anemia with nutritional recommendations, herbal tinctures or teas, and supplements.

10. *Adjustment to parenting.* This is a broad category of evaluation, but a few well-chosen questions will reveal any disturbing trends. Ask the mother how well she has been sleeping, how she and her partner are getting along, and how she is coping with the frustrations of mothering. It's wise to have the mother's partner present as you discuss these important issues, unless you have reason to believe that the mother needs privacy to express herself candidly.

HERBS AND HOMEOPATHY POSTPARTUM

by Shannon Anton

Keep the room warm immediately following the birth, and do not give a postpartum woman cold drinks. If a newly postpartum woman has to warm her body after a chill, or if she has to warm up the contents of her stomach, she is wasting vital energy. Her entire course of postpartum recovery can be greatly affected by these two factors. Her energy at this time is precious. Respect and conserve it.

Postpartum Bath

If a woman has been consistently stable in the immediate postpartum hours, I offer her a healing postpartum bath. Here is a recipe, contributed by midwife Janice Kalman and originated by the Chico midwives:

Boil one large bulb of **Garlic** in a big pot of water, for twenty minutes. Turn off flame and add dried herbs: one handful **Comfrey** leaves, one handful **Witch Hazel**, 1/2 handful **Uva Ursi** leaves, several slices of dried or fresh **Ginger** root, 1/2 handful **Yarrow** flowers, large pinch of **Rosemary**, and steep covered for at least 20 minutes. In the meantime, scrub the tub thoroughly and rinse carefully. Then paint the tub's entire surface with iodine, and let stand twenty minutes. Rinse tub completely. Run warm (not hot) water to fill, include a large handful of sea salt, and strain the herbal concoction into the tub. The mother and baby may both get in the bath, provided someone stays with them constantly.

Afterpains

These can be very painful and distracting for the new mother. Strongly brewed **Ginger** tea brings relief from afterpains. Pour one cup boiling water over three to five slices of fresh ginger and steep five to ten minutes. **Motherwort** tincture also eases afterpains—begin dosage at 1/2 dropperful and increase as needed.

Herb Pharm makes an excellent herbal compound tincture called **Hellonias Viburnum** that greatly relieves afterpains. Take one dropperful as needed.

Prolapsed Uterus/Cervix

Sometimes a woman's cervix comes down to her introitus after giving birth. If so, reglove and gently push the cervix back up to its usual position. Instruct the woman to stay in bed as much as possible, and to begin Kegel exercises. In addition, homeopathic **Sepia** 200C offers vital support.

Homeopathic **Sepia** 200C is also indicated when a woman reports feeling her insides dropping or sagging when she walks or stands. Have her take several times a day, and continue to rest in bed.

When there is uterine, bladder, or hemorrhoidal prolapse, or when a woman seems especially exhausted and compromised in the weeks postpartum, this indicates compromised Liver Chi. Refer her to a skilled practitioner of Traditional Chinese Medicine (TCM). It is worth noting that uterine prolapse at any age can usually be corrected with TCM. Recurrent yeast infections also indicate weakened Liver Chi.

Healing After Cesarean Section

Homeopathic **Staphysagria** promotes healing after a cesarean section or any surgical procedure. Staphysagria 30C taken several times a day will support full recovery. When painful symptoms ease, discontinue use.

Nipple Soreness

Expressing a few drops of **milk** and rubbing it into the areola will help sore nipples heal. Also allow nipples to air dry after nursing, or expose to sunlight. If nipples are cracked and bleeding, try homeopathic **Graphites** 30C, taken several times a day.

Milk Fever and Mastitis

Because most engorgement and milk fevers occur during nighttime hours, I ask my clients to include in their birth supplies four homeopathic remedies: **Arnica**, **Bryonia**, **Phytolacca**, and **Belladonna**, all in the over-the-counter potencies of 6x or 30C. Timely treatment demands that these be already on hand.

When the breasts are full, tender, and hot to the touch, getting the baby to nurse or expressing a bit of milk so she can latch on is crucial. In addition, try homeopathic **Bryonia** 30C and **Phytolacca** 30C, alternating the two every 20 minutes until engorgement symptoms resolve, usually in a few hours. **Echinacea** tincture—1/2 drop per pound of body weight—can be taken several times a day when the breasts are engorged to prevent the onset of mastitis.

Compresses

Compresses can stimulate the flow of milk, preventing it from backing up and becoming infected. Warm water may be used, but steamed, fresh **Comfrey** or **Cabbage** leaves, or strong **Comfrey** tea compresses, are more therapeutic. Keep compresses on for 20 minutes. During this time, a woman may cry and express concerns, disappointments, or fears. Be present and ready to listen. Also have something warm available for the mother to drink.

Fever with Engorgement

Engorgement or lumpy soreness in the breast accompanied by a rising fever can be resolved with homeopathic **Belladonna** 30C, taken every 20 to 30 minutes. Fever should reduce to normal in the next few hours, and the homeopathic remedy can be discontinued.

Meanwhile, she must also nurse and/or express the milk from congested areas. Coating the breasts with **Aloe Vera** helps reduce the risk of secondary infection. Doses of **Echinacea** tincture also support the body in healing mastitis. Make sure she is well hydrated and getting complete rest.

Building the Milk Supply

Galactagogues help women maintain an abundant supply of breastmilk. They may be helpful to any mother having a difficult time recovering from birth. A classic galactagogue is **dark beer**; have the mother drink one a day, with a raw egg mixed in. **Hops** in tincture form can also stimulate milk production.

Another old remedy is **Fennel/Barley water**: Boil 1/2 cup pearled barley in three cups water for 25 minutes. Save the barley water, and reheat it (do not boil) to make fennel tea, one cup barley water to one teaspoon fennel. Do not steep longer than 30 minutes.

Tincture of **Blessed Thistle** leaves can be taken 1/2 dropperful two to four times daily, and **Borage** leaves can be brewed as tea and drunk a few times a day.

Drying up the Milk Supply

As midwives, we eventually will help women who have miscarriages or stillbirths, or for some reason choose not to nurse their babies. Still, they will have milk. To help ease engorgement, follow the instructions above. In addition, help her bind her breasts with a long, stretchy wrap. Cold compresses also act to dry up the milk (though cold in any form undermines postpartum healing.) Drinking **Sage** tea is a dependable method for reducing milk production, and two drops daily of **Poke** root tincture minimize engorgement.

Extended Postpartum Bleeding

Some women continue bright red spotting after six weeks postpartum. To remedy this, try **Shepherd's Purse** tincture, 1/2 dropperful twice a day for up to a week. **Moxa** therapy applied midline between pubic bone and umbilicus (known as the Conception Vessel) and over the sacroiliac joints supports uterine involution. Referral for TCM is appropriate.

Umbilical Cord Care

A few drops of **Echinacea** tincture on the newly cut cord stump is a reliable way to treat the umbilical cord. You may also use **Goldenseal** tincture or honey. Treat the cord several times a day until the stump falls off.

Jaundice

Traditional Chinese Medicine offers a very effective remedy for newborn jaundice, which parents can obtain from a Chinese apothecary or herbalist. Simmer this root, and swab the liquid inside the baby's mouth. One or two applications will usually clear jaundice.

Colic

A few teaspoons of crushed **Fennel** or **Caraway** seed tea can greatly relieve the discomfort of colic. Try light pressure and warm compresses on baby's belly, or bringing his feet slowly up to his ears several times. Clockwise massage in a sweeping motion above the belly button may also be effective.

Homeopathic remedies are fairly specific. Most common is homeopathic **Chamomilla**, followed closely by **Nux Vomica** and **Mag Phos**. Highland makes a colic formula, available at most natural foods stores (their teething remedy is also excellent).

Misalignment of the skull or spine may also be implicated in colic. Have the baby see a chiropractor with pediatric expertise (newborn adjustments are more like massage than manipulations).

Some babies find great relief in this simple exercise. With the baby on her back, grasp her thighs and lift her feet towards her head, like during a diaper change. Continue to roll upward, and raise the baby until she is hanging upside down. Really! Now wait and watch her move; she will rotate her back this way and that, and when she seems finished, gently let her down. First touch her head down, then roll down shoulders, back, butt, and let her legs uncurl. Babies particularly benefit from this exercise when offered daily.

THE BABY:
COMPLICATIONS AND CONCERNS

HYPOGLYCEMIA

Hypoglycemia refers to abnormally low blood sugar levels. Fifty to 60 mg. glucose per 1 ml. blood is normal for a newborn; anything below 30 is of serious concern. Infants at risk include those large for gestational age, small for gestational age, premature, postmature, and those born to diabetic mothers. Otherwise healthy babies who became hypoxic during labor or were depressed at birth are also at risk. Symptoms of hypoglycemia include apathy, irregular respirations, inability to regulate body temperature (hypothermia), and refusal to nurse.

If a baby at risk develops any of these signs, do a dextrostix to check glucose levels. This is done by heel stick; a drop of baby's blood is collected on a special strip and tested for glucose levels. If ranging from 45 to 49, have the mother nurse the baby as often as possible, and give water with a little molasses (1 tsp. per cup) every few hours, preferably after a nursing. Rather than introducing a bottle, have her use an eyedropper, or the tip end of a small spoon.

Central nervous system damage can result if blood glucose levels are insufficient, so act on any symptoms of hypoglycemia immediately. Some babies require more aggressive treatment than fluids by mouth, such as intravenous therapy and hospital surveillance. Consult with a pediatrician if blood glucose levels dip below 45.

MECONIUM ASPIRATION

Any infant with moderate to heavy meconium at delivery is at risk for serious respiratory problems. If you are unsure that suction was sufficient to clear all meconium from the baby's respiratory passages before it began to breathe, listen carefully for any sign of lung obstruction. If the baby is breathing rapidly, be alert to other signs of **respiratory distress syndrome**. These include nasal flaring, grunting with exhale, retractions of the chest and abdomen, and cyanosis. If any of these symptoms are present, give blow-by oxygen (holding the oxygen tube to the baby's nose) and immediately contact a pediatrician to arrange for transport.

If the baby seems congested but not otherwise in critical condition, help it breathe more easily by providing steam. The easiest way to do this is to turn on the shower full force, then take the baby into the bathroom. You may also wish to apply **percussion** to release meconium from the lungs. To do this, place the baby on your lap with its head down, back exposed. Tap sharply with two or three fingertips in each quadrant of the lungs, particularly in any area you know to be obstructed.

If the baby resumes a normal breathing rhythm and is stable for several hours, you can check back with parents the next day. But if the baby remains congested despite the use of steam and percussion, contact a pediatrician immediately.

TRANSIENT TACHYPNEA

This is a temporary condition of the newborn involving abnormally rapid respirations. Normal rates are 40 to 60 breaths per minute; with tachypnea, rates may increase to 120 breaths per minute. Transient tachypnea is caused by delayed absorption of fetal lung fluid. By itself, it is not a significant problem.

But tachypnea is associated with several more serious conditions: respiratory distress syndrome, meconium aspiration, and sepsis. If the baby is not at risk for any of these, the problem is probably temporary and will resolve spontaneously with time. But if there are any predisposing factors, or tachypnea is accompanied by any sign of respiratory distress, you are obligated to take the baby promptly to the pediatrician. In any case, you cannot leave the baby until the problem is resolved or care is transferred. Once in hospital, X-rays will be performed, and the baby will be carefully monitored until it is back to normal.

NEONATAL INFECTION

If the mother is known to have group B strep, and her labor was complicated by PROM and/or signs of infection such as fever, foul-smelling amniotic fluid, or uterine tenderness, her baby should be screened for sepsis. Since blood cultures take up to

72 hours to return, antibiotics are often given to the baby prophylactically. This may seem very conservative, but consider that the first symptom of strep B infection is apnea, or cessation of breathing. This is why hospitalization is usually a good idea.

The septic baby may show a variety of symptoms: lethargy, irritability, or jitteriness. Tachypnea is a sign of sepsis, as is cyanosis. If the baby appears to be infected, cultures of the spinal fluid may be recommended to rule out meningitis.

It is important to help parents stay as close to the baby as possible in the event of continued hospitalization. Your support and reassurance can help the mother establish a good milk supply and promote continued bonding with the baby. It is more than overwhelming for new parents to face the fact that their baby may be ill, or to watch painful tests be administered repeatedly. They will need the expertise of a good pediatrician, as well as your continued presence and encouragement.

JAUNDICE

Neonatal jaundice is not the consuming concern it was a decade ago. We now recognize the vast majority of cases to be **physiologic jaundice**, unassociated with the dangerous rise in bilirubin characteristic of pathological types.

What causes physiologic jaundice? While in utero, the baby's need for oxygen is met by a high level of red blood cells in its circulation, higher than for most adults. Once the baby is born and breathing oxygen directly, excess red blood cells must be broken down and eliminated from its system. A byproduct of this breakdown is bilirubin, which imparts a yellow tinge to the baby's skin. This is physiologic jaundice. It generally manifests on the second or third day postpartum, and is remedied when the mother's milk comes in to flush the baby's system clean.

Another kind of jaundice that seldom requires treatment is due to **ABO incompatibility**. This phenomenon is similar to Rh sensitization: if blood from an O type mother transfers to her A or B type baby during delivery, the baby may develop excess bilirubin. **Breast milk jaundice** is yet another non-threatening condition caused by a hormone in mother's milk which can interfere with the baby's ability to break down bilirubin. Unlike most other varieties of jaundice, it is unique in that it manifests *after* the milk comes in.

In contrast, **pathological jaundice** is caused by obstructed bile duct, liver disease, infection, or Rh hemolytic disease. This is easy to differentiate from physiologic jaundice as it generally manifests within the first 24 hours. However, jaundice from ABO incompatibility may also appear at this time. To be on the safe side, refer any jaundice on day one to a pediatrician. If jaundice is pathological, high levels of bilirubin may be nearly impossible for the baby to eliminate and may seep into the basal ganglia of the brain, leading to **kernicterus**, or permanent brain damage.

Although physiologic, ABO, and breast milk jaundice are essentially normal and self-correcting, they can occasionally cause the baby to become lethargic and disinterested in nursing. If

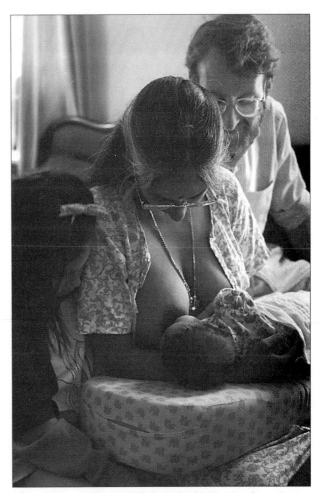

Nurse the baby frequently to help flush bilirubin from the system (note pillow support for positioning).

the characteristic yellow tinge is noted on the baby's face and neck but runs no lower than the nipple line, encourage the mother to nurse often and to expose the baby to sunshine (with its body naked and eyes protected) for 30 minutes twice daily. If the baby's extremities appear jaundiced, consult a pediatrician.

Depending on the degree and type of jaundice, the baby may be hospitalized for treatment. It will probably be placed under bili-lights, and will have blood drawn periodically to assess bilirubin levels. If bili-lights are used, it is crucial that the baby's treatment be properly supervised, as dehydration, burning, and possible genetic damage can occur with excessive exposure. Jaundiced babies also have increased risks of infection.

I've noticed that babies kept in darkened rooms for the first few days tend to have higher bilirubin levels than those liberally exposed to sunlight. Lack of light is probably a more significant factor in extreme physiological jaundice than the favored theoretical cause, late cord clamping. I always clamp the cord after it ceases pulsing, and after placing the baby on the mother's belly or chest. In all my years of practice, I've had only two home-born babies who became severely jaundiced, and in each case, lack of light seemed to be a determining factor.

Babies born to mothers whose labors have been induced or augmented with pitocin must be watched carefully. Pitocin competes with bilirubin for binding sites, rendering elimination difficult. The same is true of certain drugs, such as diazepam, sulphonamides, steroids, and salicylates.

CIRCUMCISION

Circumcision is a controversial procedure, no longer routinely recommended. The American Academy of Pediatrics now states that circumcision cannot be justified on medical grounds. Nevertheless, the practice is ancient—it is portrayed in Egyptian murals, and has long been a central rite in Jewish tradition. Circumcision was originally developed among cultures residing in hot, dry climates (with water for bathing at a premium). Today, it is a matter of custom, perpetuated primarily by fathers wishing their sons to look as they do. Parents must carefully consider the pros and cons of circumcision in order to make an intelligent decision.

Circumcision is a surgical procedure. It is done completely without anesthetic, so the baby must be strapped spread-eagled in restraints. The skin adherent to the tip of the penis is severed and cut back to completely expose the glans, then clamps are placed to control bleeding. Sometimes a plastibell device is used instead, which clamps and cuts off blood flow to the foreskin, causing gradual tissue necrosis. In either case, the pain is severe. Babies generally cry so hard with this procedure that they can scarcely breathe. Possible physical side effects include infection (several deaths have been documented), and penile sloughing necessitating reconstructive surgery.

Knowledge of the procedure is enough to persuade most parents of its dangerous and emotionally traumatic nature. Opponents of the procedure, many of whom are prominent nurses and physicians, deem it a form of sexual mutilation, or even child abuse. But what about the alternative—the uncircumcised penis? What about the supposed dangers of infection, and how about the basics of good care?

The foreskin covers and adheres to the glans penis for the first year or two of life, at which point it will be pulled back by the boy himself as he becomes aware of his genitals. Parents should not pull back the foreskin for any reason, as this can trigger a vicious cycle of bleeding and infection. Once the foreskin is movable, pulling it back in the tub or shower is sufficient to clean beneath it—it's as simple as cleaning under the fingernails, or cleaning secretions from the folds of the female labia.

There is continuing debate regarding the effect of circumcision on male sexuality. During sexual arousal, the foreskin captures the first drops of moisture secreted from the penis; as erection increases, the foreskin pulls back and the glans is automatically lubricated. Studies show that circumcised men require more stimulation to become and remain sexually aroused. This makes sense, as the foreskin preserves the sensitivity of the glans, which may be lost on the circumcised penis due to constant friction with clothing.

Returning to some fathers' concerns about their sons being different from themselves or other boys, it comes down to this—if we agree that circumcision is a violent and potentially harmful procedure, we must simply break the cycle! In all fairness, we should leave the choice to the boy himself—it's his body, and he can decide at any point in the future to have the procedure done. My personal feeling is this: if nature had intended man to be without foreskin, baby boys would be born that way.

Nervous Irritability/Colic

Dealing with a nervous or colicky baby demands the same patience, concentration, and endurance as that required for giving birth. Unfortunately, if labor has been exceptionally difficult or postpartum assistance is lacking, a fussy baby may be the last straw. Advise parents to draw again on their labor coping tools—deep relaxation, deep breathing, and touch/massage. Above all else, help them to stay objective, and avoid projecting feelings of guilt or resentment onto every anxious cry the baby utters. Reassure them that it takes a while to get to know the baby's signals—they will soon be able to differentiate fatigue-based cries of overstimulation from those demanding food, diaper changing, or simple contact.

Suggest that parents begin by noting precisely when crying spells tend to occur. Then have them identify their own tense times throughout the day, to see if there is any correlation. Crying and fretting most commonly occur around 6 P.M., when the mother typically makes dinner and tries to share the day's events with her partner, who has just finished work. The baby feels the excitement, the stress, the confusion of it all, and reacts by crying excitedly. If such is the case, perhaps evening transitions can be made more gradually, with conversation between parents saved for later in the evening. Dinner hassles can also be alleviated by relying on casseroles, soups, or stews, made while the baby naps and reheated later.

Sometimes parents try everything, but nothing seems to work. The odds are good that the baby will soon outgrow its initial crankiness. But babies' temperaments definitely differ—some are high strung and intense, others are quiet and content. Based on experience, I've come to believe a person's essential nature is evident at birth. Many times, I've met up with a family for whom I was midwife after not seeing them for many years, and sure enough, the personality and energy I remember in the baby is clearly evident in the child. Every baby has its own style of coping, its own strengths and vulnerabilities. Encourage parents to accept things as they

---

What to Do If the Baby Cries

1. Try nursing in peace and quiet, without jiggling the baby around.

2. Have the baby's bed in a quiet space that's still close to the center of activity.

3. If the baby wakes when set down, try nursing lying down, and quietly getting up once the baby is asleep.

4. Let the baby spend lots of time in a baby carrier positioned near your heartbeat.

5. Establish a ritual break period for yourself, when your partner completely takes over for an hour or so (immediately following a nursing).

6. Use that time to rest, take a shower, call a friend, or otherwise rejuvenate yourself.

7. If the baby seems to have gas (pulls its legs up sharply, stomach rumbling), try giving warm catnip tea by bottle or eyedropper.

8. If all else fails and the baby is crying hysterically, try running the shower or turning on the vacuum cleaner. High frequency sounds may be calming if the baby is very upset.

are for now, relax, and take it easy. This is especially crucial for the mother, as chronic anxiety or frustration can hinder her recuperation and sap her emotional reserves.

MINOR PROBLEMS

1. *Diaper Rash:* A good natural oil should be applied with each diaper change, following a careful cleansing of the baby's bottom. Aloe vera gel (for wet, open sores) or calendula cream (for chafing or inflammation) are also effective. Rural mothers report that "Bag Balm" (intended for use on livestock to reduce teat inflammation) is a miracle diaper salve. Sometimes diaper rash is the result of improper laundering of the diapers; ammonia residue can build up and cause repeated episodes of rash unless the ammonia is removed by bleaching. To prevent this, soak diapers in a bleach bucket immediately after rinsing, wash with plain soap flakes, and double rinse (this final step removes any bleach residue, which also can be irritating).

2. *Cradle Cap:* Apply a natural oil to the scalp before bed and leave it on all night. Scaly skin can then be removed with a soft toothbrush and natural shampoo.

3. *Heat Rash:* The obvious solution is to cool off living areas, and have the baby cozily but loosely dressed. Teach the mother to check the baby's temperature by feeling its hands and feet, which should be slightly cool to the touch.

4. *Thrush:* This mild infection can be identified by a white coating on the baby's tongue. Since thrush is caused by the same organism that causes vaginal yeast, screen the mother and treat her if necessary. The baby can be treated with topical applications of acidophilus solution, three times a day by cotton swab. Thrush may take several weeks to go away; be patient. If it is severe enough to interfere with nursing, the baby should see a physician.

In general, try to avoid synthetic, artificial substances for bathing and toileting. Baby powder is blended with talc, a substance known to be dangerous to the lungs, and most baby oils are made with a base of mineral oil which leaches vitamins from the skin. Baby shampoos claim to be mild and gentle, but are in fact complex chemical preparations rather than simple soaps. Many synthetic products also contain carcinogenic dyes which are absorbed through the skin. Suggest simple natural substances like cornstarch, olive or vitamin E oils, and liquid castile soap (which can also be used as shampoo).

THE MOTHER: COMPLICATIONS AND CONCERNS

MINOR PROBLEMS

1. *Constipation:* This complaint commonly arises immediately after delivery, particularly if labor has been prolonged. A daily serving of high-fiber bran cereal is probably the most effective and pleasant remedy. Prune juice, taken in moderation, can also be used for its softening effect. Adequate fluid intake is critical: most nursing mothers need about three quarts daily in order to meet their own needs and also produce sufficient breast milk.

2. *Hemorrhoids:* Most common immediately after delivery, these respond well to ice packs and the application of witch hazel. If rupture and bleeding occur, aloe vera gel speeds healing. Both as treatment and as a preventative measure, follow the above recommendations for constipation.

3. *Afterpains:* These commonly occur with a second or subsequent baby, and are generally experienced during nursing or immediately afterwards. Some women say they actually hurt more than labor! This may be an exaggeration, but afterpains can certainly be very uncomfortable. They are caused by loss of uterine tone with successive childbearing; if the uterus is overstretched, contractions prompting involution will hurt. Herbs such as cottonwood bark or cramp bark help tone the uterus, and black haw tincture is particularly effective.

It is crucial that the woman keep her bladder empty, as otherwise the uterus cannot fully contract. Suggest she lie face down with a pillow beneath her lower abdomen to force the uterus firmly into place—this should provide some relief. Women occasionally require pain medication for afterpains; consult a physician if the pain is debilitating or is affecting her desire to breastfeed.

HEMATOMA

Hematoma is an asymmetrical and painful swelling of the perineal area. It is usually caused by soft tissue trauma in second stage, or by a faulty repair job whereby hemostasis has not been achieved, i.e., bleeding vessels continue to seep below skin or mucosal surfaces. Although these hemorrhages almost always cease spontaneously, the blood takes time to reabsorb. Pooled blood readily permits the growth of bacteria, thus the primary danger of hematoma is infection. This can lead to breakdown of the repair, because once sepsis develops, surfaces will not adhere and close properly. Traction on the sutures from swelling is another factor in repair dehiscence.

Immediately refer any woman with signs of hematoma to a physician; she should begin antibiotics as soon as possible. To reduce swelling, have her alternate hot and cold soaks, which stimulate circulation and encourage reabsorption of the hemorrhage. Also make sure the mother pours warm water with a bit of Betadine over her vaginal area each time she uses the toilet, and remind her to dry and air her perineum thoroughly afterwards. If the repair does break down, plastic surgery may be necessary. Do your best to prevent this!

UTERINE AND PELVIC INFECTIONS

Symptoms of uterine infection include fever over 101°, pelvic pain, elevated pulse, and subinvolution of the uterus. Risk factors include PROM, prolonged labor with numerous vaginal exams, manual rotation or other manipulations of the fetus during labor, maternal exhaustion, delayed delivery of the placenta, hemorrhage, uterine exploration (as for manual removal of the placenta or sequestered clots), postpartum dehydration, or improper perineal hygiene.

In my experience, a prime cause of uterine infection is overactivity and exhaustion in the first few days postpartum. I've had only two cases in my practice; both women had other children to care for and immediately resumed normal activity after the birth. And both had notably uncomplicated deliveries, with none of the precipitating factors cited above. One woman actually went to a swap meet the day after delivery, walking around in the heat and dust with nothing to drink for many hours! Take care to warn mothers blessed with easy deliveries that bed rest is necessary postpartum not just to recover from birth, *but from the entire pregnancy.* Also reiterate that adequate rest permits oxytocin to involute the uterus, tone the vagina, and facilitate breastfeeding, whereas stress and overactivity cause counter-effects of adrenaline to slow recuperation.

Sepsis may not only affect the uterus, but pelvic ligaments, connective tissue, and/or the peritoneal cavity. These become infected only if uterine sepsis is untreated, and cause much more severe symptoms of vomiting, chills, and extreme pain. Rarely, the tubes and ovaries may also be affected, usually by a preexisting gonorrhea infection which has flared up again.

THROMBOPHLEBITIS AND PULMONARY EMBOLISM

Thrombophlebitis is the inflammation of either a superficial or deep leg vein. Women with varicosities are at greater risk. **Superficial thrombophlebitis** causes leg pain, with heat, tenderness, and redness at the site of the inflammation. Symptoms of high fever plus severe pain, edema, and tenderness along the entire length of the leg indicate **deep thrombophlebitis**. If either of these conditions develop, contact a physician immediately. Meanwhile, have the woman stay in bed and keep the affected leg elevated. And hands off the leg—if you massage it, you may loosen blood clots and cause them to enter her circulation. Should a clot lodge in her lungs, the life-threatening condition of **pulmonary embolism** will result. This is characterized by chest pain, shortness of breath, rapid respirations, and elevated pulse. If these symptoms develop, immediately call the paramedics and administer oxygen to the mother.

DIFFICULTIES WITH BREASTFEEDING

Problems with breastfeeding often spring from distraction. If a mother feels anxious about her primary relationship, worried about money matters, stressed over changes in her lifestyle, frustrated by lack of support, or impatient with her rate of recovery, she may find breastfeeding less than fulfilling.

In order to evaluate breastfeeding difficulties, we must first understand the normal physiology of the process. Each breast has approximately twenty lobes, which consist of **lobules** divided into **alveoli** and **ducts**. The alveoli contain **acini cells**, which produce the milk, and **myoepithelial cells**, which contract and propel milk from the breast. **Lactiferous ducts** carry milk from the alveoli and empty into larger ducts near the nipple, called **lactiferous sinuses** or **ampullae. Lactiferous tubules** lead to the surface of the nipple, and release the milk from the breast. The nipple itself is comprised of erectile tissue, which contracts during nursing to control the flow of milk.

The hormone oxytocin plays a role in stimulating let-down of milk, but the hormone **prolactin** is primarily responsible for milk production. Prolactin is inhibited during pregnancy by high levels of estrogen, which fall immediately after delivery to permit lactation. Continued production of prolactin and oxytocin depends on frequent, relaxed nursing sessions. The more relaxed the mother is when she nurses, the greater the release of these crucial hormones.

It is nature's design that by giving birth, a woman learns to release her inhibitions and trust her body. This is key to a successful breastfeeding experience. Disapproving relatives or unsolicited advice may, however, interfere with maternal instincts. Breastfeeding is an intimate act between mother and baby, and so requires privacy, especially in the beginning. It is also a physiologically demanding activity that can be quite exhausting unless there is good support for the woman's physical and emotional well-being. If a mother is having problems with breastfeeding unrelated to the mechanics of proper positioning, see to her needs for privacy, nourishment, and support.

Orgasmic breastfeeding is more than just an intriguing concept, it's a reality for many women. The term 'orgasmic' connotes the ability to engage oneself fully in an endeavor, to respond and let go completely. Thus it is in nursing and caring for a baby. Daily patterns vary tremendously. The baby may be easily distracted if visitors come and spend time talking with the mother. But once they are alone again, it may nurse for almost an hour, then doze off to sleep in mother's arms. Later, there may be lots of eye contact, touching, and playing between the two. Because the let-down hormone oxytocin is a precursor to orgasm, it's no wonder women sometimes feel aroused or experience orgasm when breastfeeding.

Breastfeeding has the same therapeutic value as sexual intercourse in that it affords a way for mother and baby to reaffirm their connection, to stay close and be of comfort to one another in times of change or upset. It is a gift of tenderness

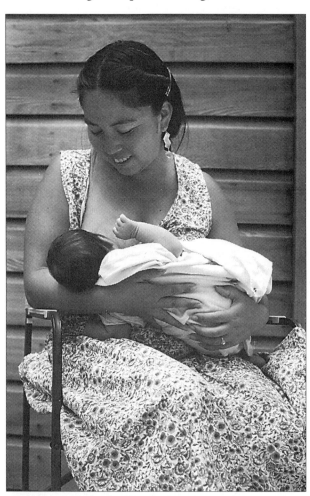

Alleviate sore nipples by lifting the baby to your breast, rather than letting him hang from your nipple.

and vitality, with the mother's urge to nurse the perfect complement to her baby's desire to suckle. Breastfeeding also provides a priceless opportunity for continued bonding and infant/child maturation. In his book, *Evolution's End*, author Joseph Chilton Pearce explains that frequent face-to-face contact with its mother is crucial for a baby's neurological development. He further suggests that the relatively low protein content of breastmilk prompts the baby to nurse almost continuously in the early weeks, precisely so it can receive this crucial growth stimulus. The more we learn about breastfeeding, the less inclined we should be to try to regulate this highly personal and richly variegated intimacy between mother and child.

Physical complications of breastfeeding include engorgement and mastitis. **Engorgement** results from an excess amount of milk relative to what the baby requires; it is normal for engorgement to occur when the milk first comes in or when the baby gives up a feeding. Engorgement may be uncomfortable, but will resolve spontaneously as the milk supply adjusts to the baby's demand. To facilitate this, apply heat, massage the breast towards the nipple, hand-express milk to start it flowing, and have the baby nurse.

If milk is left pooled in the sacs, particularly if a residual amount remains time after time, it becomes a breeding ground for any bacteria entering through the nipple. This is how **mastitis** occurs. Personal cleanliness is important in preventing mastitis, as is relaxed, unhurried, thorough nursing on demand. Of course, the mother needs adequate fluids, calories, and rest to maintain healthy resistance to infection. Mastitis can be diagnosed by fever, with sudden elevation to 103° or 104°. It is particularly likely to develop if engorgement is allowed to persist, if lumpy areas begin to redden with inflammation, or if red streaks develop. Borderline cases can occasionally be resolved with heat treatments and plenty of rest, but once fever has spiked as above, antibiotics are necessary. Dycloxicillin is generally recommended because it does not destroy intestinal flora and will not hurt the baby, although the mother may have some indigestion. However, timely treatment is critical to prevent a breast abscess from developing, which can cause even greater pain and trouble with breastfeeding.

Some mothers ask about weaning just days after starting to breastfeed. This may indicate some ambivalence about nursing, or may simply

---

10 STEPS TO SUCCESSFUL BREASTFEEDING

Excerpted from: **Protecting, Promoting and Supporting Breastfeeding:**
The Special Role of Maternity Services *(A Joint WHO/UNICEF Statement)*

1. Have a written breastfeeding policy that is routinely communicated to all health care staff.

2. Train all health care staff in skills necessary to implement this policy.

3. Inform all pregnant women about the benefits and management of breastfeeding.

4. Help mothers initiate breastfeeding within a half hour of birth.

5. Show mothers how to breastfeed, and how to maintain lactation even if they should be separated from their infants.

6. Give newborn infants no food or drink other than breastmilk, unless medically indicated.

7. Practice rooming-in—allow mothers and infants to remain together—24 hours a day.

8. Encourage breastfeeding on demand.

9. Give no artificial teats or pacifiers (also called dummies or soothers) to breastfeeding infants.

10. Foster the establishment of breastfeeding support groups and refer mothers to them on discharge from the hospital or clinic.

indicate curiosity regarding end points of the experience. Advise all mothers to let the baby be their guide; a need for solid food will be indicated by interest in what others at the table are eating (psychological readiness) and by teething (physiological readiness). Many pediatricians now believe that solid foods are unnecessary for up to nine months for a fully breastfed baby, as it takes about that long for its digestive system to mature. A relaxed approach saves parents a lot of trouble, and allows the baby to follow its natural pace of development.

POSTPARTUM BLUES AND DEPRESSION

Postpartum depression is most likely to occur in women who are not up to par physically, particularly those who have had difficult or debilitating birth experiences. For example, a mother who hemorrhaged at delivery might experience depression several weeks later, due to anemia and resulting exhaustion. Particularly if the mother has no history of emotional problems in pregnancy, look

to her current health status. Check for anemia, review her diet, and recommend supplements as indicated.

Occasionally, what appears to be postpartum anxiety may be caused by thyroid imbalance. This is surprisingly common postpartum. Hyperthyroidism, for example, has symptoms of agitation, worry, night sweats, insomnia, diarrhea, and tachycardia.

If you find no physical explanation, rest assured that minor depression is very common, and likely to affect the psyche of any sensitive, intelligent woman faced with the usual multiplicity of postpartum adjustments. As mentioned earlier, losses experienced at the onset of this new phase of life are very real. Help the mother identify and address these directly. The all-encompassing category of loss is undoubtedly loss of control. Anxiety may also spring from unprecedented emotional dependence on one's partner, family, or friends. Here's one mother's description of her postpartum struggle:

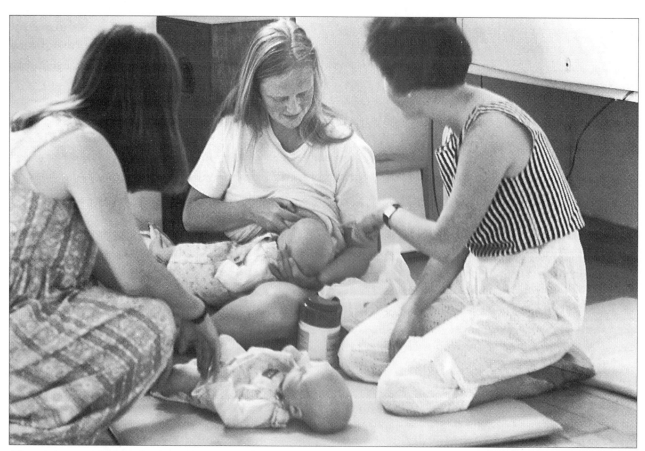

There is just no substitute for sharing concerns and insights with other new mothers.

Postpartum blues? No, not me! The joy of long awaited motherhood and the emotional stability I had achieved over the years disqualified me, I thought, as a candidate for the postpartum syndrome. But I was not immune! My "blues," however, did not fit the picture of what I had expected. In fact, I came to feel that nothing I'd read or heard had adequately prepared me, since I was not depressed according to my usual definition.

For me, the experience was one of drowning in a vacuum of mind—consumed with worry, anxiety, and uncertainty. The responsibility seemed overwhelming. In spite of reassurance from my midwives, doubts and questions plagued me . . . was my son becoming jaundiced?. . .was his cord healing properly?. . . why was his skin peeling? . . . how would I bathe and groom him? I longed for the recommended rest and would be famished, yet could not seem to coordinate time for my own needs with that of caring for him and feeding him every few hours. Trian was a good, quiet baby, but I didn't have a handle on my end at all. I felt like I was failing miserably at my goal of being a perfect mother.

Trian was several days old when I suddenly realized while nursing him that I had not leisurely touched and explored his whole body. At this moment, I knew I had been in a vacuum for days, functioning but not fully aware.

To my amazement, I just couldn't "organize" my newborn. Fifteen years of pride at being a successful organizer in my career now proved totally useless. I had to learn to simply flow with Trian, emotionally and psychically, and let go of intellectual anticipation, expectations, and planning.

My love for Trian was the grounding cord that held me together as I floundered with anxiety at the enormous task before me. When I learned to recognize my signs of postpartum syndrome—irrational fears overtaking me, heart racing, nausea, excessive perspiration and shallow breathing—I would relax, do the deep breathing I had been taught for the birthing, and concentrate on how much I loved my baby. This allowed me to center myself and deal rationally with my fears, so that I could carry on.

Remedies for postpartum blues include regular outings and dates with friends, or whatever it takes to get time away from home and the usual routine. Most babies will sleep contentedly during long car rides, out of mother's arms and in the car seat.

Frequently, what the exhausted mother needs most is physical space, a chance to get the baby off her body for a while. She should use her time alone to recuperate, letting her body rest while enjoying a favorite leisure activity.

A more serious form of postpartum blues springs from preexisting problems or conflicts that were temporarily forgotten at the time of birth, only to reemerge and intensify with the stress of parenting. Unhappiness in the primary relationship, problems with self esteem, or sexual issues may be involved. *Refer the mother to a counselor for continued support.* You may wish to help her explore her options and find emotional catharsis in the initial postpartum period, but if problems persist, send her to a specialist.

One particular type of relationship definitely predisposes to postpartum woe. The father, apathetic during pregnancy, becomes compulsively bent on proving himself in the birth or immediate postpartum, and the mother has difficulty bonding with her baby and/or trusting her instincts. She is passive-dependent; he is authoritarian, responding to the demands of fatherhood with a new set of rules regarding housework, expenditures, baby care, discipline, breastfeeding, sexuality, etc. He may also use spiritual or political beliefs to continually evaluate and judge the mother's performance. No wonder she gets depressed! I've had a few heated discussions with fathers of this temperament and find it does little good. As a typical passive-dependent, the mother will implore you for help and advice, but will seldom use it. You must extract yourself from this situation as soon as possible, and vow to be more selective henceforth in screening your clientele!

Single mothers are prone to a special brand of postpartum blues based on physical and emotional isolation. See to it that she has plenty of physical support and human contact. Try to coordinate this through her closest friend, or whoever is willing.

Sometimes suspended sexuality is a source of anxiety, especially if the new mother is made to feel that it's her job to get sex together again as her partner waits and watches impatiently (see next section for suggestions).

Another type of postpartum unhappiness difficult to clear is that resulting from a disappointing birth experience, particularly if pain medication was used or bonding disrupted. Scars from these experiences run deep, and painful memories may be especially overwhelming in the early weeks postpartum when hormones and fatigue intensify the emotions. Any mother who has transported unexpectedly should be given opportunity to go over the birth in detail, and air any misgivings or regrets. Support a woman dealing with loss of her birth dream by bearing witness to her grief. Let *her* define the issues, and ask the questions she considers important whenever she is ready. If time goes by and she becomes increasingly depressed, refer her to counseling or hypnotherapy.

On the other hand, the woman convinced perfect birth is her destiny may be quite embittered by transport, and may have trouble caring for herself and the baby once out of the hospital. Keep a close eye on her. She desperately needs contact with more even-tempered and mature mothers, whose flexibility and receptivity she can emulate. Do what you can to facilitate this.

More extreme forms of postpartum depression may border on psychosis, with overtones of violence. If you are in any way concerned that a mother is thus at risk, secure the advice and support of a family health agency before referring her to counseling.

Depression following a cesarean is in a class by itself. Women who give birth by cesarean often feel they have failed their partners, their babies, and themselves, particularly if they've had general anesthesia and missed the actual moments of birth. This is especially true of the well-prepared mother who, schooled in the importance of immediate bonding, may feel that her relationship with the baby is hopelessly and irretrievably ruined. She may also experience disturbing psychosomatic effects, as the final stages of birth have been missed. Even if she has made peace with her cesarean experience, she may still have subconscious yearnings for the climax of birth and may dream vividly of vaginal delivery, especially in the first few weeks postpartum.

What can you say to a woman struggling to reconcile a cesarean birth? The worst thing is to suggest she set it aside and be glad for what she's got. Birth is not just the act of bringing forth a baby, it's a major event in a woman's life, one which she will review and try to comprehend as long as she lives. Acknowledge her grief, and share in her feelings. There are also cesarean support groups available in most areas (see Appendix B). Refer her to counseling if her feelings threaten to overwhelm her.

SEXUAL CHANGES

Not enough has been written about postpartum sexuality, aside from the physiological aspects. Maintaining sexual communication after the birth is key to surmounting the stresses of this period. But a couple used to taking their time with foreplay or making love on the spur of the moment will find that a newborn upsets everything. Like it or not, their intimate relationship must somehow incorporate the baby.

Not to be trite, but love is the key to making this adjustment. If partners can recognize the baby as an extension of their love, and continue to uphold the primacy of their relationship, they will find their way through the disruption and frustration that characterize sex postpartum. Eventually, their intimacy will deepen. But meanwhile, fatigue, tension, loss of privacy, and feelings of isolation can make getting together difficult.

Psychological experts propose that loss of intimacy postpartum is rooted in loss of privacy as a couple. This actually begins during pregnancy, when the woman discovers that society considers her pregnant body to be public property. Perfect strangers feel free to touch, advise, and speculate. The father is likewise exhorted to support his partner appropriately, and otherwise behave himself. And once the baby is born, strangers advise and admonish with even greater zeal. These culturally inculcated behaviors are intended to uphold the most basic building block of society—the family. But it is easy to see how a couple might feel personally invaded by all this, and how their sexuality might be affected.

In reality, new fathers are often surprised to find themselves more desirous of time with the baby than they expected, and may resent the distraction of having to deal with increased financial responsibilities. For her part, the mother may feel completely overrun by turbulent emotions, contrary to the ideal of the even-tempered madonna. If the father is pushing hard at work to make ends meet, and the mother begins pulling at him for companionship and reassurance, he's going to feel torn in two, and she will feel guilty and insecure. Lesbian couples are less likely to be polarized this way, but are still susceptible to financial pressures and other interference. As if caring for a newborn wasn't enough, these additional stresses may push both parents to the breaking point. Although sex is a logical way to reunite diverging energies in a relationship, chronic fatigue and mounting resentment can definitely interfere.

There seems to be a critical point at about six weeks postpartum when expectations and disappointments run high; this is the time when the mother is supposed to be physically recovered and ready for sex again. But readiness may be tempered by the hormones of breastfeeding, which tend to repress sexual desire in many women. At six weeks, the mother is still totally absorbed with her baby; the two are almost inseparable. They are also psychically attuned, to the effect that the mother will wake seconds before her baby begins fussing, or the baby will wake crying when its mother has had a bad dream. These powerful bonds are important to the health of the family, but may also cause sex to be pushed aside indefinitely.

The best solution is to have a grandmother, other relative, or sitter take the baby for an afternoon or evening so the couple can get away together and have some time alone. Expressed breast milk can be frozen in a glass bottle, and given to the baby after reheating in a pan of water. Once in privacy, the parents should take time to relax and talk for a while before diving into sex with overloaded expectations. If getting away is impossible, second best is to make a weekly date for dinner, a video, and lovemaking in some private part of the house. Older children can spend the night with friends or relatives. And even if the baby interrupts, at least parents know their next date is only a week away!

It's important for the woman's partner to appreciate how her desire may be dampened by unsettling feelings of dependency. As one mother bluntly stated, "I realized when I was pregnant that I really needed to depend on this guy, now here I am with a little baby, and I feel so helpless. . . what if he (her partner) turns out to be a creep?" On the one hand, our culture endorses motherhood; on the other, we covet youth, freedom, sexual autonomy. No wonder the new mother feels somewhat out of place, dowdy, or invisible as a sexual being, all of which affect her desire for closeness. If her partner does little to reassure her, or teases her in any way about her body, the situation goes from bad to worse.

Again, couples must place a premium on keeping their rites of intimacy. Communication with other mothers is crucial for the woman whose self confidence is floundering. As for her partner, there are excellent books on parenting which address the sexual challenges of the postpartum period. If parents make a point of connecting daily, even if only to cuddle or kiss, they can certainly hold their ground. With time, and with intention, sex can become more meaningful, wild, and wonderful than ever before—*but it does take time.*

CONTRACEPTION

When sexual activity resumes after birth, heterosexual women must once again address contraceptive issues. It is odd to resort to birth control after not having to bother for so long, and depending on the method used, may seem just one more barrier to intimacy.

Birth control pills are not particularly suitable for breastfeeding mothers—estrogen suppresses milk production, and progesterone-only minipills are not as effective as combination formulas. The Copper 7 intrauterine device is still available, but many women find this option less than desirable for a variety of reasons, not the least of which are side effects of chronic bleeding and/or low-grade infection. The fertility awareness method is difficult to implement postpartum, as the course of lactation can cause erratic fluctuations in basal body temperature and cervical mucus. Norplant and Depo-provera both cause heavy bleeding, and can

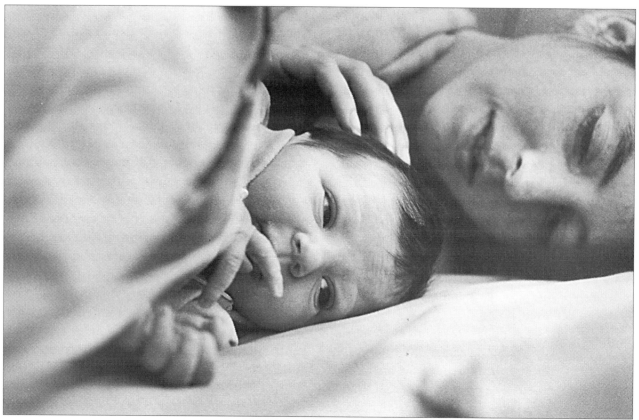

Don't forget to share the tenderness you feel for the baby with your partner.

delay the resumption of normal menses when use is discontinued. This leaves the barrier methods: condom, diaphragm, or cervical cap.

Apart from the difficulty of finding an appropriate birth control method is the difficulty of being diligent in its use. One of the more subtle conflicts affecting couples who have known the thrill of conscious conception and ecstatic childbearing is the desire for the no-barriers sexual intensity that accompanies these events, versus the desire to delay or forego having any more children. This conflict is usually unspoken, and may be set aside for some time. But after a year or so has passed and the family has stabilized, this psycho-erotic desire for conception can rise up and wreak havoc with a couple's plans for their future, as well as their compliance with birth control.

Reckoning with these feelings depends on mutual acknowledgement and communication. This is essential if contraception is to be effective, as no method will work without the mental and emotional agreement of both partners. Conception may be physically prevented, but unless conflicts regarding use of birth control are expressly cleared, a couple's intimacy will be at risk. Encourage the postpartum couple to consider contraception an open issue, one apt to arise repeatedly for review, and worthy of sensitive and candid discussion.

CHAPTER 7

Becoming a Midwife

If you are considering practicing midwifery someday, this chapter is for you. It is one thing to decide to become a midwife, but quite another to face the realities of acquiring the necessary training. As mentioned in Chapter One, current educational routes are often circuitous, and may require much determination and endurance. But what more appropriate introduction to the diligence and dedication required of the midwife? Although many women are attracted to midwifery for glory and glamour, it is undoubtedly one of the most challenging and personally demanding occupations. Even as a student, the aspiring midwife must endure long hours, intense personal interactions, and repeated sacrifice of personal and/or family time. Thus it is best if midwifery is less a career choice, and more a calling.

Should you choose to go through training to become a nurse-midwife, your course of study will be fairly well mapped out for you. See Appendix M for a list of nurse-midwifery programs, or contact the American College of Nurse-Midwives for an update. Also consult the list of direct-entry programs in Appendix M for other options.

The respective advantages and disadvantages of nurse-midwifery and direct-entry training have been partially articulated in Chapter One. To reiterate, a central advantage of becoming a nurse-midwife is legal practice anywhere in the country, and reciprocity state to state. Having utilized the political infrastructure of nursing to advance as a profession, nurse-midwifery is fairly well-positioned in our current healthcare system. But changes in this system may render certain perks of being a nurse-midwife obsolete. As HMOs seek cost containment by using midwives in high-volume clinics or labor and delivery units with little or no continuity of care, the midwifery model is subsumed by profit margins and institutional efficiency, and midwives are reduced to obstetrical technicians. In addition, CNMs are losing their collective bargaining power as HMOs systematically fire them, only to rehire them for longer hours at less pay, and without benefits. After so many years of struggling within the system and resisting the urge to relax and become complacent, will nurse-midwives have the strength to fight for autonomy of practice as their apprenticeship-trained, direct-entry sisters are now doing? Who is really ahead in this game, and who is behind? And who's running the game in the first place?

It may take some years before we have the answers to these questions. Meanwhile, we must recognize that at the root of how and what we practice, how we define ourselves both professionally and politically, is the manner in which we are educated. Most nurse-midwifery programs are housed within complex medical care delivery systems; instructor and student alike are subject to highly restrictive practice protocols. These programs are heavily weighted with theoretical instruction, but have minimal hands-on training, little or no continuity of care, and limited scope of practice. Students consequently suffer an overdevelopment of their analytical faculties at the expense of intuitive, compassionate qualities so necessary to humane caregiving. In my experience, the most common complaint of nurse-midwifery graduates is fear—fear of the responsibility of private practice, fear of being inadequately prepared

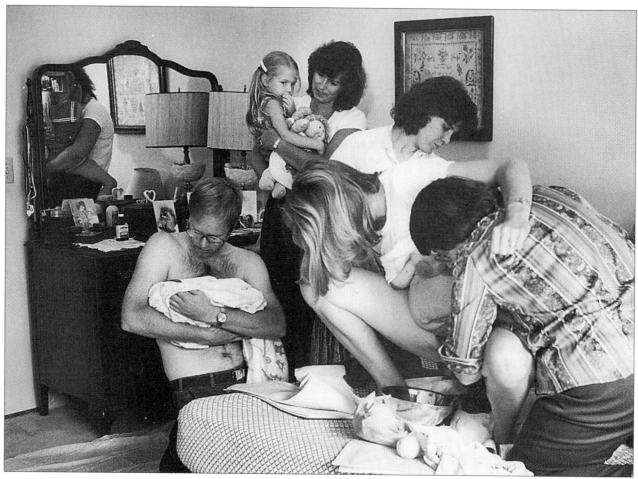

Assisting at home births affords the chance to share in a team effort and to experience birth as normal.

to work out of hospital. These fears are quite reasonable, considering what nurse-midwifery training does, and does not, accomplish.

The challenge to midwifery education today is to create curricula that develop the student as a human being, while providing supportively supervised clinical experience. All too often, the nurse-midwifery graduate has done countless rotations in clinical settings, but has never known primary responsibility for a single client from start to finish. When life-threatening complications of shoulder dystocia or hemorrhage arose in her training, she was obligated by protocol to call for help and step aside. Predictably, she feels ill equipped to practice "on her own responsibility."

In contrast, the midwife trained by apprenticeship is one-on-one with her senior midwife's clients throughout the entire perinatal cycle. She is also one-on-one with her preceptor, requiring her to develop and refine not only technical skills, but equally important abilities to communicate assertively and listen effectively. Learning takes place in context, as the senior midwife debriefs the day's events and suggests sources for further study. Student evaluation is done as much for appropriate clinical application of knowledge as for the ability to commit facts to paper. Continuity of both care and instruction force the student to put herself into her learning process, as is the case in any long term relationship. She is more likely to confronted with her technical and personal shortcomings when she has been involved in a case from start to finish, and when her interactions with her preceptor are ongoing.

Nurse-midwifery programs may come and go as funding dictates, but training by apprenticeship will endure because it is community-based, cost-effective, and perfect for women with small children who require a program with elastic time, i.e., one which allows students as much time as necessary to complete program requirements. If you are considering the apprenticeship route, check first to see if your state has any provisions for qualifying midwives. Some states require that students attend formal, on-site academic programs in conjunction with apprenticeship; others have coursework requirements that can be met at-a-distance (similar to external degree programs or independent study provisions offered by many universities). Still other states have licensing or certifying mechanisms that are entirely competency-based, with the usual requisites of documented experience, skills verification, and comprehensive exam. Several states have incorporated NARM certification requirements. Consult MANA for a list of representatives that can familiarize you with their respective states' educational and practice requirements; consult NARM for an updated listing of all states that recognize CPMs. Consult MEAC for a list of accredited direct-entry programs (see Appendix B).

If your state has no mechanism for regulating midwifery, you may wish to investigate the guidelines established by NARM for becoming a CPM, and on that basis, create your own framework for learning. Once you know the experience you must acquire, and the clinical skills and general knowledge you must be able to demonstrate, you will have some idea of how to structure your learning. Your initial efforts will probably involve: 1) studying midwifery texts; 2) participating in a group learning situation or midwifery study group; and 3) attending births as a birth assistant or labor coach.

TEXTBOOKS AND OTHER REFERENCES

Aspiring midwives with small children or those otherwise unable to be on-call for births should probably begin with book study. If you have already read extensively in general areas of prepared childbirth, breastfeeding, and parenting, concentrate on beginning midwifery texts. But if you have read very little, start with books that feature first person accounts of childbearing, in order to glean the emotional and spiritual aspects. Aspiring midwives who have not had children will invariably be confronted by skepticism regarding their suitability for this work. I too once thought

it nearly impossible for anyone who had not given birth to be truly effective as a midwife. But then, through exposure to my exceptional students, I came to appreciate the single most crucial qualification to be knowledge of one's inner resources, based on some experience of living on the edge, facing or meeting one's demons, enduring grief through personal loss, etc. Still, any aspiring midwife who has not given birth should try to attend births as early in her training as possible, so her text-acquired knowledge will not overwhelm her instinctive, intuitive abilities.

Although there are many fine books available on birth and related subjects, certain titles are classic; others are groundbreaking. Starting with the classics, Ina May Gaskin's *Spiritual Midwifery* gives a number of in-depth birth accounts from parents, with basic information for beginning midwives. Another wonderfully illuminating book is Suzanne Arms' *Immaculate Deception II* (the new, expanded edition). Any book by Sheila Kitzinger is an absolute pleasure to read—try *The Complete Book of Childbirth*, known for its lovely illustrations, or her classic, *The Experience of Childbirth*, which focuses on emotional aspects and physical sensations of giving birth. Also excellent is *The Birth Partner* (Penny Simpkin), which explains how best to assist women in labor. These books give the aspiring midwife a base of understanding from which to pursue other studies in childbirth education, breastfeeding, parenting, etc.

When you are ready to move on to midwifery or obstetrical texts, Oxorn and Foote's *Human Labor & Birth* gives basic pregnancy and birth information in a concise outline format perfect for beginners. Diagrams are abundant, clear, and easy to understand. Obstetrical emergencies and recommended treatments are also outlined step by step. The main drawback of this reference lies in its focus on obstetrical care, e.g., there are lengthy sections on the use of forceps and vacuum extraction, with virtually nothing on routine prenatal assessments. However, suggested management of complications is quite moderate, and the tone of the text is fairly respectful of mother and baby.

Probably the best text for beginners is *Myles Textbook for Midwives*, edited by Bennet and Brown.

This is the primary text for student midwives in Britain. Information throughout is detailed and complete, with a strong emphasis on caregiving. This book bears careful and repeated study, section by section. The drawings are realistic and profuse. A brief but thorough section on care of the newborn, including problems and pathology, is yet another positive feature of this text. *Like Human Labor & Birth*, this classic has been repeatedly revised; it is now in its twelfth edition.

Varney's Midwifery (Helen Varney) is a much newer text, utilized primary by nurse-midwifery programs in the United States. The strong point of this book is its clear, step-by-step instructions for performing clinical procedures like venipuncture, Pap smear, and IV infiltration. However, the scope of information is not as exhaustive as in *Myles Textbook for Midwives*, and the illustrations far less numerous than in *Human Labor & Birth*.

Although these texts were adequate for my apprenticeship period, I found I needed a more comprehensive obstetrical guide when I began giving prenatal care. Questions began to arise concerning the etiology of complications, or potential effects of certain preexisting conditions. For in-depth understanding of any pathological development, a sophisticated and exhaustive reference is essential.

Williams Obstetrics is notoriously difficult for beginners to understand, due largely to its dry, scientific style. Invest in a good medical dictionary, like *Tabers*, to help you wade through the terminology. Despite the challenges of using this text, *Williams Obstetrics* is undoubtedly the most complete reference available.

Obstetrics and The Newborn (Beischer and MacKay) is a popular, mid-level reference. It is designed specifically for medical students, complete with full color photos and study questions. Although this text is not as exhaustive as *Williams Obstetrics*, it is certainly easier to understand, and effectively fills the gap between beginning and advanced textbooks.

Another wonderful reference is *Maternity and Gynecological Care*, by Irene Bobak. This book is noted for its pro-woman voice, its broad base of information, its attention to detail, and its extensive section on women's health. This one is a gem!

When it comes to groundbreaking works, the current leader in the field is undoubtedly *Effective Care in Pregnancy & Childbirth*, by Erkin, Kerse, and Chalmers. Published by Oxford University Press, this multi-volume reference is expensive, but accomplishes what no other obstetrical text purports to do—it presents the evidence regarding the efficacy of current obstetrical practices and procedures. Evidence-based care is a foreign concept in our healthcare system, as our practice protocol is based more on liability fears than on what the research shows. But if you or your clients have questions on whether ultrasound scanning is really safe, whether screening for gestational diabetes is truly necessary, whether routine fetal monitoring improves maternal-fetal outcomes, this is your answer book. (The summary volume, *A Guide to Effective Care in Pregnancy & Childbirth*, is available at a fraction of the text's cost.)

A similar, groundbreaking work is Henci Goer's *Obstetric Myths Versus Research Realities*, which tackles such topics as routine episiotomy, screening for gestational diabetes, routine cesarean delivery of the breech, surveillance techniques for postdatism, and induction of labor for PROM. Marsden Wagner's *Pursuing the Birth Machine* covers similar material, but focuses primarily on the political underpinnings of the overuse of technology in the perinatal period.

Added to the list of groundbreaking works must be Anne Frye's latest, *Holistic Midwifery*. This is the first U.S. midwifery text written by a direct-entry midwife, and it is remarkable for its detail and thoroughness. Sections on teratogens in pregnancy, anatomy and physiology of childbearing women, and cultural sensitivity in caregiving, are just a few that stand out. Anne Frye's classic, *Understanding Diagnostic Tests in the Childbearing Year*, is yet another invaluable reference.

Of course, the list goes on. Other favorites include *Bestfeeding*, by Suzanne Arms, *The Amazing Newborn*, by Marshall and Phyllis Klaus, *Birth Reborn*, by Michel Odent, *The Wise Woman Herbal for the Childbearing Year*, by Susun Weed. Prime sources for childbirth-related books are Birth and Life Bookstore (Cascade Birthing Supplies) and ICEA Books, both listed in the Appendix.

Another important, up-to-the-minute source of information is the midwifery newsletter. The *MANA News* focuses on the political and practice issues of midwives in the U.S., Mexico and Canada. The *Journal of Nurse-Midwifery* (published by the ACNM) presents research articles and open forum. *Birth* also publishes scientific research, with a focus on humanizing obstetrics. *The Birth Gazette*, edited by Ina May Gaskin, is intended for midwives and their supporters and features human interest articles, practical advice and political updates. And *Midwifery Today* is possibly the most comprehensive and inspiring newsletter for aspiring and experienced midwives alike. *Midwifery Today* has a very active website, and organizes regular conferences in both Oregon and New York, as well as annual international conventions.

Check to see if your state midwifery association publishes a newsletter. You might also want to subscribe to newsletters from other states. Write to MANA for a list.

BIRTH ASSISTING, OR LABOR COACHING

Attending births as an assistant is an important step in midwifery training. Absolute beginners benefit immensely from discovering the extent to which birth is non-intellectual and personally transformative. Women who have already had children have opportunity to refine their understanding of the adage, "It's not my birth," as they simultaneously help women who lack support have the best possible experience.

What can you learn about midwifery by assisting births as a labor coach? If the mother's partner or other helpers are present, you will learn to coordinate your efforts and work respectfully with her intimate circle. You can suggest comfort measures, massage techniques, or certain labor positions, and offer to relieve birth team participants periodically so they can take breaks. Or, if the mother is by herself, you will quickly begin to appreciate the dedication and endurance that will one day be required of you as a midwife. Being one-on-one with the mother gives you opportu-

nity to learn precisely how women in labor like to be touched, which phrases they most like to hear, and which positions are most likely to be effective. All beginning birth assistants worry about making mistakes, about saying or doing the wrong thing, about being rebuffed or rejected by the laboring woman. But rest assured—as long as you surrender your own barriers to birth's intensity and keep pace with the mother's rhythms and needs, *you will know what to do in the moment.* Learning to speak and act spontaneously may be somewhat unnerving at first, but every student midwife must take courage and find her voice, in order to effectively encourage laboring women to express themselves freely.

Regardless of your role, the first five or six births you attend are apt to be profoundly affecting. Reverence for the power of birth, and willingness to feel it on a visceral level, are the best possible start for any aspiring midwife. But as patterns of labor and the intensity of birth become familiar, you may begin to turn your attention to the unique skills and style of the midwife or physician in attendance. It is easy to be critical at this stage, to focus on the flaws of more experienced practitioners rather than on their strengths. This may help you establish your own philosophy of practice, but take care to temper criticism with careful research, especially if you intend to assert your views. There is no point in alienating medical personnel with whom you work—you never know what special favor you may require from a certain physician or nurse some time in the future. Keep the channels of communication open, and above all, *learn from your seniors, don't merely react to them!*

BIRTH ASSISTING AT HOME

Most birth assistants work in hospital, as that is where women are least likely to have support. So if you have opportunity to attend a home birth, count your blessings! Home births generally involve minimal intervention, and provide the student unique opportunities to learn the natural rhythms of labor through pure observation. *Observe, observe, observe*—notice how different types of women respond to labor, which positions work best in each stage, which breathing patterns seem most effective, and how best to involve and integrate the rest of the family.

The latter is one of the subtler aspects of effective coaching, i.e., wisely assessing how to focus the efforts of everyone on the birth team. A competent birth assistant will discreetly direct the mother's supporters to effective and satisfying participation, based on the limit of what each can handle. An absolute beginner may be tempted to gain glory by placing the focus on her own abilities, but her real task is to empower the mother and family. Primary relationships can be greatly strengthened in labor, old wounds can be healed. All birth assistants must strive to instill enough confidence in the mother so she can relax and enjoy intimacy with her partner and other birth participants as she desires. This contributes to bonding among all involved, which in turn can ease challenging postpartum transitions.

Sometimes a midwife will use the birth assistant's "extra pair of hands" for a routine task and, sensing enthusiasm, will do a bit of teaching. I remember one midwife calling me to attention while she was suturing, telling me to "watch and learn." I had been holding a flashlight at the perineum for what seemed like forever; my arm was aching and my interest was wavering. But because of what I witnessed, I acquired a new, hands-on understanding of the repair process. Never pass up an opportunity to do technical assist, especially at home births where there is more time to ask questions, and more opportunity to follow up later.

BIRTH ASSISTING IN HOSPITAL

Hospital labor coaching offers wonderful opportunities to serve women of diverse ethnicity and learn about current obstetrical practice at the same time. It also provides a potentially shocking introduction to the political aspects of medicalized childbirth. For this reason, many women shun birth attendance in hospital, believing their personal discomfort level to be ample indication that assisting home birth is their destiny. This may result in a very long wait to attend births—a very long wait indeed. And there is much to be learned from birth in hospital; it provides rare opportunities to witness complications that seldom occur at

home, and observe medical management of preexisting pathology.

In terms of becoming a midwife, a student seeking apprenticeship (or admission to a direct-entry program) can use her birth attendance in hospital to show potential preceptors that she can handle being on call, and is willing and able to support women in labor no matter what the circumstances. I began doing hospital coaching because my home birth attendance was very sporadic. I registered as a volunteer birth assistant by calling labor and delivery at the local general hospital, and was well received due to problems with understaffing. I agreed to be available on call several nights a week, and over a ten-month period, attended nearly 50 births. On-call coaching is certainly a boon to mothers unprepared for labor, but definitely tests the mettle of the aspiring midwife!

One very unappealing aspect of hospital coaching is the environment itself. Hospital rooms are typically overheated, lack adequate ventilation, and feature annoying overhead lighting. And then, there is the package of standard obstetrical procedures to contend with. Unprepared mothers are likely to receive routine IV, fetal monitoring, and numerous unannounced vaginal exams. This bevy of interventions predisposes to pain medication, and is apt to be disturbing and oppressive to any birth assistant who has known the freedom of attending out of hospital birth. Just as the mother can be undermined by tension, so may the birth assistant, who must first overcome her own stress before she can hope to reassure her client.

Always remember when hospital coaching that an unprepared mother must contend not only with the pain of labor, but with fear. She may know nothing of the importance of relaxation, but this is no time for a lecture. If confronted with a woman who is writhing or screaming, first calm yourself, then make eye contact with her and explain that you are there to help. Women who are panicked or terrified of their sensations often breathe too rapidly, which can lead to hyperventilation. Avoid this by having her keep her breathing light, or by trying to slow it down. Getting her to slow down her breathing is a bit tricky. Begin by breathing at her rhythm, then ask her to breathe with you as you make each breath a fraction slower and deeper than the one before. Place a hand on her belly and a hand on your own, and as you look into her eyes, show her how to draw her breath down, e.g., "Try to bring your breath down to the baby." It may take some time to win her trust, so don't give up!

Once her breathing is regular, relaxation can be initiated by using touch, massage, and verbal cues. Ask her between contractions if you can rub her back, whether she would like to sit up or lean forward, etc. If she is tightening her hips or legs, a foot massage may help her let go. She may also respond to smooth firm strokes on her inner thighs, and phrases like, "let your legs feel heavy" or "let your bottom melt into the bed." I was called several times to assist Asian and Hispanic women who spoke no English, and had to rely entirely on touch and sign. It works!

Mothers without preparation often progress very slowly. More than anything else, hospital coaching will try your patience. A quote from *Childbirth Without Fear*, by Grantly Dick-Read, says it perfectly:

At the bedside of a woman in labor we have to await the will of intangible forces. The emotional conflicts and physical reactions of women present a constant stream of problems. Initiative, clear thinking and honest exposition must be at hand to control the fearful, encourage the failing and support the tired. No force of mind or body can drive a woman in labor; by patience only can the smooth course of nature be followed.

Basic to the practice of patience is validation of your own needs, both physical and emotional. If the mother is completely alone, perhaps you can bring a coaching partner with you. The two of you can alternate break times and compare notes on what is happening with the labor. Hospitals generally have a coffee room for labor and delivery staff, and while one of the nurses is busy taking vitals, you may be able to slip away for a break.

Also, be comfortable: wear something light, cool, and loose. Coaching is very demanding physically and you'll perspire a lot. You might want to bring an extra set of clothes, in case you're in the way when the woman vomits or her water bag breaks. In this age of HIV and hepatitis B, you

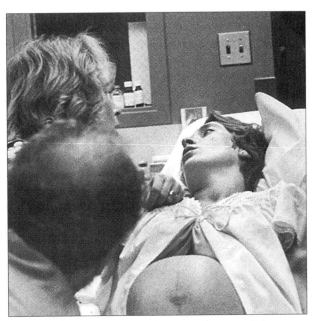

Often you are the mother's only support in hospital situations.

may wish to wear protective eyegear, and should bring gloves to wear anytime you may be in contact with maternal or newborn secretions. If you have long hair, plan to tie or clip it out of the way. Bring lip balm too, as breathing through your mouth will chap your lips; also bring some lozenges to suck on. Bring fresh fruit and bottled water or juice with you, as you will probably not have time to run to the cafeteria.

Hospital coaching will teach you that assisting births is not always easy or pleasurable. Often, you will be on your own with the mother, and may be required to make important decisions on her behalf which the staff will not support. For example, I once assisted a woman who had been pushing involuntarily and ever so slightly with each contraction from about four centimeters dilation. At six centimeters, her cervix was quite edematous, and her progress ceased for several hours. She was lying in bed with an IV, hooked to a fetal monitor, and all that was recommended was "no more pushing!" I reasoned that she needed more, not less, pressure on her cervix to thin it out, with modified chest breathing to keep her from bearing down. Once I had her breathing evenly, and had carefully disentangled the various tubes and wires to which she was connected, I had her squat and relax. Sure enough, it worked—she dilated to complete in just one hour.

Unfortunately, hospital births do not always go well. By the time you arrive, the woman may have received a mild analgesic and will be less than responsive to coaching. If she then asks for stronger pain medication, fetal distress may ensue and necessitate a cesarean. Even in this day and age, women are treated carelessly or even brutally in hospital; they are systematically disempowered in birth, which is the opposite of your intent. Much of what you see and experience will disgust you, but hopefully you will persist in your efforts, and vow to do better in your own practice someday.

The real problem for the woman birthing in hospital is that no one is really accountable for her care. Even a woman who has engaged a private physician may find her labor being managed by nurses or residents she has never seen before, and as their shifts end, new faces take their places. This may happen repeatedly in the course of a single labor, forcing the birth assistant to continually reassert the mother's wishes and needs. This raises the question of responsibility—just who is taking care of the mother, who's really in charge?

Of this, the home birth midwife has no doubt. Combining roles of nurse, obstetrician, neonatalogist, and pediatrician, she accepts responsibility for the birth from start to finish. Keep this in mind as you assist births in hospital, and utilize your experience to develop your understanding of what it means to give primary care.

Lest you think your work as a birth assistant is futile, though, rest assured that laboring women never forget an act of kindness, whether a simple touch, an encouraging word, or a compassionate look. I know this from my own experience; I had my first baby in 1972 (the dark ages of childbirth) and was utterly overwhelmed by a pitocin-induced labor of only two and a half hours (buccal pitocin was used, now contraindicated due to a high incidence of uterine rupture). My Lamaze preparation was totally useless; my contractions peaked immediately and I never had more than ten seconds' rest between them. Needless to say, I did a lot of screaming. For the most part, the nurses shunned me because I wanted a natural birth. But then, one came in and sat at the edge of my bed. She touched my arm and said quietly to me, "Let's try

to slow your breathing down a little here," showing me what to do, and letting me squeeze her arm so hard I know she had fingernail marks the next day. I can't say she made everything better, but I will never forget her sweet face, her kind intent, her caring spirit. *Women in labor are totally aware of what those around them are thinking and feeling, what they believe and what they fear.* You can't hide anything from a laboring woman; don't bother to try. By the same token, whatever you give from the heart will be deeply appreciated and always remembered.

Coaching on-call can also help prepare you for a midwife's lifestyle. You will learn to give your intimate relationships lots of special attention before leaving for a birth, and as much energy as you can muster upon your return, to compensate for your abrupt and possibly prolonged absence. You will also experience the frustration of doing hard work for minimal compensation, particularly if you are out-of-pocket for gas and babysitting expenses. As you become aware of the time and energy commitment you will make as a midwife, you may get some idea of what to charge for your services, as well as how best to arrange your personal life.

A real turning point for the birth assistant is the realization that her experience has put her in league with other medical professionals. More than once, I recall assisting a labor and delivery nurse with fetal palpation in order to best locate heart tones. My coaching partner told of a delivery she attended when, following the birth of a rather small infant, it was obvious to her by observing uterine contour that there was still another baby in utero. No one else noticed this, although the second water bag was presenting. In fact, the attending physician was busy pulling at the cord to deliver the placenta when a twin was birthed into the placenta pan! Yet another colleague gave numerous accounts of postpartum hemorrhage caused by cord traction, until she lost all reserve. The next time she encountered another "cord pulling" attendant, she firmly suggested waiting while the woman pushed her placenta out, and so it was done!

Besides volunteer coaching, what are some other ways to keep up your birth attendance?

Women who have given birth and wish to pass along their knowledge may find teaching childbirth classes to be the answer. Register your course with your local women's resource center, where you might also consider volunteering to gain exposure and make contacts. Childbirth educators are often invited to births as support persons, and thus have opportunity to observe a variety of practitioners for style and technique, at the same time establishing themselves as reasonable, helpful personalities. Teaching is a potent avenue into the birthing community.

Besides prepared childbirth classes, consider teaching prenatal exercise or yoga classes to women in early pregnancy. These can be quite informal, and may provide yet another opportunity for you to be asked to births. Community hospital prenatal clinics may be particularly receptive to having you teach "early bird" classes on health and nutrition, regardless of your credentials. If you are unfamiliar with community standards in this regard, find out which sort of childbirth prepara-

tion is preferred by maternity care providers, and to what degree teacher training is required, before you set out a schedule.

MIDWIFERY STUDY GROUPS

Participating in a study group with experienced instructors and other aspiring midwives is probably the most exciting and integrating aspect of training. Textbooks have their value, and assisting at births is crucial preparation for apprenticeship, but listening to experienced midwives discuss their case histories and management of complications is a practical education that can't be beat. Study groups also provide golden opportunities for students to get extra help in troublesome subject areas, thus tailoring their learning process to suit their needs.

I participated in a study group for over a year, and during that period went from student to primary caregiver. We had a nurse and a physician working along with us, and were therefore able to practice skills like giving injections (we practiced

---

CORE AREAS OF STUDY

General Subjects
Aseptic Technique/Universal Precautions
Human Reproduction
Anatomy of Pregnancy, Birth, and Postpartum
Physiology of Pregnancy, Birth, and Postpartum
Applied Microbiology of Pregnancy, Birth, and Postpartum
Embryology/Fetal Growth and Development
Pharmacology of Pregnancy, Birth, and Postpartum
Nutrition for Pregnancy and Lactation
Obstetrical Procedures for Complicated Pregnancy and Birth
Well-woman Gynecology and Contraceptive Care
Childbirth Education, Theory
Childbirth Education, Instruction
Infant and Child Development

Provision of Care: Antepartum Period
Risk Assessment
Comprehensive Prenatal Care
Communication and Counseling Techniques

Management of Common Complaints in Pregnancy
Charting
Interpretation of Medical History, Lab Work, and Diagnostic Testing
Complications of Pregnancy
Contraindications for Out of Hospital Birth

Provision of Care: Intrapartum Period
Management of Normal Labor and Birth
Complications of Labor and Delivery
Emergency Care
Assessment of Lacerations and Appropriate Action

Provision of Care: Postpartum Period
Immediate Care of Mother and Newborn
Newborn Assessment
Management of Normal Postpartum and Lactation
Newborn Care
Management of Common Postpartum Problems
Newborn Complications and Appropriate Action
Maternal Complications and Appropriate Action

by injecting oranges with water) and drawing blood (which we did on each other). We also learned intubation from a pediatrician. We had a few sessions on equipment, and single meetings devoted to subjects of anemia, neonatal jaundice, hypertension, fetal development, etc. Our discussions would often rove into related areas as we shared our experiences at births. During the time our group met, we all had opportunity for hands-on practice at prenatal clinics or births, under the guidance of our senior midwife instructors. Several of us formed liaisons that later blossomed into midwifery partnerships.

Starting a study group can be as easy as posting signs in birth resource centers, or any other location where new mothers or women likely to be interested in midwifery might gather. A variation of the study group learning situation can be found by attending state midwifery meetings and regional or national midwifery conferences. Contact MANA for the name of a regional representative in your area, or write *Midwifery Today* or *The Birth Gazette* for conference schedules.

APPRENTICESHIP

On occasion, I've been heavily pressured by women seeking to apprentice with me, and my invariable reaction is to suggest they look elsewhere for training. The very nature of this working relationship requires the prospective apprentice to approach with deference to the style and experience of the midwife from whom she is soliciting instruction. If she is chosen, the apprentice will not only help at births, but will share the sometimes weighty responsibilities of managing (and debriefing) emergency complications and transports. It stands to reason that the senior midwife should choose a student with whom she feels fully comfortable and compatible. Conversely, the apprentice must have respect for her senior midwife's style and philosophy of practice, seeking to complement it in all that she does.

Ideally, contacts made in study group enable the student to find a senior midwife with whom she's comfortable and vice versa, so that apprenticeship is a natural extension of an already established relationship. Apprenticeship agreements also evolve

from friendships established through local chapters of state midwifery organizations, or other birth community activities. Many students worry about their chances of finding an apprenticeship, and it is true that political and legal difficulties have caused the ranks of practicing midwives to dwindle somewhat. Nevertheless, maintaining a high profile in your midwifery community is always a step in the right direction.

How will a student know when she is ready to apprentice? There is a certain feeling of confidence that comes from having attended a number of births and from having mastered basic midwifery knowledge, often accompanied by an urge for more hands-on experience. Apprenticeship usually begins with assisting at prenatal visits, acquiring rudimentary skills of taking blood pressure, auscultating fetal heart tones, and palpating the baby. If a senior midwife is training several apprentices at once, she will probably rotate their attendance at clinic to establish which clients and students work best together, and will then arrange for those combinations at births.

For students wishing a little more structure, midwifery programs offering academic preparation and formalized apprenticeship have recently been developed. An example is the Midwifery Institute of California, which combines Heart & Hands and Study Group coursework (available on-site or at-a-distance) with apprenticeship. The intention of this program is to provide the student a solid theoretical foundation in midwifery, while helping her find apprenticeship opportunities in her own locale. She can take advantage of community-based, community-sensitive training, and be spared the considerable cost of having to relocate for schooling.

In less formal situations, the backbone of apprenticeship training is skills acquisition and evaluation. In 1995, NARM conducted a survey of midwives throughout North America to determine entry-level skills for direct-entry midwifery. The resulting practical skills list is utilized by NARM in its certification process (see Appendix B). Acquisition of these skills is outlined step by step in the *Practical Skills Guide*, by Sharon Evans and Pam Weaver. These tools can provide needed structure for senior midwife and apprentice alike. Together, they can formulate a plan to see that both skills and the experience necessary for certification or licensure are acquired by the apprentice in a reasonable amount of time.

What about cost? Apprenticeship is traditionally a relationship of exchange, whereby a master of a given trade exchanges knowledge for labor. But if part of a formal program leading directly to licensure or certification, the student can expect to pay for apprenticeship. In less structured situations, the apprentice may receive a nominal sum to cover transportation and child care, and if the midwife intends to incorporate the apprentice as a partner, she may increase her pay over time to full partnership level.

How can an apprentice best contribute to the midwife's practice? She can offer assistance with housekeeping, bookkeeping, filing, stocking supplies, public relations, errand running, etc. And how can she best serve the needs of her senior midwife at births, where the situation is ever-changing and always unique? She can provide labor coaching when the midwife is otherwise occupied with more technical duties. She can take responsibility for routine assessments of fetal heart tones, maternal blood pressure, pulse, urinalysis, etc. She can help keep charts updated during labor. She can assist delivery by opening up gauze pads, securing extra towels, bowls, etc., and by handing instruments to the midwife. She can also help in third stage by keeping an eye on the baby while the midwife sees to delivery of the placenta, or vice versa. She can assist with clean-up and care of the mother in the immediate postpartum. She can lend a hand with suturing. As she becomes more competent and self-confident, her responsibilities will increase, beginning with labor sitting and basic checks on mother and baby until the midwife arrives, and then, assisting deliveries on her own.

How will an apprentice know when she is ready to practice independently? Meeting minimum standards for skills and experience is just one aspect of her preparedness. Some students are by nature overeager and need to be repeatedly instructed in the art of caregiving; others are timid and must be given unexpected responsibilities to appreciate

their competence. If their relationship is good, an apprentice can trust her teacher's judgement regarding her readiness to practice. However, some students feel the need for experience beyond that offered by their preceptor. Senior apprentices sometimes practice briefly with other midwives, or undertake limited internships at high-volume midwifery practices or out-of-hospital birth centers in order to complete their training.

DIRECT-ENTRY MIDWIFERY PROGRAMS

There are many different types of midwifery schools and programs available for students wishing to pursue training without a nursing background. Programs offered by Maternidad La Luz and Casa de Nacimento in El Paso, Texas, serve women from Mexico who cross the border specifically to secure U.S. citizenship for their children, and to receive better care than they would at home. As many of these mothers have had no prenatal care, their births are frequently challenging or complicated. Each of these programs offers academic preparation integrated with clinical training.

Programs emphasizing a more conventional approach to learning include the Seattle Midwifery School, and the Miami-Dade program in Florida. These are both three-year programs, with extensive theoretical instruction prior to clinical training. Beyond these options, investigate other training opportunities by consulting the list in the Appendix, and writing programs for current catalogues.

Perhaps the best guideline for a student unsure of which sort of program to select is to consider her learning style. Ask yourself if you need lots of structure in order to master academic material, i.e., plenty of written assignments, quizzes, tests, etc. Or are you a self-starter, capable of working autonomously and without much guidance to keep you on track? Most students are a combination of the two, and need a program that will provide both structure and freedom. If you are somewhat hesitant to begin hands-on work for fear you don't "know enough," you may need a program that provides theoretical preparation prior to, and distinct from, clinical training. If you feel you learn best by doing, look for a program that will integrate practice with theory right from the start.

Any program you consider should have some mechanism of providing student feedback to potential enrollees. Also take every opportunity to query recent graduates or beginning midwives for their opinions of their training.

NURSE-MIDWIFERY PROGRAMS

Nurse-midwifery programs also vary tremendously in terms of structure and prerequisites. Some require a bachelor's of science in nursing (BSN) for admission; others, an RN certificate only. There are a handful of master's level programs for students with either BA or BS degrees, which incorporate nursing studies within CNM training—in three years, you get a RN, MSN, and CNM. These are programs the ACNM considers "direct-entry."

Many CNM programs are focused on efficiency, rather than on the art of midwifery. One way to identify a program's philosophy of teaching is to see what type of clinical settings are involved. If most or all are tertiary, high-tech medical centers, you will get more active management, interventive obstetrical training than woman-centered caregiving. Programs that offer training in birth centers or hospitals known for expectant management will teach you more about the art of midwifery than the strictly scientific or medicalized model.

EPA (Educational Program Associates) and CNEP (Community-Based Nurse Midwifery Education Program) allow students to precept in their own communities. Programs at San Francisco General Hospital and at the University of California, San Francisco, emphasize progressive midwifery. When applying to a program, always ask to speak to a current student or recent graduate to get a better sense of what is being offered.

Chapter 8

The Midwife's Practice

As a midwife's status changes from apprentice to primary caregiver, great changes take place in the rest of her life as well. Her focus shifts from the thrill of catching babies to her new professional responsibilities. In order to practice successfully, she must effectively combine demands of her work with those of her personal life. Putting together a cohesive practice is difficult for most beginning midwives.

As you prepare to set up a practice, begin by articulating your intention, i.e., your philosophy of caregiving. This is the linchpin on which many other work-related decisions will be based. Your philosophy of practice should incorporate your beliefs regarding optimal care and responsibility in childbearing. If your philosophy is clearly stated, it will define your purpose. For example, if your philosophy states that midwifery must serve the needs and desires of childbearing women, your purpose is clearly to support women in choosing how they wish to give birth. From this point forward, the structure of your practice should at all times and in all ways uphold your philosophy and express your purpose.

It might seem that all midwives share a similar philosophy. But one has only to look at the services and clientele of several different midwifery practices to see that this is not the case. If you are unclear on your philosophy or intention, you may wish to try this simple exercise I give my midwifery students.

Begin with the following statements: "A pregnant woman should always..." or, "A pregnant woman should never..." or, "A pregnant woman's partner should always..." or "A pregnant woman's partner should never..." Choose any one of these, then write your response as spontaneously and exhaustively as you can, not censoring anything, just jotting down your thoughts. You may have a lengthy list when you are finished, but will probably find that one "should" or "shouldn't" really stands out—it is highly charged for you. Then, in the same spontaneous way as before, write again regarding all possible reasons why this is such an issue for you. Finally, recognize this issue for the bias or prejudice it is, and look closely at how it might interfere with the integrity of a potential client's experience.

Were you to do this exercise in a group, you might be surprised to discover that other participants hold biases in direct contrast to your own. The same is true of practicing midwives—they all have their biases, and on that basis, make decisions on who they will, and will not, care for. If they are wise, they readily refer prospective clients to midwives who are likely to work well with women they themselves find trying or difficult. The point is that our biases determine, to a large extent, our philosophy and capabilities for caregiving.

As regards matching your practice structure with your philosophy of care, there is much to consider. You must consolidate your backup arrangements, define your working relationship with partners or other assistants, choose an office location, name your business, establish your financial structure, create promotional materials and marketing strategies, etc., based on the needs and desires of your anticipated clientele.

Even with careful planning, beginning practice is difficult. Will your initial client volume be adequate to pay the bills? Would it be better to have an office in your home for a while, to keep overhead low until you get things going? Is your personal life stable enough to withstand these start-up stresses? Your first clients seem to take all of your energy, as you work to make the best impression and agonize over every detail lest anything be overlooked. Your family life may well begin to show some strain, which of course puts an extra burden on you.

The important thing to remember is to take one challenge at a time, and your life, one day at a time. Step back to reflect on your progress once in a while. In fact, most experienced midwives schedule regular weekly meetings with their partners to go over practice issues, attend to business matters, and otherwise clear the air. Consider having these meetings in retreat settings once in a while. Especially in the beginning, your aim is to stay alert enough not to miss anything, and calm

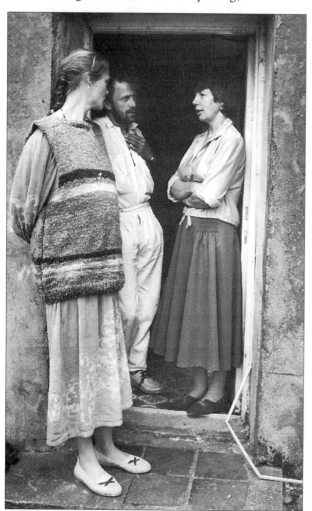

An Irish midwife responding to the call of a woman in early labor

enough to observe congruity and resonance in order to consolidate your efforts.

LOCATION: URBAN OR RURAL PRACTICE?

Urban practice has its ease in the availability of emergency medical facilities, good support from other midwives, and easy access to consultation. Home birth is a very safe alternative in an urban setting—transport time is minimal, and intensive care services are available at need. However, close contact with the medical community demands that you establish and maintain good professional relationships. Difficulties with urban practice depend largely on the politics surrounding out of hospital birth. It remains difficult, if not impossible, for many midwives to secure physician backup for home birth in many parts of the country. But if tolerance prevails in your community, you may be able to practice and transport openly, with good support from hospital staff.

A midwife who practices in a hostile legal environment will eventually find herself in the untenable position of having to transport and face the consequences of inadequate or nonexistent backup. On the one hand, she is obligated to relay case details that necessitated transport in the first place, but on the other, she knows if she provides this information, she fully incriminates herself. A midwife working thus must be discreet, keep her practice quiet, get plenty of support from her peers, and gain clear agreements with her clients as to the limits of her responsibility and liability. It seems that urban midwives have more difficulty in this respect than their rural sisters, whose home birth practices may be viewed as a necessary alternative for women far from the nearest hospital. Economic competition between doctors and midwives is also a crucial factor in cities. Consumers are well aware of the padding involved in hospital costs, and, if paying out of pocket, are serious about getting their money's worth. Midwives spend more time, and give more personal attention before, during, and after the birth than virtually any obstetrician. And they further threaten the local obstetrical community by offering sliding scale fees, or rock-bottom prices. (More on this in sections on Medical Backup and Public Relations, forthcoming.)

Urban practice may be hindered by urban lifestyle more than anything else. A common problem is finding adequate time to really get to know your clients. The environment itself is stressful, the air polluted, the pace harried and intense. None of this is particularly conducive to good health. Urban midwives have the challenging task of modulating energy levels during prenatal visits to induce comfort and ease, so as to show parents what is most essential in preparing for birth, i.e., they must slow down and let pregnancy determine their lifestyle, rather than the other way around.

Sometimes a city will have several competitive midwifery practices. In the past, midwives have succumbed to factionalism, and have discredited one another's work. Such power struggles are self-defeating; they are also evidence that the "divide and conquer" strategy of American Medical Association politics has succeeded. But the more organized and powerful midwives become, the more they realize that cooperation is imperative. Only by sharing resources, exchanging information, and passing clients along can they hope to generate the broad base of strength necessary to cope with challenges of limited scope of practice, lack of autonomy, and the need for public education.

The real competition for city midwives is in hospital-based alternative birth centers. Women who might otherwise investigate home birth may be quite impressed with the "home-like atmosphere" of nicely furnished, decorator birthing rooms—an undeniable improvement over the stark white of traditional labor and delivery. What is not immediately obvious is that regardless of which room she occupies, any woman in hospital is subject to standard obstetrical risk guidelines, which in turn are influenced by liability concerns. Transfer to labor and delivery facilities is apt to occur with even the slightest hint of a complication. Yes, the rooms are lovely—but easy chairs and flowered sheets cannot substitute for the comfort of one's own home, or the freedom to negotiate with one's caregiver in borderline situations. Unfortunately, a woman may be aware of all this and yet be bound by economic considerations to choose hospital birth. Insurance coverage for hospital birth is standard, whereas coverage for home birth depends on the backup physician's willingness to assist with billing, which is limited (once again) by liability concerns.

An alternative to this dilemma is the freestanding birth center. Although backup may still be difficult to obtain, it is certainly easier to secure for birth in this setting than for birth at home. Midwives at work in freestanding birth centers are generally subject to more stringent practice guidelines (as per backup) than are home birth midwives. However, they are ultimately accountable to accreditation standards for out of hospital, not hospital birth, which can be beneficial to them and their clients. Working in a freestanding birth center can also provide the midwife relief from the woes of private practice, particularly if her work has involved nearly continuous on-call availability.

Thus the urban midwife's practice situation is complex, and yet, with good standing in her community and supportive backup, opportunities for professional growth are tremendous. Training and working in the city can take a midwife across class and cultural boundaries, fostering adaptability in practice while providing the pleasure of getting to know all sorts of people intimately.

The main benefit of **rural practice** is the environment itself. Open space, clean air and a relaxed lifestyle are obvious benefits for the rural midwife and her clients. Working in conjunction with nature and the seasons is a definite source of strength for women living rurally. There is also more tendency for women in rural areas to feel a part of their community, which makes it much easier for new mothers to find support regardless of the distances that separate them. Birth in a rural setting is usually an extended family event, in contrast to the couple-oriented style of birthing endemic to the urban woman's social isolation.

Problems with rural practice are generally caused by geographical isolation. Although it makes sense to give prenatal care at a central location and to schedule checkups on certain days each week, this may not be workable in rural areas. If you are detained at a birth or someone goes into labor on your clinic day, clients already en route to prenatals may be quite disgruntled to have come so far only to find you unavailable when they arrive.

Rural midwives often end up doing a lot of home care, unless they have an extra assistant, or backup from other midwives.

In fact, what rural midwives seem to miss the most is contact with others in practice. Midwifery is an interactive profession, not a circumscribed batch of skills. Midwives need regular opportunities to share experiences, to participate in peer review, and to undertake continuing education. If these opportunities are not available locally, the rural midwife may have to travel to an urban location, or be content with periodic attendance at midwifery conferences.

In addition, good medical backup and consultation may be limited in rural areas. It can be very difficult to get a second or third opinion, and transport time may be considerable. Thus any midwife practicing more than half an hour from the nearest hospital will need advanced skills and equipment. She should be trained to administer an IV in case of severe hemorrhage, and should be certified in neonatal resuscitation (including intubation) in case of neonatal asphyxia.

EQUIPMENT

Most beginning midwives take great pleasure and pride in their growing treasury of equipment. It's usually best to purchase equipment slowly during the apprenticeship period, so you can try out various brands and see which suits you best. This bit-by-bit method is also a lot easier on the pocketbook. A complete midwife's kit, including bag and oxygen system, can run around $2700. Fortunately, birthing supply houses such as Cascade Birthing Supplies (see Appendix B) cater to midwives and home birth couples, reducing costs for those who buy in bulk.

Take a look at the supply list in Appendix L. Certain basics like urine sticks, nonsterile exam gloves, Betadine antiseptic, sterile gauze pads, underpads, and bulb syringes can be purchased at your local drugstore.

When students ask which equipment to purchase first, I usually suggest they start with a fetascope. This tool for auscultating fetal heart tones can be your ticket to interaction with pregnant women, and will give you opportunity to develop a trained ear before you begin primary practice. Mothers in your childbirth classes or those whose births you plan to assist are usually eager to have you listen to the baby, and may also want you to palpate for position, size, etc. The best fetascope currently available is the Allen Series 10, which features an amplification unit in the horn. For best results, avoid Allen-type economy models.

If you decide to purchase a Doppler, the best starter model is Pocket-Dop One. This comes with both 3 MHz and 2 MHz probes, the former used for early pregnancy, the latter during late pregnancy and labor. Purchasing different intensity probes is important, as your goal is to minimize exposure to ultrasound by using the lowest megahertz possible. Or, you can step up to Pocket Dop OB, which filters background noise so heart tones are clearer (select the two-probe option).

Other items such as the sphygmomanometer (blood pressure cuff) should be purchased by comparison shopping, your goal being quality without tinsel. Blood pressure cuffs are sporting some stylish colors of late, but apart from looks, the most valuable and important component of your unit is the gauge. The cuff, bladder, and tubing are readily and cheaply replaced, but the gauge should be built to last. Make sure it has no automatic pin stop to prevent it from showing need for adjustment. The unit should come with a warranty of at least three years, and the gauge should be certified (you can see a register number stamped on the face of any decent gauge).

Although your lab will supply everything you need for doing blood draws, consider purchasing a hemoglobinometer for office use. These currently run about $200—much less expensive than a centrifuge. You might also wish to invest in a blood glucose monitor; Cascade Birthing Supplies sells a fully equipped model called Accu-Chek III for about $100.

Beyond what your lab provides, you should stock disposable items for urinalysis, pH assessment, and pregnancy testing. Your resuscitation equipment should include De Lee suction devices, pocket masks for mouth-to-mouth, oxygen tanks and regulator, adult oxygen mask for the mother, bag-mask unit for the baby, and, if you are trained to use them, laryngoscope and endotracheal tubes. The Spur Disposable bag-mask costs around $40, and may be a wise choice for the midwife with a small practice. For a more permanent investment, both the Hudson Lifesaver Infant Resuscitator or the Ambu Baby Resuscitator are excellent choices; the latter meets and exceeds all standards for neonatal/infant resuscitation.

Make sure your instruments are 100 percent stainless steel. It's especially important that your blunt scissors and curved hemostats be top quality, as you'll be using them repeatedly for cutting the cord. It is also wise to get a good needle-holder, as the precision work of suturing is best accomplished with a quality tool. The finest instruments are made in Germany by Medline and Miltex; both come with lifetime guarantees. A less expensive grade made in Pakistan is entirely adequate for instruments like ring forceps or mosquito forceps that you will rarely use.

Last but not least are the restricted items: suture material and syringes. If you have authorization to purchase these items in your state, no problem. Otherwise, you may be able to enlist the help of a friend or colleague with the proper credentials. Many student midwives wonder how they will be able to obtain oxytocic drugs and other medications when they are in practice. It all depends on your legal status—if you have a physician willing to help you, count your blessings; otherwise, you must rely on assistance from other midwives. Stock up whenever you have the opportunity.

SETUP AND ADMINISTRATION

In terms of physical setup, you have a number of choices. You can do clinic visits in your home, using a bedroom for exams and living room for waiting. You might prefer to see clients in their homes (some midwives do this exclusively). Or you may decide to rent an office, with exam room, separate waiting area, restroom, and storage space. It depends on your practice. If you set up a freestanding birth center, all the above plus birth rooms can be housed under one roof.

Seeing clients in your home may appeal to them—the setting is relaxed and conducive to inti-

macy. The obvious drawback is having to keep everything neat and clean on a regular basis. This can be especially challenging if you've come in from a birth at 3 A.M., and your clinic day starts in a few hours. Lack of privacy is yet another issue—there may be strenuous objections from your partner if he/she needs extra sleep or solitude. If the cost of renting an office is prohibitive, consider sharing office space with other midwives or health providers in your area.

Whatever you decide, your exam room should be arranged for both comfort and efficiency. Most women would rather be examined on a bed than an exam table. Choose a firm mattress, large enough for you and your assistant to sit comfortably on either side of the mother. Another possibility is a chaise couch, or antique "fainting sofa" with chairs set around it. If space permits, you may also want to have an exam table (minus the stirrups) as backup for problematic pelvic assessment. The drawers and cabinets in the base are perfect for storing medical supplies. You may be able to obtain a used one from a medical supply house, or might try soliciting a donation from a sympathetic doctor or clinic. Convert a walk-in closet or corner of the room for lab equipment, and you've got your exam room ready to go.

In the waiting area, there should be adequate seating for family and friends, toys for small children, birth pictures on the wall, and photo albums readily available. Post all pertinent documents here, like the WHO/UNICEF Breastfeeding Resolution, the WHO Resolution on Midwifery, and the Patient's Bill of Rights in your state of practice. Have a bookcase with lending library in or near the waiting area.

How about supplies? What will you need, and how much should you keep in stock? Besides your permanent essentials, various disposable items must be kept on hand. Underpads may be purchased in bulk for economy—the small, 17" X 23" size is fine for doing internal exams. Exam gloves, lubricating jelly, urine testing strips, long-handled cotton swabs for cultures, cotton balls and Band-aids for venipuncture, paper cups for urinalysis, and lots of toilet paper should be kept in stock at all times. Take inventory of these items weekly.

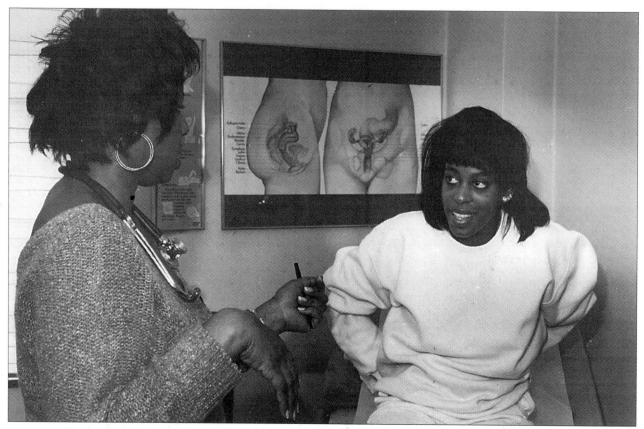

This midwife provides care in a comfortable office, in an informal manner.

You must also keep tabs on your stock of forms, and make sure you have other office supplies necessary for filing, bookkeeping, and correspondence. Have ample cartridges for your printer, disks for your computer, etc. It never hurts to post a running list of your needs, with highlighted priorities. Whatever your level of practice, keep it organized.

What about the actual structure of caregiving? How much time should you schedule for initial, follow-up, and routine visits? That depends on your style and volume of practice. If you assist four to six births per month, you can probably limit yourself to two clinic days per week. Schedule a minimum of two hours for the initial visit, and one and a half hours for the visit immediately after, to allow for routine assessments plus medical history intake and review, consent to care, nutritional counseling, complete physical assessment and/or pelvimetry, and evaluation of the mother's emotional state. Even routine checkups may take 45 minutes or so, figuring 25 minutes for physical assessment and another 20 minutes for discussion.

If topics of conversation result in controversy or upset, or if physical findings are questionable, a visit may run over. This is why you need a well-stocked library in the waiting area, and might also want to have tea and healthy snack foods available. When a visit is running over, make sure to explain the situation to mothers waiting their turn, and if anyone is on a tight schedule, have your partner or apprentice start initial physical assessments. Women due around the same time can be scheduled so their appointments overlap, giving them opportunity to meet or even share in one another's checkups. This principle of overlap can also be used to bring partners/fathers together.

Some midwives have extended this concept of overlap to the provision of group prenatal care. This requires a large block of time, perhaps four or five hours, when a number of clients come together for prenatals. Women due at the same time particularly benefit from the opportunity to socialize and learn from each other. They may also enjoy carpooling together, especially if coming from some distance. Often, they spontaneously participate in one another's clinical assessments. If you decide to try group prenatal care, you'll need ample assistance in order to provide technical instruction and facilitate group discussion. California midwife June Whitson swears by this system as the best possible way to help mothers find postpartum support and autonomy.

Apart from client visits, you may also want to schedule weekly business meetings with your colleagues to go over finances, marketing, special events, etc. This is also a good time to consider purchasing new reference books or supplies, refurnishing your facility, organizing public outreach, etc. These meetings may rove into case review, but it is better to make separate time for this. Consider dividing your weekly meeting into two segments; the first part for business, the second, for airing interpersonal concerns. The latter is crucial for the psychological health of your practice. Occasionally, or perhaps initially, an outside facilitator may be helpful.

Also plan a comprehensive annual review of all aspects of your business: facilities, organization, location, image, competition, finances, marketing strategies, and community and professional relationships. This provides an opportunity to create long-term goals for your organization, in contrast to the short-term, problem-solving focus of your weekly meetings. In so doing, continually refer back to your most basic premise of operation— your intention, as expressed in your statement of philosophy. *Are all components of your business still in keeping with this document?* If so, all is well; if not, you may need to do some restructuring.

Be sure your filing system is at all times in order. In California, medical records must be kept for 21 years (although laws vary from state to state). File charts alphabetically, and by year in which the mother gave birth. This allows you to access files with ease, and to move sections to more permanent storage from time to time. You may need to hire an accountant, or at least consult with one, to educate you on tax laws and organizational options relevant to small business owners. A good reference on this subject is *The Business of Midwifery*, by Suellen Miller.

GENERAL PRESENTABILITY AND PERSONAL HYGIENE

A midwife in private practice must realize that some of her clients may have trouble adjusting to care in a casual setting. Particularly if she is seeing clients in her home, it is important that the midwife present herself professionally.

This requires some attention to her personal appearance. Most working women carefully plan their wardrobes for a variety of business occasions; there is no reason the midwife should not do the same. Clothes suitable to wear to births should be readily washable; dark-colored pants are most practical. Tops should be layered, as the amount of warmth required upon arrival will be way too much once the birth room is adequately heated for delivery. Some midwives prefer to wear special aprons in the final stages of labor. Apron or no, you must have a change of clothes with you at all times. It is not unusual to be soaked with amniotic fluid, or stained with blood at some point during the birth. You certainly cannot go out in public or transport to the hospital in this condition.

One of the reasons there is less infection attendant to home birth is that the mother has resistance to microorganisms in her environment. She may not, however, have resistance to what you bring in from outside. This is why your clothes should be completely clean and fresh, and why you should always wash your hands upon arrival and before examining the mother.

When doing prenatals, keep in mind that pregnant women are exceedingly sensitive to smell, thus you should avoid wearing perfume or cologne. Observe proper aseptic technique, and always wash your hands before and after each prenatal. This is important in the postpartum period as well: wash your hands before examining the mother, and again before handling the baby.

To return to wardrobe, consider several highly presentable outfits for greeting the public. Midwives are increasingly called to political work in the legislature or the public arena, for which you will need a suit, heels, the whole bit. Don't be put off by the notion of dressing to fit the part. If life is a stage, then it pays to have your costumes in order.

FEES

A midwife's fee should be fair and reasonable, which should make it affordable for most parents. Beyond that, a sliding scale policy makes way for exceptions. For example, of a total fee of $2000-$2800, clients can be asked to pay anything in that range which seems appropriate to their financial situation. Many midwives report great success with this system.

Once you've made peace with your fee, explain to your clients the services it includes and how you would like it to be paid. Some midwives prefer to work with fee schedules, and have mothers bring a payment to each visit. This system may provide some protection against rip-offs, but may be challenging for clients who have erratic work/pay schedules. And too, if a mother is short of funds but feels pressed to bring money to her next prenatal, she may cancel the visit, or if she does come, anxiety regarding her finances may overshadow other important health or personal issues. Most clients are happy to bring a little money each time, barring any extenuating circumstances. If the mother is clearly behind in payments at 28 weeks, firm up future payments more precisely. Most midwives prefer to be paid in full by 36 weeks.

Midwives in rural practice usually have no trouble receiving payment. One reason may be physical proximity to their clients; another may be less opportunity for clients to drain financial resources on city-based spending sprees or diversions. Rural midwives may also derive benefit from taking certain services or goods in trade for their work.

A word now about outside work. Beginning midwives sometimes plan to supplement their income with another, part-time occupation. Well, never mind that idea, unless you have a highly flexible, home-based sideline. Regularly scheduled employment is really out of the question; no employer will tolerate an employee apt to run off at any moment, and likely to phone in sick the next day. Midwifery practice is much more time and energy consuming than you might imagine. And it just won't do for you to be preoccupied with extraneous, work-related concerns, or wound up by tensions that disrupt your concentration on clients about to give birth.

Midwifery requires abundant energy and tremendous personal commitment. Try to take a realistic, long-term view of your needs right from the start, then design your practice in a way that will keep you financially solvent and anxiety free. No one wants a tense, worried midwife to assist them. It's up to you to set up a midwifery business that suits your style, reflects your beliefs, and accommodates your personal limitations.

PUBLIC RELATIONS AND EDUCATION

The first step in public relations is to become visible. List your service with women's agencies and resource centers. Then methodically contact all prominent alternative health care providers in your area—homeopathists, acupuncturists, herbologists, woman-centered therapists, massage therapists—to announce your new practice. Some of these may want to contact former clients for their opinions of your care. Once on file, client feedback may be made available to the general public, which can boost your professional profile and credibility.

Midwives occasionally have opportunity to combine a presentation on birth with an introduction to their services. Consider hosting a slide show and information night for the general public, with business cards or brochures ready for the taking. Even small, informal slide shows for clients and their friends will keep your name circulating and bring you business by word-of-mouth.

Film or video showings featuring well-known speakers can be organized to focus on themes of alternatives in childbirth, family participation in the birth process, breastfeeding and adjustment to parenthood, etc. Panel discussion is another format interesting to the public. These public events take effort to coordinate, and require plenty of advance publicity to assure good attendance. Although sometimes profit-generating, their main benefit is to expose a large, diverse audience to the benefits of midwifery, and more specifically, to your services.

You might also consider renting a booth at the county or city fair. Our local midwifery organization has done this for several consecutive years, with great success. We show birth videos right at

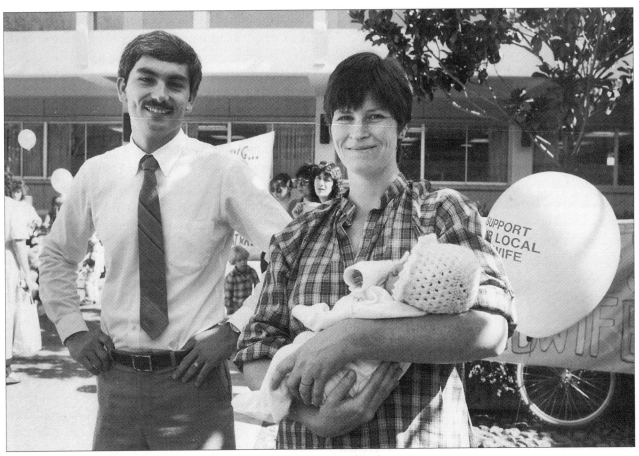

It pays to keep an updated client list, so support can be rallied in time of need.

the booth to attract the passersby, and have T-shirts, flyers, and a directory of local midwives available.

Television and radio appearances can further enhance public awareness of midwifery, but adequate preparation is essential. Have statistics on the tip of your tongue, in anticipation of questions you are likely to be asked. And remember—you always have the option of responding to an unappealing question with one you prefer to answer, as the media savvy do. For example, if an interviewer asks, "Is homebirth safe?" you might respond with, "Well, who says hospital birth is all that safe?" and launch into a discussion of iatrogenic complications. If you are being taped for either radio or television, it's wise to prepare a series of simple statements virtually impervious to an editor's distortion. The same goes for statements you make to journalists, although liability concerns increasingly prompt editorial departments to fact-check before they go to print. Don't let yourself be badgered,

and don't get flustered—just calmly return to your key position statements, or raise a new issue more to your liking.

Midwife Diane Barnes has built a remarkably successful freestanding birth center practice, and claims great success with television advertising spots on cable networks. She cautions that success takes time—just as the ad salespeople say, don't quit on your spot if response is not forthcoming in two or three months. In her case, calls started to pour in after about six months. The obvious advantage of paying for advertising is that you get to say, and portray, exactly what you want the public to know about you and your services.

Remember that your words and appearance reflect on midwives everywhere. Dress for the part, prepare carefully, consult with your colleagues, and ask for feedback on your presentations. Promotional packets of information are often available from state midwifery organizations, or contact MANA for information.

MEDICAL BACKUP AND CONSULTATION

By grace, faith, or the law of averages, the first births usually go well for the beginning midwife. But with additional experience, the unusual and unexpected begin to manifest, along with the desire for more in-depth medical consultation and assistance.

In areas where midwifery is illegal or unregulated, the new midwife may be hesitant to search out medical backup. But there is obvious need for a relationship between her home birth practice and the local hospital, if she expects to maintain the integrity of a birth experience if and when she must transport. Her first priority is to keep birth woman-centered, and to see that parents' most basic rights are preserved. She too must be recognized and respected, so that her recommendations will be appreciated and incorporated by the attending physician.

My partner and I began working on backup long before we became midwives. We slowly and carefully developed good relationships at a progressive hospital where we worked as birth assistants. Later, as apprentices, we transported clients there with our senior midwife. We were already respected as birth assistants, and so were well received by the hospital staff. We used the "iron fist in a velvet glove" approach, maintaining a low profile while persistently advocating our clients' wishes.

Once in practice for ourselves, we won the confidence of staff physicians by being clearheaded and articulate regarding our own transports, and by presenting complete and well-organized client records. After several more drop-in transports, the head obstetrician called and asked if we would like his assistance on a continuing basis, and we formalized our backup relationship.

If you must transport a mother to a hospital where you don't have backup, it is crucial to maintain an open, adaptable, friendly attitude. The staff will probably be suspicious, but may be more accepting if you behave responsibly and present the details of your case intelligently. Some physicians persist in defining midwives as kindly but decidedly naive women, whereas others are outright condescending or openly hostile. A few

are curious to learn just what it is that midwives do, and may therefore provide you opportunities to demonstrate your skills and knowledge.

Particularly if you have no backup arrangement, it helps to understand the psychology of labor and delivery personnel. Staff nurses are frequently overworked, underpaid, and underacknowledged. Why not offer your assistance and gain their cooperation? Don't attempt to usurp routine vital assessments, as the nurse is held responsible for these. But do empty the bedpan, fetch drinking water and linens, and change bedding for your client. When the birth is over and you are preparing to leave, go out of your way to personally thank every nurse who participated.

If your transport hospital trains residents, you'll have a challenging but promising situation on your hands. Fresh out of school, their heads crammed with information, medical residents are primed to answer questions. In fact, speculative discourse is their forte, and your key to forging a connection. If you acknowledge the resident's authority in the realm of information as you project authority in action, you two will be perfect complements. Pose a question on episiotomy, for example, and the resident may be only too happy to discuss the data as you do perineal massage. Suddenly, the baby is crowning, and the two of you are catching it together!

Residents are also unbelievably overworked and almost always exhausted. A former apprentice of mine would offer mints or gum to break the ice, then provide a vigorous shoulder rub to the resident on duty as I went ahead and attended our client. Again, always remember to be generous with appreciation and praise before you leave, establishing yourself as an appreciative colleague.

The attending obstetrician is often in and out of the mother's room before you have a chance to say a word. Immediately step out in the hall to converse, and begin by asking whether he/she has reviewed the chart or would like to see it. Then ask his/her opinion in the case. Listen respectfully, chime in agreement whenever you can, but assume a collegial air as you discuss your client in as technical a manner as possible.

If the physician suggests a course of action with which you don't agree, never confront him/her directly. Reiterate his/her recommendations, then offer to present these to the parents. Once alone with them, inform them of their options. You will, of course, submit your own opinion—that's why they hired you. After they decide what they want to do, present the physician with their decision. This strategy works in two ways: 1) it upholds principles of woman-centered birth, and 2) it keeps you from direct confrontation with the physician. Even if the physician is entirely disinterested in you and your ideas, he/she will generally honor the parents' wishes for fear of future malpractice liability.

If you are in very good standing with one particular hospital, you may link up with several doctors, and if problems arise in the future you can choose your consult at your discretion. A midwife in the early stages of establishing backing may actually need to distribute her clients among various practitioners so as not to overwhelm or intimidate any of them. Make your decision on whom to consult according to what is required. For example, if you suspect twins and need a sonogram, have it ordered through the obstetrician most likely to support vaginal birth of twins. Then again, if you need a sonogram to accurately date the pregnancy of a latecomer client with uncertain menstrual history, you might want to have a general practitioner do the authorization, as there is no reason to involve an obstetrician at this point. Refer minor questions to a friendly resident, obstetrical nurse, or midwife colleague.

Of course, if you are legally licensed or certified to practice in your state, your backup arrangement will be more or less defined by law. In some states, the midwife must have a relationship with a particular physician, who usually has a cap on how many midwives he/she may assist. Sometimes midwife and physician are constrained to practice under written guidelines, which tends to discourage physicians from offering backup for out of hospital birth due to liability concerns. Nurse-midwives may be similarly affected by a lack of physician backup for out-of-hospital birth.

An entirely different approach to backup is to have your clients negotiate their own. This may be especially wise if you practice in a conservative area. A physician unwilling to back you personally might feel more comfortable backing your client as his/her private patient. Advantages of this arrangement are: 1) the midwife is free to practice according to midwifery guidelines; 2) the client is free to choose her own physician, instead of being funneled into the care of a certain practitioner; and 3) liability for the physician, both professionally and politically, is reduced. This approach to backup is in keeping with the original *MANA Standards and Practice Statement*, which asserts that requiring the midwife to have a relationship with a particular physician is at odds with parents' rights to self-determination, and the International Definition's affirmation that the midwife "conducts deliveries on her own responsibility."

These difficulties are nonexistent in health care systems like that in the Netherlands, where midwives are the gatekeepers of maternity care. Every woman begins care with midwives, and only if she is determined to have risk factors requiring the care of a specialist is she referred to an obstetrician—referred by the midwife! In any case, midwives must have medical consultation to practice safely. Collaborative relationships insure continuity of care when a client becomes high-risk, whether in pregnancy or during labor. The ideal is to have backup at every hospital where client insurance might necessitate transport.

In areas where the political climate is very oppressive and the "old boys" are out to get you, your task is especially difficult. Explore each and every inroad to the medical establishment. For example, if you can't find a sympathetic doctor, perhaps you can find a progressive labor and delivery nurse who might give advice, and then put in a good word for you at the hospital. This takes time and is more than a little humiliating, but you owe it to your clients.

Here is a story of acquiring backup on the spot. This was a first birth, and after many hours of ineffectual labor and resulting maternal exhaustion, we all agreed on transport. The usual backup physician was not available, and so we were forced to take "OB potluck." As the mother curled up contentedly on her hospital bed, it was obvious that she had deep ambivalence about home birth only now coming to the surface. But after nearly 48 sleepless hours, my partner and I felt only relief. Our rapport with the nurses had always been great, and tonight, even the head nurse (who was usually a bit disapproving) seemed sympathetic and supportive.

Progress with pitocin was much more rapid than anyone expected. Braving disapproval, my partner donned sterile gloves and checked the mother. She was fully dilated, so I began doing a bit of internal massage. By the time the head nurse came back, the baby's head was beginning to show. She paused, and took it all in before going to get the doctor. As the doctor (a woman) came in and the nurses gathered around, the head was close to crowning. My partner was checking fetal heart tones, and I was supporting the perineum. When a nurse brought the instrument tray and asked the doctor where she wanted it, she said, motioning to us, "Ask them, I don't have anything to do with it." It was placed at the end of the bed, and after an awkward moment, someone unwrapped it for us. Good thing, too, for just then, a lovely baby girl delivered. The doctor stepped up to help me check for tears; the perineum was intact but there was an internal muscle split. "She may need a few stitches there," she commented.

"No," I said, "just press down with some gauze and it will stop bleeding." She did so and watched, waited a moment, and concurred as I told her, "Those little tears heal fine if the mother keeps her legs together."

After some time had passed, she motioned me to come outside with her. "Uh oh," I thought, "This is it. I'm busted." Instead, she held up the birth certificate and asked me uncertainly, "Do you sign this, or should I?"

In my amazement, I uttered, "I consider it a privilege to be able to work here, so just do whatever makes it smoothest for you."

"Then I'll sign it," she said. "You know, this is the first time I've ever done this." Then came a marvelous exchange of warmth and appreciation, with good feelings all around.

Whatever the genesis of your consulting relationship, you must continue to cultivate good communication. Periodic chart review, and disclosure of any revisions in your practice protocol, is critical to maintaining a solid working relationship. Friendly lunch dates are a good idea, too. Trust between you and your backup associates makes all the difference in crisis situations.

MEDICAL RECORDS, CHARTING, AND INFORMED CHOICE/CONSENT

This section will focus on the midwife's responsibility to document all aspects of caregiving. Accurate and appropriately detailed medical records are essential in professional practice. The forms in the Appendix are intended not as models, but as samples you may freely adapt to your own needs.

As her training nears completion, it is a good idea for the apprentice to begin evaluating the forms of various practicing midwives so she can decide what suits her. The medical history form will vary most dramatically, depending on whether

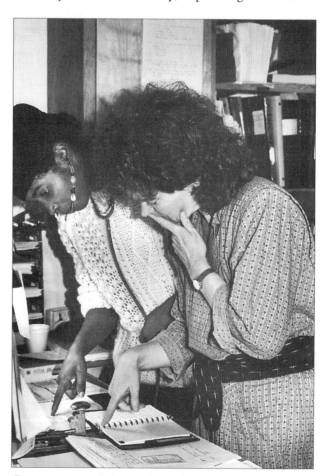

Partners review their records together.

it is formatted for take-home use or interview. Don't hesitate to patch together sections or components of various forms to create your own unique adaptations. And plan to revise your forms periodically, perhaps with your annual review of practice.

The importance of complete and accurate charting cannot be overemphasized. *A medical chart is a legal document.* In the event of a civil or malpractice suit, your chart may be your only witness to thorough and responsible caregiving. For this reason, you must carefully record everything you say and do, every assessment and recommendation, as well as all pertinent discussions between you and the parents, you and your backup physicians, you and the hospital staff.

Certain types of charting are considered the most legally defensible. For example, all your commentary should be on lined paper, and your notes should be continuous, broken only by the date and time of each assessment. Do not leave any part of a line blank; in fact, if your forms are designed with areas that might be just partially filled out, a court could find your entire chart invalid, as nothing would have prevented you from going back and adding to your notes at a later date. And never white-out or cross out information on a chart so it is unintelligible—put a straight line through it, write "error" above it, date and initial it. All contributors to a chart must identify their notes by adding their signature (first initial, last name) at the end of their entry.

There is a particular format for note-taking that is commonly taught medical students, called **SOAP charting**. These initials respectively stand for *subjective*, *objective*, *assessment*, and *plan*—all crucial aspects of caregiving essential to document.

For example, say you are confronted with a client at 26 weeks complaining of middle back pain. First, cite the mother's report as your S (subjective) finding. Then make an O (objective) determination, based on what you note by examination or observation, e.g., CVAT is present. Your A (assessment) notation would probably be suspected kidney infection, and your P (plan) would list treatment steps of urinalysis, consultation with your backup physician, follow-up appointment, etc. In some cases, SOAP may be extended to SOAPIER charting: I (implementation) refers to steps the mother will take to enact the plan; E (evaluation) is your follow-up determination; and R (reassessment) includes any recommended modifications to the plan, based on evaluation.

And yet, even SOAPIER charting may cause omissions of crucial information. Remember that it is also necessary to chart every interaction between you and the parents, your backup associates, hospital staff, and other allied health professionals. This includes not only personal interactions, but phone consultations and discussions. You must also make certain not only to chart recommended procedures or tests, but information you provided regarding attendant benefits and risks. If parents decline a suggested procedure, ask them to review your notes to that effect, and sign to verify that your notes are accurate. Some midwives work with special forms for this purpose (see forthcoming section on Informed Consent).

When doing prenatal care, be sure to make notes during each visit, rather than after it ends. Yes, this can be distracting in the midst of a passionate discussion, but unless you stop and make concrete notes in the moment, you will inevitably forget important details later on.

Keeping up with note-taking is even more difficult during labor. There may come a time in late second stage when it is virtually impossible to continue charting. Midwife Tish Demmin suggests putting strips of masking tape on your pants, jotting notes there, then transferring them to the chart as soon as possible. It is particularly important to note both time and findings of all fetal heart tone assessments.

In the event of transport, make certain to update the chart completely before arriving at the hospital. Your chart will be carefully scrutinized, possibly photocopied and made part of the woman's hospital record. It also serves as a testament to your professionalism, or lack thereof. Protect yourself by noting when you first contacted the hospital, to whom you spoke, and what they recommended. And definitely continue to make notes once you arrive—you cannot assume the hospital's charting system to be unbiased, or as accurate and complete as your own. Again, this is for your protection, though it will also be important to the parents later for purposes of debriefing their experience.

Informed consent is another crucial aspect of documentation, certainly whenever you suggest a particular test or diagnostic procedure and it is declined. Your form or statement should include: 1) risks and benefits of the suggested test or procedure; 2) alternatives, with possible consequences; 3) parents' response and plan; and 4) their signature. For example, if you recommend a non-stress test, inform the mother of risks and benefits, and chart. If she declines, chart this too, as well as all you have told her regarding risks attendant to her refusal. And should you recommend fetal kick-counts as an alternative, again list all possible risks/benefits, plus her response and plan.

Yes, this is complicated, even overwhelming for a beginner. But in our litigious society, even birth assistants have begun charting their care in hopes of protecting themselves. Why is this so important? Imagine yourself in court, facing the parents of a stillborn, postmature baby who claim, "She told us we needed a non-stress test, but didn't tell us that this might happen if we said no." Of course, none of us think this could happen to us. We tell ourselves that we screen more carefully, and maintain higher standards for communication and caregiving than the "average" midwife. But believe me, I've seen it happen to the most experienced, dedicated, and highly competent midwives, and the effects are devastating.

To this end, many midwives additionally have parents sign a *Professional Disclosure/Consent to Care* statement at the onset of the caregiving relationship. (See Chapter Two, Initial Visit, for details.) The statute of limitations runs a full three years for criminal charges, much longer for civil/malpractice suits. People change, so be prepared just in case.

However, lest we dismiss midwifery wisdom entirely, it does make a significant difference if we cultivate the best possible relationships with our clients, especially if we put them in charge of perinatal decision-making right from the start. This is now common knowledge in medical circles, and medical textbooks increasingly allude to the importance of good practitioner-patient relations in avoiding litigation.

Another important way to uphold good relations with your clients is to respect their **confidentiality** at all times. This is challenging if one of your clients hears that another had a difficult birth, and asks you to talk about it. Particularly if there is some question of why you handled the case as you did, the temptation to explain and/or defend your actions may be very strong. But nothing is worse for a woman than having her birth discussed at large! The only ethical response is to refer the curious client directly to the mother, who can tell her whatever she chooses.

Midwifery students or other associates in the practice must also agree to uphold your confidentiality policy.

PARTNERSHIP

No matter where you are located, working with a partner is the best way to practice. Midwives who work alone are very rare. If such is their style, they must prepare the mother's partner or other attendant to assist in the event of an emergency. If partnership opportunities are available, I cannot imagine why a midwife would choose to work alone unless for purely financial reasons.

Partnership is a safer way of practicing. A normal labor and delivery can be managed by one person, but if complications arise, an extra pair of skilled hands is essential. Long or difficult labors, for example, often produce a tired, mildly depressed baby and tired mother/tired uterus predisposed to hemorrhage. How well can the solitary midwife deal with both of these complications simultaneously? How can she possibly do mouth-to-mouth resuscitation on the baby and bimanual uterine compression on the mother at the same time?

Other benefits of partnership include increased comfort and ease in practicing. Partners can spell one another at births, they can fill in emotionally for each other in times of personal crisis, and they can give each other days or weeks off once in a while. Best of all, they have the opportunity to share their mutual passion for midwifery. To work in collaboration with a partner you know and trust gives you confidence in your opinions, and also

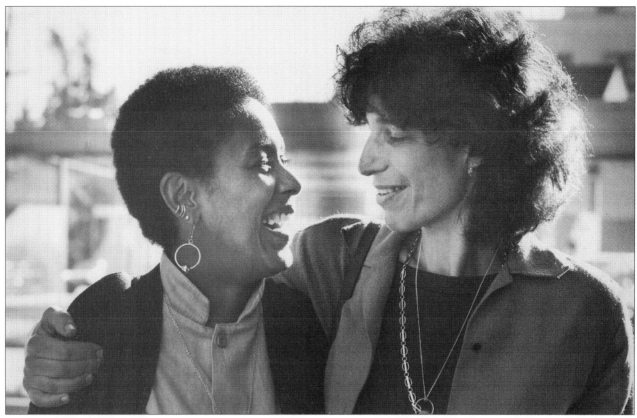

Much like a successful marriage, partnership needs nourishing.

helps you identify areas where you have trouble being objective or assertive. Working with an equal to evolve and implement creative responses to problematic situations is the supreme pleasure and power of partnership.

Of course, partners do not always agree. One may become passionately involved with a mother that the other, taking a more pragmatic view, considers at risk. Ironing out these disagreements will teach each of you about your biases and prejudices, and will help keep humility a constant for you both.

Partners need good humor and sound judgment to make their practice work. They need to respect one another's intimacies with various clients, and take pleasure in both high and low profile roles. In a successful partnership, midwives truly enjoy one another's company and respect each other, weak or strong. This sets a good example for the parents (and their supporters) who depend on them.

Let's take a look at the fiscal bottom line again, and consider several ways to make partnership work financially. One possibility is to have a student apprentice assist with prenatals, so partners can alternate their attendance. This frees each up to spend time on other activities, which may be profit-generating for them personally, or money-saving to the practice. As the apprentice becomes increasingly skilled, she can accompany one partner to births, with the other free to arrive just as delivery approaches. Alternating full-time attendance at births may not save a lot of money, but definitely saves partners time and energy.

Another possibility is to work collectively. Principles of partnership can be incorporated in a larger group practice of four or more midwives. The Bay Area Homebirth Collective in my locale is a good example. This group of five midwives each take clients of their own. They each have at least one apprentice. At the beginning of pregnancy, clients have the opportunity to meet the other partners, and to choose one as second midwife for their birth. This midwife will come to a few prenatals—definitely to the home visit with the rest of the birth team—but is not expected to attend the birth until delivery is imminent. Payment is received by the primary midwife, who uses it to handle her own business expenses and pay the second midwife several hundred dollars for her assistance.

Financial benefits of this collective structure are obvious. And think of the possibilities for taking time off! However, communication can be tricky with so many partners involved. Regular meetings are essential in order to air grievances, clear up misunderstandings, and make decisions by consensus.

TRAINING THE STUDENT/APPRENTICE

Why bother with the added responsibility of training an apprentice? There are several reasons, the most obvious being help with your practice. An apprentice can save you time and energy by monitoring early labor, assisting at prenatals, running errands, doing bookkeeping and filing, or keeping the office clean and tidy. With studies fresh in her mind, she can offer new, interesting bits of information to you and your clients. And when you are tired or worn thin, she can lend you some of her beginner's stamina and passion. With just a little guidance on your part, her enthusiasm can literally revitalize your practice.

Other benefits are less tangible, but more personally affecting. There can be deep satisfaction in transmitting your knowledge, sharing all you know. And it is quite stimulating to tailor your information to a student's needs and degree of readiness as you observe her growth. Above all, training an apprentice allows you to play a pivotal role in preserving this traditional entry route to our profession. Those of us trained by apprenticeship know that it has many advantages over other educational models. The learning process is more integrated and therefore more complete. If, as is often the case, the apprentice trains in a community where she will one day practice, she is well prepared to field the health needs and issues of her future clientele. And too, the inter-dependency of teacher and student fosters an intimacy that can be a great pleasure.

It can also be a mighty challenge. Training an apprentice requires top-notch communication based on an understanding of the developmental phases inherent in the process. Not to condescend, but the stages of parent-child relationship are remarkably similar to those of the senior midwife-apprentice configuration. They are:
1) infancy—being one;
2) childhood—being together;
3) adolescence—breaking away and being separate;
4) adulthood—being together again.

For the apprentice, the stages of falling in love are also relevant:
1) infatuation;
2) disillusionment and struggle;
3) communication and compromise;
4) mature love.

In the beginning, teacher and student are mutually pleased with the promise and excitement of their new relationship. But gradually, their differences arise; the apprentice may be disappointed that her teacher doesn't have all the answers, may not seem open to experimentation, or will not give her as much responsibility as she thinks she can handle. The senior midwife may feel that her student lacks humility or genuine dedication, expects too much too soon, or is neglecting basic chores that she did so willingly in the beginning. Power struggles may then erupt and threaten the relationship.

This adolescent phase is undoubtedly the most difficult. The apprentice may openly contradict her senior in the presence of clients, the senior may respond by withdrawing privileges, and the apprentice may threaten to leave. But if the two can hold to their original commitment, and articulate their expectations, disappointments, and needs, they may be able to see things through until the apprentice strikes out on her own. Through communication and compromise, the relationship can mature into one of mutual respect and understanding. Many a former apprentice of mine has phoned in the early months of private practice to say that she finally understood the degree of responsibility I carried, and why I was so conservative at times. At this point, teacher and student are equals.

The trouble is that many midwife/apprentice relationships never survive the adolescent/struggle phase and reach resolution. When mothering two teens, I was repeatedly advised that no matter how insulting and critical they became, I should do everything in my power to keep communication channels open. It is likewise crucial to help "adolescent" students find appropriate outlets for fulminating energies. Give your apprentice new responsibilities at this point—perhaps just a bit beyond her immediate grasp—to teach her humility and let her know her limits. At the same time, consider taking on a junior apprentice. The senior apprentice can teach the junior what she has learned; this is a perfect opportunity for her to test her wings while still being supervised.

The dynamics of this arrangement work quite well. All three attend births together, and soon, the senior apprentice begins doing deliveries under supervision, while the junior assists. This gives the senior midwife a well-deserved rest!

This break is unfortunately short lived, as the junior apprentice still has much to learn from the senior midwife. Once the senior apprentice has completed her training, you may need to set a graduation to encourage her to get out on her own. Plan to celebrate with her when she passes her licensing/certification exam. And once she is in practice, refer a few clients to her to help her get started. Or, if she decides to relocate, recommend her to other midwives or health workers in her new locale.

Growing pains are natural in the apprenticeship process. But if emotional upheaval reigns, consider implementing some structure. The Midwifery Institute of California offers a blueprint to help midwife and apprentice develop realistic timelines for skills and knowledge acquisition, with guidelines for communication and feedback. If you have no such blueprint, create your own. Give your apprentice reading and research assignments, and have her write up analyses of particularly difficult cases. Test her by oral, written, or practical examination. Your student must have ample opportunity to demonstrate her learning, so you and she can evaluate her progress at regular intervals.

In any case, it will help your apprentice tremendously if you meet with her weekly to discuss current learning objectives, and identify those that have already been met. Remember that your apprentice is there to learn, not to practice! Her responsibilities should change continuously so she can achieve proficiency in all areas.

Every senior midwife should be familiar with the various learning styles and types of intelligence she may expect to encounter in her students. As author Howard Gardner reveals in his book, *Frames of Mind*, we tend to approach our learning by employing one or more of eight intelligences. These are:

1. *verbal/linguistic*—this is learning through written and spoken language.
2. *logical mathematical*—this is deductive reason, recognition of abstract patterns.
3. *intrapersonal*—this is learning based on self-awareness, metacognition, intuition.
4. *interpersonal*—this is learning in relationship to others, based on communication.
5. *musical/rhythmical*—this is learning based on sound, tonal patterns, rhythm.
6. *body/kinesthetic*—this is body-based knowing, learning through movement.
7. *visual/spatial*—this is learning based on sight, and an ability to visualize.
8. *natural*—this is learning based in nature, on observation of natural occurrences.

With this in mind, consider presenting material to students in a variety of ways. For example, when teaching fetal heart tone patterns common during labor, provide students with written information, use diagrams to illustrate as you explain, sound out various rhythms, and suggest that students tap along to feel the beat. You probably cover these bases automatically if you have taught for a while. Interpersonal learning is facilitated by group discussion, whereas work involving student insight or self-reflection stresses intrapersonal learning. To better delineate the faculties of reason, intuition, and compassion, and to help students appreciate the interplay of these in midwifery work, read *Emotional Intelligence*, by David Goleman.

It is also important that instruction be as student-centered as possible, considering the weighty responsibilities attendant to midwifery practice. From the beginning, do whatever it takes to put the student in charge of her own learning process!

Ask her how she learns best, and whether she needs more or less structure to meet her learning objectives. Continually give her opportunities for self-evaluation. Whether one-on-one or teaching in groups, let your students be teachers. If, for example, you are explaining techniques for intramuscular injections, have your student demonstrate as you talk her through the steps, rather than doing the procedure yourself. Encourage students to be hands-on from the start!

Also thoroughly debrief students after caregiving, especially after births, by asking their experience of the event. Did anything happen that they didn't understand, or feel should have been handled differently? Challenge them to think as equals, and take the time to carefully provide both detailed information and context for their learning.

As mentioned earlier, the structure of a practice also affects the learning dynamic. There are a variety of possible practice arrangements; here is a sampling, with pros and cons:

1) *Senior midwife and single apprentice.*
   It is undeniably economical for the midwife to practice solo and pay an apprentice a slowly increasing sum concomitant to her level of responsibility. But this arrangement is extremely stressful in the early stages, when the student is new.

2) *Senior midwife and two apprentices, one senior and one junior.*
   This arrangement has been discussed already as per its value in helping the senior apprentice consolidate her learning by teaching the junior apprentice. The downside is that the two may occasionally conspire against the teacher. And training two students at once is ultimately more work and more responsibility than training just one, even though there is more opportunity to receive assistance.

3) *Two midwives and one apprentice.*
   This can be a confusing arrangement, especially if the midwives have marked differences in how they practice. Then again, the contrast can be instructive for the student, as it may keep her

from getting locked into one way of thinking or operating. Still, it is best that the apprentice be trained by one midwife primarily. It can be awfully hard on the partnership if the student attempts to curry favor by pitting her instructors against each other.

A distinct benefit of this setup is that the apprentice is strictly a student. The midwives already have the support of one another; they need not saddle the apprentice with responsibilities she may not yet be ready to handle. By the same token, they must make sure that she has ample opportunity to demonstrate her learning, and to advance at a reasonable pace.

4) *Two midwives and two apprentices.*
   This arrangement is optimal in several respects. Students not only have opportunity to observe differing styles of practice, but to compare notes. Midwives also benefit from an opportunity to compare notes, and double check their evaluations of the students. The main drawback is the complex interpersonal dynamic inherent in a practice this size. Again, it usually works best if each of the midwives takes primary responsibility for a particular student.

If you do train an apprentice from a solitary practice, you might enhance her learning by asking another midwife who is unencumbered to take her to a few births. This is especially important if you have a small practice, or if your apprentice is pressing for more experience. If you are training your apprentice through a formal program, you will need to make the appropriate arrangements for this addendum to her training. And of course, both you and the student need to discuss her goals and accomplishments with the other midwife, so everyone knows what to expect.

Training an apprentice is a lot of work, but well worth it. Once you experience the joy of teaching this way, you will probably decide to continue. In so doing, you will also make an invaluable contribution to the international effort to keep community-based apprenticeship alive and growing.

PEER REVIEW

Peer review provides a mechanism for midwives to get together and review their work. In a larger sense, peer review promotes quality assurance for consumers by encouraging safe and responsible caregiving. Exposure to the standards and practices of others in the field motivates participants to continually upgrade their knowledge and skills, so that they not only become accountable to one another, but to the profession at large.

Peer review is also known as chart review because it revolves around the discussion of difficult or challenging cases. This involves debriefing of troubling outcomes, but also presentation of unusual cases in progress. In the event of a tragic occurrence like fetal death, emergency peer review may also serve to forestall litigation and/or the spread of rumors throughout the community.

All it takes to begin peer review is a group of midwives committed to regular attendance every six to eight weeks. Six to eight participants is ideal; ten is probably maximum. Here is a description of how each midwife participates:

1. She states the number of normal births attended since the last meeting;
2. She reports fully on any births with complications, including her assessment of what might have been done differently;
3. She mentions all prenatal cases with risk factors, including those referred to another provider;
4. She takes feedback from the group.

Since quality assurance is a major goal of peer review, it may be necessary to schedule educational workshops as follow-up.

Probably the greatest benefit of peer review is self-regulation, i.e., it provides a way for the midwifery profession to take care of itself. Many states offering midwifery licensing or certification either require or recommend peer review on an ongoing basis. This is because discipline through state bureaucratic channels is notoriously slow and encumbered by red tape. Peer review has also become increasingly popular with physician groups, in response to the malpractice crisis. It is one way to weed out incompetent or irresponsible providers.

Peer review may also help defend a midwife who has been unjustly accused of malpractice or other wrongdoing. My local group once called an emergency meeting to address a case where the parents were dissatisfied with their outcome and had threatened to sue the midwife. After receiving written testimony from both sides, we found in favor of the midwife, at the same time making recommendations to help her avoid a similar occurrence in the future. We then issued a public statement supporting her management of the case, and no further action was taken by the parents. This process is particularly efficacious if dissatisfied clients are talking around town.

On the other hand, lack of consumer participation in peer review may be seriously at odds with our goal of woman-centered caregiving. New Zealand midwife and political activist Joan Donely has espoused the merits of involving consumers in virtually every aspect of midwifery regulation, including annual review of standards, chart review, conflict resolution, and disciplinary proceedings. She considers this essential to counteract the historical tendency of professions that self-regulate to become self-serving and elitist.

It takes some courage to participate in peer review at first, especially if you have been isolated in your work. It is normal to fear that no other midwife thinks or does as you do, when in fact most midwives operate from a common base of knowledge and experience. Peer review will improve both your practice and your communication with other midwives.

Student Evaluation: Assessment and Management Abilities

Antepartum Management

A. *Obtains and records all data necessary for evaluation and risk assessment of the client/couple:*

1. menstrual history _____

2. medical, surgical history _____

3. family history _____

4. obstetrical history _____

5. current medications _____

B. *At each prenatal visit, reviews chart for:*

1. previous findings _____

2. laboratory data _____

3. treatment and effectiveness of previous management. _____

C. *Evaluates the present status of client including:*

1. determination of emotional well-being _____

2. laboratory data _____

3. recognition of need for genetic counseling _____

4. obtaining and interpreting appropriate laboratory and
   diagnostic tests and procedures _____

D. *Assumes direct responsibility for the development of a comprehensive, supportive plan of care for the client, with the client's participation* _____

E. *Implements plan of care:*

1. Interprets findings to client accurately, and in a way
   comprehensible to client _____

2. Determines client's reaction to findings _____

3. Acquaints client with alternative plans when possible
   and determines client's preferences _____

4. Encourages client to assume responsibility for her own health _____

5. Prepares a defined needs/problems list with participation from client _____

6. Evaluates, with corroboration from client, the achievement of
   health care goals and modifies plan of care appropriately _____

7. Consults, collaborates with, and refers to appropriate members
   of the health care team _____

Management of Labor and Delivery

A. *Obtains history since last prenatal visit completely and accurately* _____

B. *Assesses maternal condition:*

    1. Differentiates phases of labor by observing client _____

    2. Shares information with client about care provided:

        a. explains examination procedures _____

        b. preparation for exams _____

        c. interpretation of clinical findings _____

    3. Provides appropriate support for each stage of labor _____

    4. Recognizes abnormal progress in labor _____

    5. Consults with appropriate members of the health care team regarding any abnormalities during the course of labor _____

C. *Recognizes emergency situations and responds effectively:*

    1. Initiates emergency measures _____

    2. Reevaluates and modifies emergency treatment as indicated _____

    3. Transports in a professional manner _____

Immediate Postpartum

A. *Assesses maternal condition, including:*

    1. Emotional status/bonding _____

    2. Physical stability _____

    3. Initiation of breast-feeding _____

B. *Assesses newborn condition, including:*

    1. Physical adjustment _____

    2. General appearance and behavior _____

C. *Develops a plan of comprehensive, supportive care with client/family during the immediate postpartum period* _____

D. *Implements plan of care:*

    1. Provides complete postpartum instructions _____

    2. Supports initial family adjustments _____

    3. Leaves a stable environment _____

E. *Recognizes signs of maternal and/or neonatal abnormality and consults or refers to appropriate members of the health care team* _____

Subsequent Postpartum

A. *Facilitates postpartum adjustments and continues to provide supportive, responsive care:*

1. Makes follow-up visits as frequently as indicated _____

2. Performs maternal exam at appropriate intervals to insure normalcy and healing, including involution and lochia flow _____

3. Makes appropriate suggestions for minor postpartum problems _____

4. Supports mother and baby in establishing breastfeeding and makes appropriate recommendations and referrals _____

5. Recognizes problems with breastfeeding and makes appropriate recommendations and referrals _____

6. Provides support and guidance for postpartum emotional changes and makes appropriate referrals _____

B. *Helps client/family identify postpartum health care needs and discusses with them the following:*

1. Aspects of sexuality during the postpartum period _____

2. Available methods of contraception, with referrals _____

3. Newborn care _____

4. Community resources available to new families _____

C. *Demonstrates understanding and supportive skills necessary to help families cope with malformed infants, mental retardation, fetal or neonatal death* _____

Recording and Charting

A. *Enters notations accurately and completely* _____

B. *Enters notations concisely and legibly* _____

C. *Clearly communicates plan of management to other appropriate care providers* _____

_____

CHAPTER 9

The Long Run

This final chapter will focus on the midwife again, this time in terms of the many adaptations involved in continued practice. No doubt about it, midwifery is a way of life, both grueling and transformative. The intensive and unpredictable nature of this work soon persuades the novice that midwifery is much more than the joy of catching babies. It works a woman on all levels, either disintegrating her or bringing her to essence.

In optimal caregiving, the assessment process works both ways. In order to entrust themselves to her care, the parents will scrutinize the midwife most carefully: her appearance, personality, and character. At the same time, she works to address their needs, and encourage their disclosure by being candid and forthcoming. Thus each prenatal visit provides an opportunity to deepen communication and develop trust by sharing impressions, thoughts, and feelings. But this doesn't afford the midwife much privacy, and so can be draining at times.

In contrast, an overzealous beginner may get so carried away by the thrill of caregiving that she intimidates clients with her thoughts and opinions. There is a big difference between compulsive caregiving and genuine service, the latter being based on discretion and appropriate involvement. In order to render service, the midwife must be sensitive enough to pick up her cues and respond without ego. She must also have a healthy sense of self unrelated to the practice of midwifery.

Take this premise a step further, and observe the difference between making assessments and passing judgment. It is easy to pass judgement at the threshold of our limitations, particularly on some-

one who inadvertently reveals them by leaving our expectations unmet. In contrast, a clear-headed ability to make assessments has no strings attached, and is the key to a sane and enduring practice.

Midwives sometimes play roles of ascetic, madonna, or super-sleuth in the attempt to sustain an unselfish orientation to their work. A steady diet of spontaneity and discretion demands maturity; it helps if the midwife has faced some of her demons and has developed a sense of humor. Still, many fine midwives struggle with some role-playing in the beginning, and quickly outgrow it as they are increasingly thrown back on their own resources.

What many beginners don't realize is that midwifery will affect every aspect of their lives. There may be major upheavals in love, particularly if the midwife's partner does not feel ready or willing to communicate in ways she finds imperative in order to practice effectively. Men often feel the midwife's intensity as pressure to go deeper, look further, be more involved in life than they might otherwise desire, implicit in her character and way of speaking, touching, nurturing. It's been said repeatedly that "midwifery is the acid test of a relationship," and there is certainly truth in this.

The midwife's partner sometimes feels jealous or threatened if his/her way of making a living seems less principled or dynamic than hers. This may necessitate a review of their personal and professional goals, both long and short term. By the same token, it is crucially important that the midwife acknowledge the incredible demands her work places on her partner, as well as the stresses placed on her family. Running off at inopportune

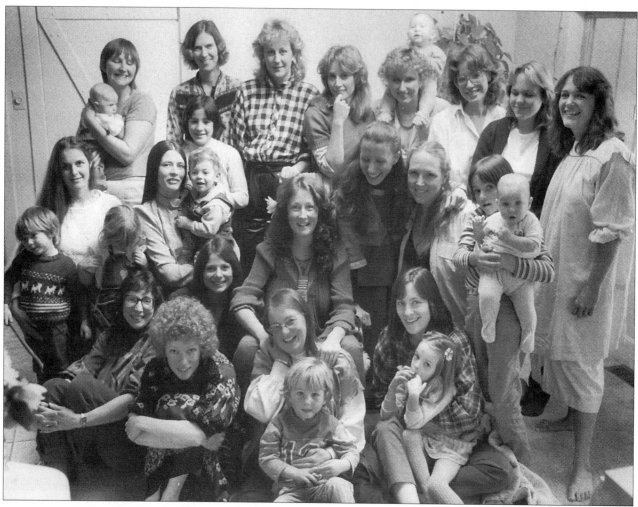

A pregnant midwife, surrounded by friends and former clients at a celebration in her honor.

moments can be hard on small children, and really rough on the nursing baby. Not to mention the obvious; more than once I've been interrupted by an emergency phone call in the middle of a love-making that was fantastic, or sorely needed. In fact, the phone rings constantly, much to the chagrin of my family. Occasionally I've found myself saying as I reach for the receiver, "Don't let this be a heavy one" or even half seriously, "I hope no one's in labor." Usually this is because my children need attention, my partner needs love, I have shopping, cleaning, or paperwork to do, or want simply to relax without interruptions. Being on-call means keeping one's self, home, and family in a constant state of readiness. All midwives should consider (and reconsider) limiting their practice to a level that is workable overall. If doing home births, this is generally around four to six births a month,

which allows time to integrate the lessons of each birth experience, catch up on sleep, get the family back in order, and generally rejuvenate before going on.

It's interesting to note how principles of smooth labor and birth also apply to smooth practice. The plateau phenomenon, or stopping to integrate, is basic to midwifery work. The frustration of trying to make labor fit a preconceived pattern is similar to that experienced by the midwife if she tries to make her practice develop quickly, or be of a certain size. And just as there comes a time with delivery when the mother must stop pushing, the midwife must also know when to ease up and let life happen. Even though birth teaches potent lessons in this regard, there is a continual battle of impatience versus forbearance at play in the midwife's psyche.

Every midwife needs some way to help herself when she is floundering. She needs to learn how to take as well as give, to humble herself to wise counsel, to be receptive to her partner, and to listen well to the experience of other midwives. Mostly though, she needs to be able to heal herself through her own recuperative powers. Intrinsic to midwifery practice is the development of self-reflective and intuitive abilities. At first, the midwife may feel rather uncomfortable as hunches and precognitions play themselves out in her work and life. But this is part of a long tradition of women's ways of knowing, crucial for handling the challenges of safe and individualized care.

Part of the task of nurturing psychic faculties and protecting the delicacy in oneself as these emerge is to take time for relaxation and emotional free-flow in day-to-day life. Finding time for solitude and reflection may be difficult with young children, but may be easier to manage if incorporated from the beginning. A student of mine recently shared a memory of how her mother routinely sent her and her siblings off for naps after lunch, no matter how old they got. Eventually, it dawned on her that no one was sleeping, that her mother knew this and it was alright. She soon learned to treasure the total privacy of this time, and the freedom to do whatever she wanted. Meanwhile, her mother was reading, relaxing, and otherwise taking care of herself.

In other words, midwifery practice requires the art of energy conservation. Otherwise, the midwife may find herself in a tough situation where the appropriate course of action is perfectly clear, but she lacks the strength to carry it out. It is said that for human beings, power is a natural enemy; in midwifery practice, it is power derived from increasing clarity that can lead us beyond our capacity.

Overextension, even when the calling is clear, is bound to create trouble. To avoid this pitfall, cultivate the ability to delegate responsibility to students, apprentices, and other midwives. Opportunities for involvement will only increase as you become more powerful and articulate. Learn to work to your capacity, and then, to say no.

Another way to conserve energy is to pass clients along whenever you find yourself at case load capacity. Be aware that the number of clients you can handle will vary from time to time, depending on other obligations. Learn to recognize signs of burnout, such as faulty communication with your clients or peers, general distraction or absent-mindedness, or in progressed cases, borderline hysteria. Without exception, midwives need regular vacations! In order to get away, you must set up a support system strong enough to allow for your absence. But if you are tired and run down, nothing can take the place of a good long escape from the beeper, phone, or piled-up correspondence.

It is also important for the midwife to develop her professional identity. Join local, state, and national midwifery organizations, and participate on a regular basis. This can help you overcome feelings of isolation, particularly if you practice rurally. Or if you work in a competitive or combative environment, contact with a larger circle of midwives can help you rise above petty concerns and recall your original dedication to your work. I remember the first time I attended a national midwifery convention—what an incredible awakening of identity and purpose! It was also reassuring to find that midwives had similar levels of passion and commitment, no matter where they lived.

As states continue to formalize standards for continuing education, attendance at midwifery conferences becomes mandatory. This benefits the midwife by helping her stay abreast of the latest information, which may inspire her to try new approaches in her work.

Another possible solution for burnout is to try a new form of practicing. Particularly if you have been working with an assistant only, consider forming a partnership or joining a group practice. This can alleviate stress and help you regain your strength and perspective.

Sometimes midwives forget to use their knowledge of health-promoting practices in their own lives. For example, nutrition should be optimal on clinic days, and in the midst of a long labor watch. Sometimes the mental deliberations regarding a complicated pregnancy or forthcoming labor can take so much energy that extra sleep is required.

Stress reduction techniques, relaxant herbal remedies, massage therapy, and regular exercise all have an important place in the midwife's daily life.

Maintaining yourself in a healthy condition also means learning to separate threads of your personal problems from those belonging to others. Often, this happens less by rational process than by contemplative reflection. If your mind is fully relaxed, revelations are apt to occur. And this brings us to the crux of the matter—the need for midwives to "bottom out" and get down to essence periodically.

Emptying yourself of thoughts and feelings makes room for insight and new direction. This is so important! Although midwifery is ideally a blend of service and self-expression, the high-stress demands of practice definitely interfere with healthy narcissism. Developing personal interests, new skills, talent, and artistry is simply essential. A midwife's prime offering to others is her unique-

ness, her independent perspective. In order to keep this alive, it must be nourished. The midwife should take pleasure in many things, and have the ability to relate broadly. She must be willing to be repeatedly reborn, to be both transformed and transformer.

Take care not to become jaded as you become seasoned in practice. Just when you think you have seen it all, some totally new configuration occurs to set you back on your heels, and teach you humility all over again. Tune up your sensitivities so intuitive directives keep coming through, and be grateful for higher intelligence.

In the end, what is at the heart of our work? What makes the difference in crisis, and keeps us coming back for more? Pure and simple, it is the transformative power of love. No matter where midwifery takes you, do not forget this! Be who you are, and do what you can to keep your love alive.

SUPPORT YOUR LOCAL MIDWIFE!

Here are some suggestions for keeping midwifery alive in your community:

1. Since the midwife's fee is usually modest, consider giving her a bonus if you can possibly afford it. All told, the average midwife makes less than ten dollars an hour! In contrast, consider the astronomical amount charged for a physician's limited services. Particularly if your midwife assisted you above and beyond her usual duties, pay her accordingly.

2. If you cannot afford to pay extra, you might offer to help your midwife with childcare, clerical work, or housekeeping. In the past, midwives were totally supported by their communities, with all their personal and material needs completely met. Traditionally, midwives have been older women, already past childbearing and unburdened with family responsibilities. But today, due to the practice's recent resurgence, midwives are coming from the younger generation. This is why helping them with housework or childcare is so important. Even if

you are only able to volunteer once, it will be greatly appreciated.

3. Understand that in many states, midwives are under fire politically and may need support for legislative efforts. Contact your local or state midwifery association to see how you can help. Perhaps you can send a note to your local Congressional representative, make a donation, write a letter to the editor of your newspaper, or help organize a public event. Let everyone know how much having a midwife meant to you!

4. Tell your friends all about midwifery and out of hospital birth. Read to them from books or articles, and refer them to appropriate reading material. Solicit their questions, and inspire them with your passion. Move them to investigate alternatives, and make informed decisions. With your help, midwifery will not only survive, but flourish!

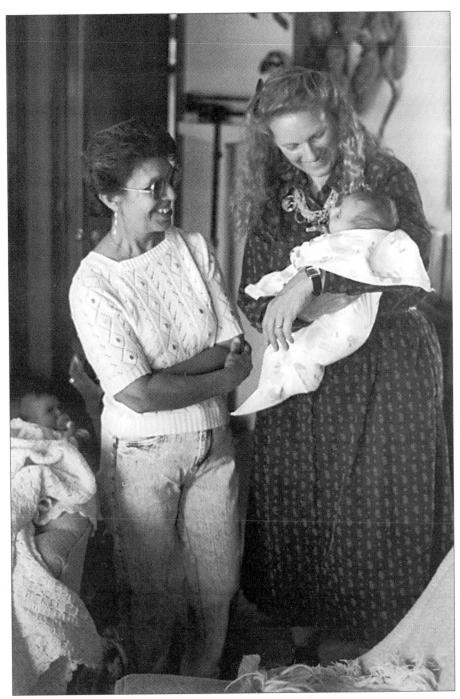

Midwife Elizabeth Gilmore, cradling a baby born at her birth center.

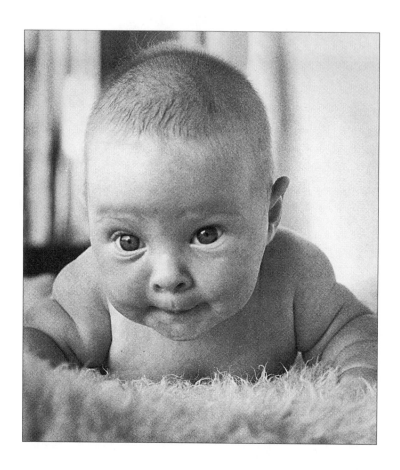

APPENDIX A

The MANA Statement of Values and Ethics

We, as midwives, have a responsibility to educate ourselves and others regarding our values and ethics and to reflect them in our practices. Our exploration of ethical midwifery is a critical reflection of moral issues as they pertain to maternal/child health on every level. This statement is intended to provide guidance for professional conduct in the practice of midwifery, as well as for MANA's policy making, thereby promoting quality care for childbearing families. MANA recognizes this document as an open, ongoing articulation of our evolution regarding values and ethics.

First, we recognize that values often go unstated and yet our ethics (how we act), proceed directly from a foundation of values. Since what we hold precious, that is, what we value, fuses and informs our ethical decisions and actions, the Midwives Alliance of North America wishes to explicitly affirm our values[1] as follows:

I. Woman as an Individual with Unique Value and Worth
A. We value women and their creative, life-affirming and life-giving powers which find expression in a diversity of ways.
B. We value a woman's right to make choices regarding all aspects of her life.

II. Mother and Baby as Whole
A. We value the oneness of the pregnant mother and her unborn child; an inseparable and independent whole.
B. We value the birth experience as a rite of passage; the sentient and sensitive nature of the newborn; and the right of each baby to be born in a caring and loving manner, without separation from mother and family.
C. We value the integrity of a woman's body and the right of each woman and baby to be totally supported in their efforts to achieve a natural, spontaneous vaginal birth.
D. We value the breastfeeding relationship as the ideal way of nourishing and nurturing the newborn.

III. The Nature of Birth
A. We value the essential mystery of birth.[2]
B. We value pregnancy and birth as natural processes that technology will never supplant.[3]
C. We value the integrity of life's experiences; the physical, emotional, mental, psychological and spiritual components of a process are inseparable.
D. We value pregnancy and birth as personal, intimate, internal, sexual, and social events to be shared in the environment and with the attendants a woman chooses.[4]
E. We value the learning experiences of life and birth.
F. We value pregnancy and birth as processes which have lifelong impact on a woman's self esteem, her health, her ability to nurture, and her personal growth.

---

[1] *The membership largely agrees with the values that follow. However, some may word them differently or may leave out a few. This document is intended to prompt personal reflection and clarification, not to represent absolute opinions.*

[2] *Mystery is defined as something that has not or cannot be explained or understood, the quality or state of being incomprehensible or inexplicable; a tenet which cannot be understood in terms of human reason.*

[3] *Supplant means to supersede by force or cunning; to take the place of.*

[4] *In this context internal refers to the fact that birth happens within the body and psyche of the woman; ultimately she and only she can give birth.*

IV. The Art of Midwifery

A. We value our right to practice the art of midwifery. We value our work as an ancient vocation of women which has existed as long as humans have lived on earth.

B. We value expertise which incorporates academic knowledge, clinical skill, intuitive judgment and spiritual awareness.[5]

C. We value all forms of midwifery education and acknowledge the ongoing wisdom of apprenticeship as the original model for training midwives.

D. We value the art of nurturing the intrinsic normalcy of birth and recognize that each woman and baby have parameters of well-being unique unto themselves.

E. We value the empowerment of women in all aspects of life and particularly as that strength is realized during pregnancy, birth and thereafter. We value the art of encouraging the open expression of that strength so women can birth unhindered and confident in their abilities and in our support.

F. We value skills which support a complicated pregnancy or birth to move toward a state of greater well-being or to be brought to the most healing conclusion possible. We value the art of letting go.[6]

G. We value the acceptance of death as a possible outcome of birth. We value our focus as supporting rather than avoiding death.[7]

H. We value standing for what we believe in in the face of social and political oppression.

V. Woman as Mother:

A. We value a mother's intuitive knowledge of herself and her baby before, during and after birth.[8]

B. We value a woman's innate ability to nurture her pregnancy and birth her baby; the power and beauty of her body as it grows and the awesome strength summoned in labor.

C. We value the mother as the only direct care provider for her unborn child.[9]

D. We value supporting women in a non-judgmental way, whatever their state of physical, emotional, social or spiritual health. We value the broadening of available resources whenever possible so that the desired goals of health, happiness and personal growth are realized according to women's needs and perceptions.

E. We value the right of each woman to choose a care giver appropriate to her needs and compatible with her belief systems.

F. We value pregnancy and birth as rites of passage integral to a woman's evolution into mothering.

G. We value the potential of partners, family and community to support women in all aspects of birth and mothering.[10]

---

[5] *An expert is one whose knowledge and skill is specialized and profound, especially as the result of practical experience.*

[6] *This addresses our desire for an uncomplicated birth whenever possible and recognizes that there are times when it is impossible. That is to say, a woman may be least traumatized to have a cesarean and a live birth, but a spontaneous vaginal birth, in this case, is not possible. We let go of that goal to achieve the possibility of a healthy baby. Likewise, the situation where parents choose to allow a very ill, premature or deformed infant to die in their arms rather than being subjected to multiple surgeries, separations, and ICU stays. This too, is letting go of the normal for the most healing choice possible within the framework of the parent's ethics given the circumstances. What is most healing will, of course, vary from individual to individual.*

[7] *We place the emphasis of our care on supporting life (preventative measures, good nutrition, emotional health, etc.) and not pathology, diagnosis, treatment of problems, or heroic solutions in an attempt to preserve life at any cost of quality.*

[8] *This addresses the medical model's tendency to ignore a woman's sense of well-being or danger in many aspects of health care, but particularly in regard to her pregnancy.*

[9] *This acknowledges that the thrust of our care centers on the mother, her health, her well-being, her nutrition, her habits, her emotional balance and, in turn, the baby benefits. This view is diametrically opposed to the medical model which often attempts to care for the fetus/baby while dismissing or even excluding the mother.*

[10] *While partners, other family members, and a woman's larger community can and often do provide her with vital support, in using the word potential we wish to acknowledge that many women find themselves pregnant and mothering in abusive and unsafe environments.*

VI. The Nature of Relationship:

A. We value relationship. The quality, integrity, equality and uniqueness of our interactions inform and critique our choices and decisions.

B. We value honesty in relationship.

C. We value caring for women to the best of our ability without prejudice against their age, race, religion, culture, sexual orientation, physical abilities, or socioeconomic background.

D. We value the concept of personal responsibility and the right of individuals to make choices regarding what they deem best for themselves. We value the right to true informed choice, not merely informed consent to what we think is best.

E. We value our relationship to a process larger than ourselves, recognizing that birth is something we can seek to learn from and know, but never control.

F. We value humility in our work.

G. We value the recognition of our own limits and limitations.

H. We value direct access to information readily understood by all.

I. We value sharing information and our understanding about birth experiences, skills, and knowledge.

J. We value the midwifery community as a support system and an essential place of learning and sisterhood.

K. We value diversity among midwives; recognizing that it broadens our collective resources and challenges us to work for greater understanding of birth and each other.

L. We value mutual trust and respect, which grows from a realization of all of the above.

Making decisions and acting ethically:

These values reflect our feelings regarding how we frame midwifery in our hearts and minds. However, due to the broad range of geographic, religious, cultural, political, educational and personal backgrounds among our membership, how we act based on these values will be very individual. Acting ethically is a complex merging of our values and these background influences combined with the relationship we have to others who may be involved in the process taking place. We call upon all these resources when deciding how to respond in the moment to each situation.

We acknowledge the limitations of ethical codes which present a list of rules which must be followed, recognizing that such a code may interfere with, rather than enhance, our ability to make judgments, and we must have adequate information; with all of these an appeal to a code becomes superfluous. Furthermore, when we set up rigid ethical codes we may begin to cease considering the transformations we go through as a result of our choices as well as negate our wish to foster truly diversified practice. Rules are not something we can appeal to when all else fails. However, this is the illusion fostered by traditional codes of ethics.[11] MANA's support of the individual's moral integrity grows out of an understanding that there cannot possibly be one right answer for all situations.

We acknowledge the following basic concepts and believe that ethical judgments can be made with these thoughts in mind:

• Moral agency and integrity are born within the heart of each individual.

• Judgments are fundamentally based on awareness and understanding of ourselves and others and are primarily derived from ones own sense of moral integrity with reference to clearly articulated values. Becoming aware and increasing our understanding are on-going processes facilitated by our efforts at personal growth on every level. The wisdom gained by this process cannot be taught or dictated but one can learn to realize, experience and evaluate it.

---

11 Hoagland, Sarah, paraphrased from her book *Lesbian Ethics.*

- The choices we can or will actually make may be limited by the oppressive nature of the medical, legal or cultural framework in which we live. The more our values conflict with those of the dominant culture, the more risky it becomes to act truly in accord with our values.
- The pregnant woman and midwife are both individual moral agents unique unto themselves, having independent value and worth.
- We support ourselves and the women and families we serve to follow and make known the dictates of our own conscience as our relationship begins, evolves and especially when decisions must be made which impact us or the care being provided. It is up to all of us to work out a mutually satisfactory relationship when and if that is possible.

It is useful to understand the two basic theories upon which moral judgments and decision making processes are based. These processes become particularly important when one considers that in our profession, a given woman's rights may not be absolute in all cases, or in certain situations the woman may not be considered autonomous or competent to make her own decisions.

One of the main theories of ethics states that one should look to the consequences of the act (i.e. the outcome) and not the act itself to determine if it is appropriate care. This point of view looks for the greatest good for the greatest number. The other primary ethical theory states that one should look to the act itself (i.e. type of care provided) and if it is right, then this could override the net outcome. This is a more process oriented, feminist perspective. As midwives we weave these two perspectives in the process of making decisions in our practices. Since the outcome of pregnancy is ultimately an unknown and is always unknowable, it is inevitable that in certain circumstances our best decisions in the moment will lead to consequences we could not foresee.

In summary, acting ethically is facilitated by:

- Carefully defining our values.
- Weighing our values in consideration with those of the community of midwives, families, and culture in which we find ourselves.
- Acting in accord with our values to the best of our ability as the situation demands.
- Engaging in on-going self-examination and evaluation.

There are both individual and social implications to any decision making process. The actual rules and oppressive aspects of a society are never exact, and therefore conflicts may arise and we must weigh which choices or obligations take precedence over others. There are inevitably times when resolution does not occur and we will be unable to make peace with any course of action or may feel conflicted about a choice already made. The community of women, both midwives and those we serve, will provide a fruitful resource for continued moral support and guidance.

Bibliography:
Cross, Star, MANA Ethics Chair, 1989, unpublished draft of MANA Ethics code.
Daly, Mary, *GynEcology: The Metaethics of Radical Feminism*, Beacon Press, Boston, 1978.
Hoagland, Sarah Lucia, *Lesbian Ethics: Toward New Value*, Institute of Lesbian Studies, Palo Alto, CA, 1988.
Johnson, Sonia, *Going Out of Our Minds: The Metaphysics of Liberation*, Crossing Press, Freedom, CA 1987.

MANA CORE-COMPETENCIES FOR MIDWIFERY PRACTICE

Guiding Principles of Practice

The midwife provides care according to the following principles:

A. Midwives work in partnership with women and their chosen support community throughout the care-giving relationship.

B. Midwives respect the dignity, rights and the ability of the women they serve to act responsibly throughout the care-giving relationship.

C. Midwives work as autonomous practitioners, collaborating with other health and social service providers when necessary.

D. Midwives understand that physical, emotional, psycho-social and spiritual factors synergistically comprise the health of individuals and affect the childbearing process.

E. Midwives understand that female physiology and childbearing are normal processes, and work to optimize the well-being of mothers and their developing babies as the foundation of care-giving.

F. Midwives understand that the childbearing experience is primarily a personal, social and community event.

G. Midwives recognize that a woman is the only direct care provider for herself and her unborn baby; thus the most important determinant of a healthy pregnancy is the mother herself.

H. Midwives recognize the empowerment inherent in the childbearing experience and strive to support women to make informed decisions and take responsibility for their own well-being.

I. Midwives strive to ensure vaginal birth and provide guidance and support when appropriate to facilitate the spontaneous processes of pregnancy, labor and birth, utilizing medical intervention only as necessary.

J. Midwives synthesize clinical observations, theoretical knowledge, intuitive assessment and spiritual awareness as components of a competent decision making process.

K. Midwives value continuity of care throughout the childbearing cycle and strive to maintain continuous care within realistic limits.

L. Midwives understand that the parameters of "normal" vary widely and recognize that each pregnancy and birth is unique.

General Knowledge and Skills:

I. The midwife provides care incorporating certain concepts, skills and knowledge from a variety of health and social sciences, including but not limited to:

A. Communication, counseling and teaching skills.

B. Human anatomy and physiology relevant to childbearing.

C. Community standards of care for women and their developing infants during the childbearing cycle, including midwifery and bio-technical medical standards and the rationale for and limitations of such standards.

D. Health and social resources in her community.

E. Significance of and methods for documentation of care through the childbearing cycle.

F. Informed decision making.

G. The principles and appropriate application of clean and aseptic technique and universal precautions.

H. The selection, use and care of the tools and other equipment employed in midwifery care.

I.   Human sexuality, including indications of common problems and indications for counseling.
J.   Ethical considerations relevant to reproductive health.
K.   The grieving process.
L.   Knowledge of cultural variations.
M.   Knowledge of common medical terms.
N.   The ability to develop, implement and evaluate an individualized plan for midwifery care.
O.   Woman-centered care, including the relationship between the mother, infant and their larger support community.
P.   Knowledge of various health care modalities[12] as they apply to the childbearing cycle.

Care During Pregnancy

II. The midwife provides health care, support and information to women throughout pregnancy. She determines the need for consultation or referral as appropriate. The midwife uses a foundation of knowledge and/or skill which includes the following:

A.   Identification, evaluation and support of maternal and fetal well-being throughout the process of pregnancy.
B.   Education and counseling for the childbearing cycle.
C.   Preexisting conditions in a woman's health history which are likely to influence her well-being when she becomes pregnant.
D.   Nutritional requirements of pregnant women and methods of nutritional assessment and counseling.
E.   Changes in emotional, psycho-social and sexual variations that may occur during pregnancy.
F.   Environmental and occupational hazards for pregnant women.
G.   Methods of diagnosing pregnancy.
H.   Basic understanding of genetic factors which may indicate the need for counseling, testing or referral.
I.   Basic understanding of the growth and development of the unborn baby.
J.   Indications for, and the risks and benefits of bio-technical screening methods and diagnostic tests used during pregnancy.
K.   Anatomy, physiology and evaluation of the soft and bony structure of the pelvis.
L.   Palpation skills for evaluation of the fetus and uterus.
M.   The causes, assessment and treatment of the common discomforts of pregnancy.
N.   Identification of, implications of and appropriate treatment for various infections, disease conditions and other problems which may affect pregnancy.
O.   Special needs of the Rh- woman.

Care During Labor, Birth and Immediately Thereafter

III. The midwife provides health care, support and information to women throughout labor, birth and the hours immediately thereafter. She determines the need for consultation or referral as appropriate. The midwife uses a foundation of knowledge and/or skill which includes the following:

A.   The normal processes of labor and birth.
B.   Parameters and methods for evaluating maternal and fetal well-being during labor, birth and immediately thereafter, including relevant historical data.

---

[12] *Health care modalities may include but are not limited to such practices as bio-technical medicine, homeopathy, naturopathy, herbology, Chinese medicine, chiropractic, etc.*

C. Assessment of the birthing environment, assuring that it is clean, safe and supportive, and that appropriate equipment and supplies are on hand.

D. Emotional responses and their impact during labor, birth and immediately thereafter.

E. Comfort and support measures during labor, birth and immediately thereafter.

F. Fetal and maternal anatomy and their interactions as relevant to assessing fetal position and progress of labor.

G. Techniques to assist and support the spontaneous vaginal birth of the baby and placenta.

H. Fluid and nutritional requirements during labor, birth and immediately thereafter.

I. Assessment of and support for maternal rest and sleep as appropriate during the process of labor, birth and immediately thereafter.

J. Causes of, evaluation of and appropriate treatment for variations which occur during the course of labor, birth and immediately thereafter.

K. Emergency measures and transport procedures for critical problems arising during labor, birth or immediately thereafter.

L. Understanding of and appropriate support for the newborn's transition during the first minutes and hours following birth.

M. Familiarity with current bio-technical interventions and technologies which may be commonly used in a medical setting.

N. Evaluation and care of the perineum and surrounding tissues.

Postpartum Care:

IV. The midwife provides health care, support and information to women throughout the postpartum period. She determines the need for consultation or referral as appropriate. The midwife uses a foundation of knowledge and/or skill which includes but is not limited to the following:

A. Anatomy and physiology of the mother during the postpartum period.

B. Lactation support and appropriate breast care including evaluation of, identification of and treatment for problems with nursing.

C. Parameters of and methods for evaluating and promoting maternal well-being during the postpartum period.

D. Causes of, evaluation of and treatment for maternal discomforts during the postpartum period.

E. Emotional, psycho-social and sexual variations during the postpartum period.

F. Maternal nutritional requirements during the postpartum period including methods of nutritional evaluation and counseling.

G. Causes of, evaluation of and treatment for problems arising during the postpartum period.

H. Support, information and referral for family planning methods as the individual woman desires.

Newborn Care:

V. The entry-level midwife provides health care to the newborn during the postpartum period and support and information to parents regarding newborn care. She determines the need for consultation or referral as appropriate. The midwife uses a foundation of knowledge and/or skill which includes the following:

A. Anatomy, physiology and support of the newborn's adjustment during the first days and weeks of life.

B. Parameters and methods for evaluating newborn wellness including relevant historical data and gestational age.

   C. Nutritional needs of the newborn.

   D. Community standards and state laws regarding indications for, administration of and the risks and benefits of prophylactic bio-technical treatments and screening tests commonly used during the neonatal period.

   E. Causes of, assessment of, appropriate treatment and emergency measures for newborn problems and abnormalities.

Professional, Legal and Other Aspects:

VI. The entry-level midwife assumes responsibility for practicing in accord with the principles outlined in this document. The midwife uses a foundation of knowledge and/or skill which includes the following:

   A. MANA's documents concerning the art and practice of midwifery.

   B. The purpose and goal of MANA and local (state and provincial) midwifery associations.

   C. The principles and practice of data collection as relevant to midwifery practice.

   D. Laws governing the practice of midwifery in her local jurisdiction.

   E. Various sites, styles and modes of practice within the larger midwifery community.

   F. A basic understanding of maternal/child health care delivery systems in her local jurisdiction.

   G. Awareness of the need for midwives to share their knowledge and experience.

Well-Woman Care and Family Planning:

VII. Depending upon education and training, the entry-level midwife may provide family planning and well-woman care. The practicing midwife may also choose to meet the following core competencies with additional training. In either case, the midwife provides care, support and information to women regarding their overall reproductive health, using a foundation of knowledge and/or skill which includes the following:

   A. Understanding of the normal life cycle of women.

   B. Evaluation of the woman's well-being including relevant historical data.

   C. Causes of, evaluation of and treatments for problems associated with the female reproductive system and breasts.

   D. Information on, provision of or referral for various methods of contraception.

   E. Issues involved in decision-making regarding unwanted pregnancies and resources for counseling and referral.

APPENDIX A

MANA STANDARDS AND QUALIFICATIONS FOR THE ART AND PRACTICE OF MIDWIFERY

The midwife recognizes that childbearing is a woman's experience and encourages the active involvement of family members in her care.

1. **Skills:** Necessary skills of a practicing midwife include the ability to:

    -   Provide continuity of care to the woman and her family during the maternity cycle, continuing inter-conceptionally throughout the childbearing years;
    -   Assess and provide care for healthy women in antepartal, intrapartal, postpartal and neonatal periods;
    -   Identify and assess deviations from normal;
    -   Maintain proficiency in life-saving measures by regular review and practice; and
    -   Deal with emergency situations appropriately.
    -   In addition, a midwife may choose to provide well-woman care.

    It is affirmed that judgment and intuition play a role in competent assessment and response.

2. **Appropriate equipment:** Midwives are equipped to assess maternal, fetal and newborn well-being; to maintain a clean and/or aseptic technique; to treat maternal hemorrhage; and to resuscitate mother or infant.

3. **Records:** Midwives keep accurate records of care provided for each woman such as are acceptable in current midwifery practice. Records shall be held confidential and provided to the woman on request.

4. **Data Collection:** Midwives collect data for their practice on a regular basis. It is highly recommended that this be done prospectively, following the guidelines and using the data form developed by the MANA Statistics and Research Committee.

5. **Compliance:** Midwives will inform and assist parents regarding the Public Health requirements of the jurisdiction in which the midwifery practice will occur.

6. **Medical consultation and referral:** All midwives recognize that there are certain conditions when medical consultations are advisable. The midwife shall make a reasonable attempt to assure that her client has access to consultation and/or referral to a medical care system when indicated.

7. **Screening:** Midwives respect the woman's right to self-determination within the boundaries of responsible care. Midwives continually assess each woman regarding her health and well-being relevant to the appropriateness of midwifery services. Women will be informed of this assessment. It is the right and responsibility of the midwife to refuse or discontinue services in certain circumstances. Appropriate referrals are made in the interest of the mother or baby's well-being, or when the required or requested care is outside the midwife's legal or personal scope of practice as described in her protocols.

8. **Informed choice:** Each midwife will present accurate information about herself and her services, including but not limited to:

- Her education in midwifery
- Her experience level in midwifery
- Her protocols and standards
- Her financial charges for services
- The services she does and does not provide
- The responsibilities of the pregnant woman and her family

9. **Continuing education:** Midwives will update their knowledge and skills on a regular basis.

10. **Peer review:** Midwifery practice includes an on-going process of case review with peers.

11. **Protocols:** Each midwife will develop protocols for her services that are in agreement with the basic philosophy of MANA and in keeping with her level of understanding. Each midwife is encouraged to put her protocols in writing.

(revised October, 1996)

References:

American College of Nurse-Midwives' documents

ICM membership and joint study on maternity, FIGO, WHO, etc. revised 1972

New Mexico regulations for the practice of lay midwifery, revised 1982

North West Coalition of Midwives Standards for Safety and Competency in Midwifery

Varney, Helen, *Nurse Midwifery*, Blackwell Scientific Pub., Boston, MA 1980.

RESOURCES

American Academy of Husband-Coached
Childbirth
P.O. Box 5224
Sherman Oaks, CA 91413
(800) 423-2397

American College of Nurse-Midwives
818 Connecticut Ave. NW #900
Washington, DC 20006
(202) 728-9860

Association of Labor Assistants and Childbirth
Educators (ALACE)
P.O. Box 382724
Cambridge, MA 02238-2724

ASPO/Lamaze
1200 19th St. NW Ste. 300
Washington, DC 20036-2401
(800) 368-4404

Association for Pre and Perinatal Psychology
and Health (APPPH)
340 Colony Rd. Box 994
Geyserville, CA 95441
(707) 857-4041

Association of Radical Midwives (ARM)
c/o Ishbel Kagar
62 Greetby Hill
Ormskirk L39 2DT
ENGLAND

Birth
238 Main St.
Cambridge, MA 02142
(800) 215-1000

Birth Gazette
42 The Farm
Summertown, TN 38438

Birthworks
42 Tallowood Dr.
Medford, NJ 08055
(609) 953-9380

Cascade Birthing Supplies
(Moonflower, Birth and Life Bookstore)
141 Commercial St. NE
Salem, OR 97301
(800) 443-9942

Citizens for Midwifery (CfM)
c/o Susan Hodges
P.O. Box 82227
Athens, GA 30608-2227
(316) 267-7236

The Compleat Mother
P.O. Box 209
Minot, ND 58702

Doulas of North America (DONA)
1100 23rd Ave. E
Seattle, WA 98112
Fax (206) 325-0472

Global Maternal/Child Health Association
Waterbirth Information and Referral Center
P.O. Box 366
West Linn, OR 97068
(503) 682-3600

Informed Homebirth/Informed Birth and
Parenting (IH/IBP)
P.O. Box 3675
Ann Arbor, MI 48106
(313) 662-6857

Internation Association of Infant Massage
1720 Willow Creek Circle, #516
Eugene, OR 97402
(800) 248-5432

International Cesarean Awareness Network
(ICAN)
P.O. Box 276
Clarks Summit, PA 18411
(717) 585-4226

International Childbirth Educators Association
(ICEA)
Box 20048
Minneapolis, MN 55420-0048
(612) 854-8660

International Confederation of Midwives (ICM)
10 Barclay Mow Passage
Chiswick, W4 4PH
ENGLAND

Journal of Nurse-Midwifery
67 Tarryhill Rd.
Tarrytown, NY 10591-6511

La Leche League, Int. (LLLI)
P.O. Box 1209
Franklin Park, IL 60131
(708) 455-7730

Midwifery Education Accreditation Council
(MEAC)
c/o Mary Anne Baul
318 W. Birch, Ste. 5
Flagstaff, AZ 86001
(510) 214-0997

Midwifery Today
P.O. Box 2672
Eugene, OR 97402
(800) 743-0974
midwifery@aol.com

Midwives Alliance of North America (MANA)
P.O. Box 175
Newton, KS 67114
(316) 283-4543

Midwives International Research Service
(MIDIRS)
9 Elmdale Rd.
Clifton, Bristol BS8 1SL
ENGLAND

Mothering
P.O. Box 1690
Santa Fe, NM 87504
(800) 827-1061

National Association of Childbearing Centers
(NACC)
3123 Gottschall Rd.
Perkiomenville, PA 18074
(215) 234-8068

National Association of Childbirth Assistants
205 Copco Ln.
San Jose, CA 95123

National Association of Parents and Professionals
for Safe Alternatives in Childbirth
(NAPSAC)
Route 1, Box 646
Marble Hill, MO 63764
(314) 238-2010

National Association of Postpartum Care Services
(NAPCS)
8910 299th Pl. SW
Edmonds, WA 98026

National Organization of Mothers of Twins Clubs
P.O. Box 23188
Albuquerque, NM 87192-1188
(505) 275-0955

Naturopath
1410 NW 13th St., Ste. 2
Gainsville, FL 32601

NOCIRC
P.O. Box 2512
San Anselmo, CA 94979
(415) 488-9883

North America Registry of Midwives (NARM)
c/o Ann Cairns
Education Advocacy
1033 Woodlawn
Iowa City, IA 52245
(319) 354-5365

MEDICAL/HEALTH HISTORY

Please fill out this medical and personal history very carefully. When you come for your next visit we will go over the history together and discuss any questions that you might have. Just leave blank any technical terms or questions with which you are not familiar.

Personal Information

Date _____

Your name _____

Phone _____

Address _____

Birth date _____ Height _____

Usual Weight _____

Partner's name _____

Birth Date _____

Address _____

Emergency contact person _____

Phone _____

Who referred you to me? _____

Insurance _____

Pediatrician _____

Do you have any drug allergies or sensitivities? _____

Menstrual History

When do you think you may have conceived? _____

How long is your menstrual cycle? _____

LMP—last menstrual period _____

○ Yes ○ No Was it normal in length and heaviness of flow?

○ Yes ○ No Did you have a pregnancy test?

○ Yes ○ No Was this a planned pregnancy?

PMP—previous menstrual period _____

How old were you when you began menstruating? _____

Were you using birth control when you conceived?
  ○ Yes ○ No What kind? _____

Any complications after abortion or miscarriage?
  ○ Pain   ○ Infection   ○ Incomplete   ○ Emotional trauma

If Rh negative, did you receive RhoGAM? ○ Yes ○ No

Please list information about your previous births:

Obstetrical History

Total pregnancies: _____

Full term: _____

Premature: _____

Abortion: _____

Ectopic: _____

Miscarriage: _____

Twins: _____

Living children: _____

Cesarean section: _____

VBAC: _____

Date Mo/Yr.	# of Weeks	Length Labor	Birth Weight	Sex M/F	Place of Birth	Comments/Complications

Medical History

Please check if you have had any of the following conditions. In the space below, record date, treatment, and any follow-up you received. Also feel free to list any other important conditions/concerns.

○ Kidney disease
○ Diabetes
○ Hypertension
○ Epilepsy
○ Heart disease
○ Thyroid problems
○ Blood clotting problems
○ Asthma
○ Anemia
○ Hepatitis

○ Liver problems
○ Tuberculosis
○ Urinary tract surgery
○ Pelvic/back injuries
○ Stomach problems
○ Bowel problems
○ Skin problems
○ Bladder infection
○ Hospitalizations
○ Seizures

○ Surgeries
○ Hemorrhage
○ Allergies
○ Severe headaches
○ Ear/hearing problems
○ Dental problems
○ Eye/vision problems
○ Phlebitis/Varicosities
○ Hemorrhoids

_____

_____

_____

_____

_____

Is there any hereditary disease or condition in your family such as diabetes, cancer, heart disease, hypertension? (List, and indicate in which relative.)

_____

_____

_____

Lab Work (please leave blank)

INITIAL LABS	DATE	RESULT
BLOOD TYPE	/ /	A B AB O
D (Rh) TYPE	/ /	
ANTIBODY SCREEN	/ /	
HCT/HGB	/ /	_____ % _____ g/dL
PAP TEST	/ /	NORMAL/ABNORMAL/_____
RUBELLA	/ /	
VDRL	/ /	
URINE CULTURE/SCREEN	/ /	
HBs Ag	/ /	
HIV COUNSELING/TESTING	/ /	❏ POS. ❏ NEG. ❏ DECLINED
PPD	/ /	
CHLAMYDIA	/ /	
GC	/ /	
TAY-SACHS	/ /	
OTHER	/ /	

8–18-WEEK LABS	DATE	RESULT
AFP	/ /	
AMNIO/CVS	/ /	
24–28-WEEK LABS	**DATE**	**RESULT**
HCT/HGB	/ /	_____% _____g/dL
DIABETES SCREEN	/ /	1 HOUR_____
GTT (IF SCREEN ABNORMAL)	/ /	___FBS ___1 HOUR ___2 HOUR ___3 HOUR
D (Rh) ANTIBODY SCREEN	/ /	
32–36-WEEK LABS	**DATE**	**RESULT**
HCT/HGB	/ /	_____% ___g/dL
GROUP B STREP (35–37 WKS.)	/ /	

○ Yes ○ No   Have you or the father of your baby ever had a baby with a birth defect or mental retardation?

○ Yes ○ No   Do you or the father of your baby have any family members with birth defects or conditions diagnosed as genetic or inherited?

○ Yes ○ No   Are you and the father of your baby related by blood? (e.g. cousins)

○ Yes ○ No   Are you or the father of your baby from any of these ethnic/racial groups?
     ○ Jewish   ○ Black/African   ○ Asian   ○ Aleutian   ○ Mediterranean

How many times was your mother pregnant? _____

How many children did she have? _____

Did she have any miscarriages? _____

Were there any complications in any of her pregnancies? _____

How long were her labors? _____

Did your mother take DES while she was pregnant with you? _____

How much did you weigh at birth? _____

○ Yes ○ No   Do you have any unresolved emotional problems?

○ Yes ○ No   Do you think, or has anyone ever told you, that you have used drugs/alcohol excessively?

○ Yes ○ No   Have you ever experienced dramatic fluctuations in your weight?

○ Yes ○ No   Have you ever had anorexia, bulimia, or eating problems?

○ Yes ○ No   Have you ever been in an abusive relationship, including now, or been abused in the past (physically and emotionally intimidated, beaten, or injured)?

○ Yes ○ No   Have you ever had non-consensual sex?

○ Yes ○ No   Have you ever used any drug intravenously (IV)?

○ Yes ○ No   Have you ever had a blood transfusion?

○ Yes ○ No   Do you think you are at increased risk for HIV/AIDS?

○ Yes ○ No   Do you want information about safer sex practices?

How would you describe your usual diet? _____

What do you generally do for exercise? _____

Gynecological/Contraceptive History

When was your last Pap smear? _____

Have you ever had an abnormal Pap? If so, when? _____

Do you do self breast exam? _____

Please check if you've ever had any of the following:

○ Yeast   ○ Chlamydia   ○ Genital sores
○ Bacterial vaginosis   ○ PID   ○ Condyloma (warts)
○ Syphilis   ○ Oral herpes   ○ HPV (human papilloma virus)
○ Genital herpes   ○ Cervical surgery   ○ Cervical polyp
○ Cervicitis   ○ Fibroids   ○ Endometriosis
○ Ovarian cyst   ○ Uterine surgery   ○ Breast lumps
○ Abnormal bleeding   ○ Infertility   ○ Other reproductive
○ Breast surgery   ○ Gardnerella   problems/ conditions
○ Trichomonas   ○ Gonorrhea

○ Yes   ○ No   Have you ever used birth control? If so, what kind? Problems/complications?

_____

Current Pregnancy

What prenatal care have you had up to the present? Please list doctors, clinics, and hospitals where you have had care, what was done, and especially if you have had any lab work or special testing done.

_____

_____

_____

Please check if you've had any of the following problems during this pregnancy:

○ Nausea   ○ Vomiting   ○ Fever
○ Headache   ○ Dizziness   ○ Indigestion
○ Leg cramps   ○ Rash   ○ Backache
○ Swelling   ○ Constipation   ○ Diarrhea
○ Urinary problems   ○ Abdominal/pelvic pain   ○ Loneliness
○ Vaginal discharge   ○ Bleeding gums   ○ Relationship problems
○ Hemorrhoids   ○ Vaginal bleeding/spotting ○ Depression
○ Family problems   ○ Varicose veins   ○ Work problems

Have you used or been exposed to any of the following:

○ Tobacco   ○ Viruses   ○ Herbs
○ Caffeine   ○ Measles   ○ Vitamins
○ Alcohol   ○ Cats   ○ Non-prescription drugs
○ Marijuana   ○ Vaccinations   ○ Prescription drugs
○ Cocaine   ○ Ultrasound   ○ Fumes/Sprays
○ Street drugs   ○ X-rays   ○ Other environmental hazards

How do you feel about this pregnancy? _____
_____

How does your partner feel about this pregnancy? _____
_____

Do you feel that your sexual relationship has changed appreciably since you became pregnant? _____
_____

Do you plan to breast feed this baby? If so, for how long do you think you'll nurse? _____
_____

Are there any particular ethnic, cultural, or religious preferences for your care that you'd like to discuss?
_____
_____

Do you feel you have adequate resources, i.e., food, shelter, money, for this pregnancy? _____
_____

Do you have a car seat for the baby yet? _____
Please list the people you plan to invite to your birth _____
_____

Have you faced any opposition to your plans for home birth? _____
_____

Please give some thought to the following questions and write your ideas. If you and your partner are together, each of you should answer. Read all questions before answering.

Why do you want to have this baby at home? _____
_____
_____

Partner: _____
_____
_____

What do you see as the duties or responsibilities of your midwife? _____
_____
_____

Partner: _____
_____
_____

There are some things that can go wrong without previous warning during labor and birth and after. If you are a low risk woman, the chances of unpredictable complications are low. However, if such complications should occur, you or your baby might be at greater risk because of being at home. There are risks involved with childbirth just as there are with driving a car. Some of these risks will probably never be eradicated no matter what our state of technology. There is a certain subset of risks involved in having your baby in a hospital as well as in your home (or in an alternative birth center or birthing house). If you opt for the risks involved in birthing at home you need to find out what they are and how they can be dealt with. Please comment on what you know about risks and complications and how you feel about them:

_____

_____

_____

Partner: _____

_____

How do you feel about going to the hospital to deliver if your midwife feels that complications are arising?

_____

_____

Partner: _____

_____

How do you think you might deal with the problem of a baby or mother who suffered permanent injury or died at home? _____

_____

Partner: _____

_____

What do you think are the benefits of having your baby at home? _____

_____

Partner: _____

_____

Please add any comments or thoughts that you think might be important for your midwife to know about you:

_____

_____

_____

_____

_____

_____

_____

_____

_____

_____

_____

PRENATAL CARE RECORD

Name _____ Phone _____

LMP _____ EDD _____

Visit	Date	Weeks Gestation	Urine	Weight	Pulse/BP	FHR	Presentation/ Position	Fundal Height	Internal Exam	Next Appt.	Provider (Initials)

APPENDIX D

PRENATAL CARE PROGRESS NOTES

Name _____ EDD _____

_____

_____

_____

_____

_____

_____

_____

_____

_____

_____

_____

_____

_____

_____

_____

_____

_____

_____

_____

_____

_____

_____

_____

_____

_____

_____

_____

_____

_____

_____

_____

_____

_____

_____

_____

_____

_____

_____

LABOR RECORD

Name _____ Date _____

Labor onset: Latent _____ Active _____

Baby's position _____ EDD _____

Membranes _____ Usual FHT _____

Concerns _____ Midwife _____

Observations on arrival _____

Time	BP/Pulse	Fetal Heart Tones	Urinalysis	Contractions	Internal Exam

Labor Progress Notes

Name _____ EDD _____

_____

_____

_____

_____

_____

_____

_____

_____

_____

_____

_____

_____

_____

_____

_____

_____

_____

_____

_____

_____

_____

_____

_____

_____

_____

_____

_____

_____

_____

_____

_____

_____

_____

_____

_____

TRANSPORT RECORD FROM HOME DELIVERY

Midwife _____ Date/Time _____

Mother's Name _____ Partner's Name _____

Address _____

EDD _____ Mother's Age _____ Gravida _____ Para _____

Prenatal History

Gestational age 1st visit _____ Weight gain _____ Usual BP _____

Urine _____ Edema _____ Pelvimetry _____ Fundus_____

HCT/HGB _____ ABO & Rh _____ GBS _____ at _____weeks _____ HBsAg _____

Comments _____

_____

Labor History

Began labor _____ Initial events _____ Midwife arrived at _____

General observations _____ Vaginal exam _____

Comments _____

_____

Course of Labor

Inactive labor _____ Active labor _____ Pushing _____

Ruptured membranes _____ How? _____ Meconium? _____

Fetal response to labor _____

_____

Comments _____

_____

Reasons for Transport _____

_____

_____

_____

_____

_____

_____

_____

_____

_____

_____

BIRTH RECORD: MOTHER

Name _____

Phone _____ Age _____

Address _____

Gravida_____ Para _____ EDD_____ Date of Birth _____ Time_____

Labor Summary

Latent _____ hrs.

1st stage _____ hrs.   2nd stage _____mins.   3rd stage _____mins.

Membranes ruptured at _____ Spontaneously ____ Surgically ____ Clear ____ Stained ____

GBS _____ at _____

Estimated Blood Loss _____ Treatment _____

Comments/Problems _____

_____

Placenta

Size _____ Adherent clot _____

Method of delivery _____ Missing cotyledons _____

Infarcts _____ Calcifications _____ Succenturiate lobe _____

Time cord cut _____ Number of vessels in cord _____

Perineum

Lacerations _____ Repairs _____

Immediate Postpartum

BP _____ Pulse_____ Fundus _____

Shower _____ Urination _____ Food/Drink _____

Stable at _____

BIRTH RECORD: BABY

Name _____ Sex _____ Weight _____ Length _____ Chest _____ Head _____

Apgar   1 minute _____   5 minutes _____ Suctioning _____

Resuscitation _____

Molding, Caput, Hematoma _____ Eye Medication _____ Vitamin K _____

Nursing _____

Unusual Behavior Problems or Abnormalities _____

_____

_____

If problems develop and you call in, give time of birth, sex, weight, Apgar, respirations per minute, temperature, heart rate and describe symptoms.

Newborn Examination

DATE _____

SEX _____   WT. _____

AXILLARY TEMPERATURE

_____

TOTAL LENGTH _____

HEAD (O.F.) _____

CHEST _____

APGARS (one minute_____) (five minutes_____)

APGAR	0	1	2
Heart rate	Absent	Under 100	Over 100
Respirations	Absent	Slow (Irr.)	Good (cry)
Muscle tone	Limp	Some flexion	Active
Color	Blue/white	Blue hands or feet	Pink totally
Response to nasal catheter	None	Grimaces	Sneeze or cough

1. GENERAL APPEARANCE _____
   (Activity, tone, cry, edema)

2. SKIN _____
   (Color, desquamation, birth marks)

3. HEAD, NECK _____
   (Molding, caput, fontanelles)

4. EYES _____
   (Red spots, medication instilled)

5. ENT _____
   (Lips, palate, ear placement)

6. THORAX_____
   (Retractions)

7. ABDOMEN _____
   (Cord, masses)

8. HEART_____
   (Femoral pulses)

9. GENITALS _____
   (Testes descended, clitoris)

10. REFLEXES _____
    (Moro, grasp, sucking, swallowing)

11. SPINE/ANUS _____
    (Sinuses, anus patent)

12. LUNGS _____
    (Rales, grunting, cry)

13. EXTREMITIES _____
    (Clavicles, hip abduction)

COMMENTS _____

_____

_____

CLINICAL ESTIMATION OF GESTATIONAL AGE
An Approximation Based on Published Data*

PATIENT'S NAME _____

⌂ Examination First Hours

WEEKS GESTATION: 20 21 22 23 24 25 26 27 28 29 30 31 32 33 34 35 36 37 38 39 40 41 42 43 44 45 46 47 48

PHYSICAL FINDINGS	Description across weeks gestation
VERNIX	APPEARS → COVERS BODY, THICK LAYER → ON BACK, SCALP, IN CREASES → SCANT, IN CREASES → NO VERNIX
BREAST TISSUE AND AREOLA	AREOLA & NIPPLE BARELY VISIBLE, NO PALPABLE BREAST TISSUE → AREOLA RAISED → 1-2 MM NODULE → 3-5 MM / 5-6 MM → 7-10 MM → 7-12 MM
EAR — FORM	FLAT, SHAPELESS → BEGINNING INCURVING SUPERIOR → INCURVING UPPER 2/3 PINNAE → WELL-DEFINED INCURVING TO LOBE
EAR — CARTILAGE	PINNA SOFT, STAYS FOLDED → CARTILAGE SCANT, RETURNS SLOWLY FROM FOLDING → THIN CARTILAGE SPRINGS BACK FROM FOLDING → PINNA FIRM, REMAINS ERECT FROM HEAD
SOLE CREASES	SMOOTH SOLES NO CREASES → 1-2 ANTERIOR CREASES → 2-3 ANTERIOR CREASES → CREASES ANTERIOR 2/3 SOLE → CREASES INVOLVING HEEL → DEEPER CREASES OVER ENTIRE SOLE
SKIN — THICKNESS & APPEARANCE	THIN, TRANSLUCENT SKIN, PLETHORIC, VENULES OVER ABDOMEN, EDEMA → SMOOTH THICKER NO EDEMA → PINK → SOME DESQUAMATION PALE PINK → THICK, PALE, DESQUAMATION OVER ENTIRE BODY
NAIL PLATES	AP-PEAR → NAILS TO FINGER TIPS → NAILS EXTEND WELL BEYOND FINGER TIPS
HAIR	APPEARS ON HEAD → EYE BROWS & LASHES → FINE, WOOLLY, BUNCHES OUT FROM HEAD → SILKY, SINGLE STRANDS LAYS FLAT → PRECEDING HAIRLINE OR LOSS OF BABY HAIR, SHORT, FINE UNDERNEATH
LANUGO	AP-PEARS → COVERS ENTIRE BODY → VANISHES FROM FACE → PRESENT ON SHOULDERS → NO LANUGO
GENITALIA — TESTES	TESTES PALPABLE IN INGUINAL CANAL → IN UPPER SCROTUM → IN LOWER SCROTUM
GENITALIA — SCROTUM	FEW RUGAE → RUGAE, ANTERIOR PORTION → RUGAE COVER → PENDULOUS
GENITALIA — LABIA & CLITORIS	PROMINENT CLITORIS, LABIA MAJORA SMALL WIDELY SEPARATED → LABIA MAJORA LARGER NEARLY COVERED CLITORIS → LABIA MINORA & CLITORIS COVERED
SKULL FIRMNESS	BONES ARE SOFT → SOFT TO 1" FROM ANTERIOR FONTANELLE → SPONGY AT EDGES OF FONTANELLE, CENTER FIRM → BONES HARD, SUTURES EASILY DISPLACED → BONES HARD, CANNOT BE DISPLACED
POSTURE — RESTING	HYPOTONIC LATERAL DECUBITUS → HYPOTONIC → BEGINNING FLEXION THIGH → STRONGER HIP FLEXION → FROG-LIKE → FLEXION ALL LIMBS → HYPERTONIC → VERY HYPERTONIC
RECOIL - LEG	NO RECOIL → PARTIAL RECOIL → PROMPT RECOIL
ARM	NO RECOIL → BEGIN FLEXION NO RECOIL → PROMPT RECOIL MAY BE INHIBITED → PROMPT RECOIL AFTER 30" INHIBITION

POSTPARTUM CARE

NAME _____ PHONE _____

	1st HOME VISIT Date_____	2nd HOME VISIT Date_____
Breasts/Nipples & Breastfeeding		
Perineum Sutures		
Lochia		
Uterus		
Baby's cord		
Jaundice/ Baby Behavior		

SUGGESTIONS: _____

_____

FIRST PHONE CALL _____

DATE _____ _____

SECOND PHONE CALL _____

DATE _____ _____

	3 WEEK CHECKUP Date_____	6 WEEK CHECKUP Date_____
Breastfeeding		
Uterus		
Vaginal exam Cervix Muscle tone		
Lochia		
Parenting		

BIRTH CONTROL? _____

Postpartum Instructions

1. Let us know if you soak more than one pad in 20 minutes—massage your uterus firmly to re-contract it, and if bleeding doesn't stop, contact us at once or seek emergency care.

2. Check your uterus for firmness and/or tenderness several times a day, for 3 days at least.

3. Notice if your flow has any bad odor (it should smell like your period)—and report to us.

4. Take your temperature twice daily for at least four days.

5. Drink lots of water (about three quarts daily to establish milk flow) and make one quart of that a mixture of shepherd's purse and comfrey tea (for healing and bleeding control).

6. If you've had stitches, soak them in (or use compresses of) comfrey, goldenseal, and ginger tea—three or four times daily. Report any pain.

7. Clean your baby's cord stump carefully with hydrogen peroxide or alcohol every few hours (or at each diaper change). Pay special attention to the folds where cord joins skin.

8. Don't hesitate to call us if the baby seems disinterested in nursing, listless, or irritable.

9. Get lots of rest, sleep when the baby sleeps, eat lots of good food with plenty of iron to replenish lost blood, and ask visitors for real help—like doing your dishes or laundry. Work into activity slowly, and you won't have any sudden breakdowns later.

10. Try to take the parenting one day at a time—call if you need to.

The Midwife's Kit

fetascope

Doppler (optional)

watch, with second hand

blood pressure cuff

stethoscope

2 curved hemostats

1 pair scissors with blunt points

1 pair scissors with sharp points

1 needleholder

3 mosquito forceps

1 ring forceps

stainless steel cord clamps (Hazeltine)

stainless steel instrument tray with cover

sterile gloves (elbow-length and wrist-length)

regular exam gloves

disposable underpads

lubricating jelly

5cc syringes

3cc syringes

1 1/2-inch, 21-gauge needles (injections)

1/2-inch, 23-gauge needles (suturing)

suture material (3-0 chromic)

lidocaine anesthetic

pitocin

methergine

tetracycline or erythromycin eye drops

vitamin K for baby

nitrazine paper

urine testing sticks

pregnancy tests

plastic disposable amnihooks

DeLee mucus traps

cord blood tubes

bulb syringe

Betadine solution

alcohol prep pads

4 x 4 sterile gauze pads, or topper sponges

water bottle

heating pad

light (and extension cord) for suturing

plasticized or fiberglass tape measure

infant scales (hanging fish-scale type)

oxygen system with infant resuscitation unit (Hudson Lifesaver or Ambu Baby Resuscitator)

pocket masks for resuscitation (newborn and adult)

IV equipment (optional)

hemoglobinometer (optional)

herbs: shepherd's purse, comfrey, blue cohosh, liquorice root, hops, skullcap, chamomile

herbal tinctures: shepherd's purse, blue cohosh, angelica

Care and Preparation of Instruments

Most of the instruments require no special care, except for those which must be scrubbed and sterilized repeatedly. Careful cleansing immediately after use is a good idea; dried blood cakes up the hinges and is difficult to remove. Use scouring pads to clean blood from the grooved blades of the forceps and needleholder.

The first method for sterilizing your instruments is by boiling. Boil instruments and instrument tray in a large pot of water for 25 minutes. Be sure to remember to sterilize the tongs that you will use for removing instruments from the water, and be sure to place them in the water with handles up. Once the 25 minutes have passed, let the pot cool off a bit and then remove the tray with your tongs. Open some packets of sterile gauze, put on a sterile glove, and line your tray with the gauze. Then use the tongs once again to place the instruments in the tray, and cover (either drip-dry the cover as it's removed or blot with sterile gauze). Place in a doubled paper bag, wrap it up snugly, tape and date it.

A simpler method is the baking method. All you have to do is bake your double-wrapped package of tray, liner, and tools for one hour in a 250-degree oven. Be sure to add a pan of water so the bag doesn't scorch. Simply remove, cool, and store.

Repeat sterilization every two weeks.

PARENTS' SUPPLY LIST

Betadine solution

olive oil

bulb syringe (rubber ear type, 3 oz.)

4 x 4 sterile gauze pads (two dozen)

cotton balls

hydrogen peroxide

oral thermometer

bendable straws

plastic drop cloth and tape, or plastic sheet

bleach

plastic trash bags

disposable underpads (at least 20)

sanitary napkins (heavy and mini-pads) plus belt

4 sheets, 4 washcloths, 4 towels, 8 receiving blankets—all dried in hot dryer for ten extra minutes and bagged in plastic, then taped shut

herbs: shepherd's purse, comfrey, ginger root, etc.

plastic eye dropper

DIRECT-ENTRY MIDWIFERY EDUCATION PROGRAMS

The following programs are MEAC accredited (*) or pre-accredited (**).

Birthingway Midwifery School**
5731 N. Williams
Portland, OR 97217
503-283-4996

Maternidad La Luz*
Deb Kaley
1308 Magoffin
El Paso, TX 79901
915-532-5895

Midwifery Institute of California**
Elizabeth Davis & Shannon Anton
3739 Balboa #179
San Francisco, CA 94121
415-248-1671

North East College of Healing Arts & Sciences**
Elizabeth Mazenac
P.O. Box 250
Bellows Falls, VT 05101

Oregon School of Midwifery**
P.O. Box 40591
Eugene, OR 97404
541-689-0464

Seattle Midwifery School*
JoAnne Myers-Ciecko
2524 16th Ave. South #300
Seattle, WA 98144
206-322-8834

Utah School of Midwifery*
P.O. Box 412
Springville, UT 84062
801-489-4254
800-372-8255

Some of the programs listed below are recognized by the state in which they are located; others receive no recognition at all.

Academy of Midwifery Arts
Jeanie Rosburg
330 "A" Utah, #133
Colorado Springs, CO 80903

Apple Tree Family Ministries
P.O. Box 2083
Artesia, CA 90702-2083
310-925-0149

Ancient Art of Midwifery
Carla Hartley
P.O. Box 788
Claremore, OK 74018-0788

Artemis
Nan Koehler
13140 Fratilane
Sebastopol, CA 95472
707-829-1131

Association of Texas Midwives Training Program
603 West 13 #1A SC202
Austin, TX 78701
512-928-2311

BirthRight Education Center
Dee Anne Dominick
P.O. Box 276
Madisonville, LA 70477

Birthwise Educational Program
Heidi Fillmore-Patrick
P.O. Box 360
Denmark, ME 04022
207-452-2547

Cilia Bannenberg
P.O. Box 381
Barrington, NH 03825
603-332-7766
(Practical course with midwife in Holland—
maximum time 2-3 weeks)

Connecticut Friends of Midwives
54 Fairview Dr.
Madison, CT 06443
(Apprenticeships available, no formal classes
presently)

Family Birth Services
Helen Jolly
814 Dalworth
Grand Prairie, TX 75050
214-263-0299

The Farm
Christine Schoenbrun
156 Drakes Ln.
Summertown, TN 38483

Florida Institute of Acupunture & Midwifery
Jennie Joseph
P.O. Box 622105
Oviedo, FL 32762-2105
407-366-8615

Florida School of Traditional Midwifery, Inc.
P.O. Box 5505
Gainesville, FL 32602
904-338-0766

Frazier Valley School of Midwifery
c/o MTF
Box 65343, Station S
Vancouver, BC Canada V5N 5P3

Hygieia College
Jeanine Pavarti Baker
Box 398
Monroe, UT 84754
801-527-3738 or 801-527-3219

Imani Family Life Center
39 Dracut St.
Dorchester, MA 02124-3818

Informed Homebirth
Rahima Baldwin
Box 3675
Ann Arbor, MI 48106
313-662-6857

International Center for Traditional Childbearing
(ICTC) African-Centered
Training
Shafia M. Monroe
3507 NE MLK Jr. Blvd. Suite A33
Portland, OR 97212
503-288-3315

Lisa Hines
Correspondence Course
2901 Larkhall Rd.
Columbia, SC 29223

Lisa Lawrence
1008 Illinois St.
Bedford, IA 50833
(Correspondence Course)

Massachusettes Midwives' Alliance
MMA Study Course
368 Village St.
Millis, MA 02054

Miami-Dade Community College
Allied Health Technologies
c/o Justine Clegg
950 NW 20th St.
Miami, FL 33127
305-237-4234

Michigan School of Traditional Midwifery
Casey Makela
P.O. Box 162
Mikado, MI 48745
517-736-6583

National School of Technology, Inc.
16150 NE 17th Ave.
N. Miami Beach, FL 33162
305-945-9500

New Life Birth Services
MariMikel Penn
2311 west 9th
Austin, TX 78703
512-477-5452

Northern New Mexico Midwifery Center &
National College of Midwifery
Elizabeth Gilmore
Drawer SSS
Taos, NM 87571
505-758-1216

Re-Creation Training
P.O. Box 1653
Pahoa, HI 96778

Resourcing Birth
Terra Richardson
P.O. Box 3146
Boulder, CO 80307-3146

Sage Femme Midwifery School
Patty Craig
P.O. Box 2014
Clackamas, OR 97015
800-786-1460

Sherry Willis
HC 64 Box 85
Woodville, VA 22749

Spiritual and Scientific Non-Medical Midwifery
Mister Midwife
315 Sampson
San Diego, CA 92113

Vermont Midwives' Association
Maryanne Toronto
P.O. Box 9364
South Burlington, VT 05407
802-860-9364

Via Vita Health Project, Inc.
Vicki Penwell
600 3rd St. - Graehi
Fairbanks, AK 99701

Mexico

CASA Midwifery School
Umaran #62
San Miguel de Allende, GTO
37700 Mexico

Clinical Site of Midwifery Students in Mexico City
Contact Elizabeth Gilmore
Drawer SSS
Taos, NM 87571
505-758-1216

APPENDIX M

NURSE-MIDWIFERY EDUCATION PROGRAMS

(ACNM Accredited or Pre-Accredited)

Certificate Nurse-Midwifery Programs

Baystate Medical Center Nurse-Midwifery
Education Program
689 Chestnut St.
Springfield, MA 01199

Charles R. Drew University of Medicine & Science
Nurse-Midwifery Education Program
1621 E. 120 St.
Los Angeles, CA 90059

Education Program Associates
Midwifery Education Program
1 West Campbell Ave.
Campbell, CA 95008

Frontier School of Midwifery & Family Nursing
CNEP
P.O. Box 528
Hyden, KY 41749

Institute of Midwifery, Women and Health
c/o Philadelphia College of Textiles and Science
Room 220 Hayward Hall
School House Ln. and Henry Ave.
Philadephia, PA 19144

Parkland School of Nurse-Midwifery
UTSW Medical Center at Dallas
5201 Harry Hines Blvd.
5th Floor, WCS Dept.
Dallas, TX 75235

State University of New York Midwifery
Education Program
Box 1227, 450 Clarkson Ave.
Brooklyn NY 11203

UCSF/SFGH
Interdepartmental Nurse-Midwifery Education
Program (Certificate Track)
SFGH, Ward 6D, Rm 21
1001 Potrero Ave.
SF, CA 94110

University of Medicine and Dentistry of New
Jersey Nurse-Midwifery Program
65 Bergen St.
Newark, NJ 07107-3001

University of Southern California Nurse-
Midwifery Education Program
Women's Hosptal Rm. 8K5
1240 North Mission Rd.
Los Angeles, CA 90033

Master's Nurse-Midwifery Programs

Baylor College of Medicine Nurse-Midwifery
Education Program
Dept. of Ob/Gyn
6550 Fannin, Ste. 901
Houston, TX 77030

Boston University School of Public Health
Nurse-Midwifery Education Program
80 East Concord St., Room A-207
Boston, MA 02118

Case Western Reserve University
Nurse-Midwifery Program
10900 Euclid Ave.
Cleveland, OH 44106-4904

Columbia University
Graduate Program in Nurse-Midwifery
630 W 168 St.
NY, NY 10032

East Carolina University
Nurse-Midwifery Program
School of Nursing
Greenville, NC 27858

Emory University
Nell Hodgson Woodruff School of Nursing
Atlanta, GA 30322

Georgetown University School of Nursing
Graduate Program in Nurse-Midwifery
3700 Reservoir Rd. NW
Washington, DC 20007

Marquette University College of Nursing
Nurse-Midwifery Program
P.O. Box 1881
Milwaukee, WI 53201-1881

Medical University of South Carolina
Nurse-Midwifery Program
171 Ashley Ave.
Charleston, SC 29425

New York University Graduate Program in Nurse-Midwifery
50 W 4th St., 429 Shimkin Hall
NY, NY 10012

Oregon Health Sciences University
School of Nursing Nurse-Midwifery Program
3181 SW Sam Jackson Park Rd.
Portland, OR 97201

SDSU/UCSD Nurse-Midwifery Program
UCSD School of Medicine
9500 Gilman Dr.
LaJolla, CA 92093-0809

State University of New York at Stony Brook
School of Nursing
Stony Brook, NY 11794-8240

UCI/UCLA Nurse-Midwifery Education Program
5-631 Factor
Box 956919
LA, CA 90095-6919

or
UCI College of Medicine
101 The City Dr., Bldg. 41
Orange, CA 92668

UCSF/SFGH
Interdepartmental Nurse-Midwifery Education
Program
SFGH, Ward 6D, Rm. 21
1001 Potrero Ave.
SF, CA 94110
or
UCSF School of Nursing
N411X Box 0606
SF, CA 94143-0606

UCSF/UCSD Intercampus Graduate Studies
UCSD School of Medicine
9500 Gilman Dr.
LaJolla, CA 92093-0809
or
UCSF School of Nursing
N411X Box 0606
SF, CA 94143-0606

University of Colorado Health Science Center
Nurse-Midwifery Option
4200 East 9th Ave.
Denver, CO 80262

University of Florida Health Science Center
Nurse-Midwifery Program
653 West 8th St., Bldg. 1, 2nd Floor
Jacksonville, FL 32209-6561

University of Illinois at Chicago
Nurse-Midwifery Program
845 South Damen Ave.
Chicago, IL 60612

University of Kentucky
College of Nursing
760 Rose St.
Lexington, KY 40536-0232

University of Miami School of Nursing
5801 Red Rd.
P.O. Box 248153
Coral Gables, FL 33124-3850

University of Michigan Nurse-Midwifery Program
400 North Ingalls, Rm. 3320
Ann Arbor, MI 48109

University of Minnesota School of Nursing
6-101 Unit F
308 Harvard St., SE
Minneapolis, MN 55455

University Missouri-Columbia
Nurse-Midwifery Program
Columbia, MO 65211

University of New Mexico
Nurse-Midwifery Program
Albuquerque, NM 87131-1061

University of Pennsylvania School of Nursing
420 Guardian Dr.
Philadelphia, PA 19104-6096

University of Rhode Island
Graduate Program in Nurse-Midwifery
Kingston, RI 02881-0814

University of Rochester School of Nursing
601 Elmwood Ave., Box SON
Rochester, NY 14642

University of Texas at El Paso
Collaborative Nurse-Midwifery Education
Program
Texas Tech University HSC, Dept. OB/GYN
4800 Alberta Ave.
El Paso, TX 79905

University of Texas Medical Branch at Galveston
School of Nursing
301 University
Galveston, TX 77555-1029

University of Utah
Nurse-Midwifery Program
25 South Medical Dr.
Salt Lake City, UT 84112

University of Washington
Nurse-Midwifery Program
Box 357262
Seattle, WA 98195-7262

Vanderbilt University
Nurse-Midwifery Program
400B Godchaux Hall
21st Ave. S
Nashville, TN 37240-0008

Yale University Nurse-Midwifery Program
100 Church St.
New Haven, CT 06536-0740

Pre-Certification Nurse-Midwifery Programs

North Central Bronx Hospital
3424 Kossuth Ave.
Bronx, NY 10467

Ramsey Clinic
640 Jackson St., Ste. 5
St. Paul, MN 55101

University of Miami/Jackson Memorial Medical
Center
Women's Hospital Center
East Tower, 3003
1611 NW 12th Ave.
Miami, FL 33136

Additional

State University of New York
Midwifery Education Program
Box 1227, 450 Clarkson Ave.
Brooklyn, NY 11203

APPENDIX M

REFERENCES

Arms, Suzanne. *Adoption: A Handful of Hope.* (Berkeley, CA: Celestial Arts, 1990).

Arms, Suzanne. *Bestfeeding: Getting Breastfeeding Right for You.* (Berkeley, CA: Celestial Arts, 1989).

Bates, Barbara. *A Guide to Physical Examination and History Taking,* 6th Ed. (Philadelphia, PA: JB Lippincott, 1995).

Bennet, V. Ruth and Brown, Linda, eds. *Myles Textbook for Midwives,* 12th Edition. (New York: Churchill Livingston, 1993).

Beischer, Norman and Mackay, Eric. *Obstetrics and the Newborn, 2nd Edition* (Philadelphia, PA: W.B. Saunders, 1991).

Bobak, Irene, et.al. *Maternity and Gynecological Care,* 5th Edition. (St. Louis, MO: Mosby, 1993).

Brewer, Tom. *Metabolic Toxemia of Late Pregnancy.* (New Canaan, CT: Keats Publishing, 1982).

Cunningham, MacDonald & Gant. *Williams Obstetrics,* 19th Edition. (Norwalk, CT: Appleton-Century-Crofts, 1993).

Davis, Elizabeth. *Women's Intuition.* (Berkeley, CA: Celestial Arts, 1989).

Davis, Elizabeth. *Women, Sex & Desire: Exploring Your Sexuality at Every Stage of Life.* (Alameda, CA: Hunter House Publications, 1995).

Davis, Elizabeth and Leonard, Carol. *The Women's Wheel of Life: Thirteen Archetypes of Woman at Her Fullest Power.* (New York: Viking/Penguin, 1996).

Davis, Laura and Bass, Ellen. *The Courage to Heal.* (New York: Harper & Row, 1988).

Dick-Read, Grantly. *Childbirth Without Fear.* (New York: Harper & Row, 1959).

Ehrenreich, Barbara and English, Deirdre. *Witches, Midwives and Nurses: A History of Women Healers* . (New York: Feminist Press, 1973).

Erkin, Kerse & Chalmers. *A Guide to Effective Care in Pregnancy, 2nd Edition.* (Oxford: Oxford University Press, 1995).

Frye, Anne. *Holistic Midwifery,* Volume I. (Portland, OR: Labrys Press, 1995).

Frye, Anne. *Understanding Diagnostic Tests in the Childbearing Year,* 5th Edition. (Portland, OR: Labrys Press, 1995).

Gaskin, Ina May. *Spiritual Midwifery, 3rd Edition.* (Summertown, TN: The Farm Publishing Co., 1990).

Goer, Henci. *Obstetric Myths Versus Research Realities: A Guide to the Medical Literature.* (Westport, CT: Bergin & Garvey, 1995).

Hatcher, Robert, et.al. *Contraceptive Technology*, 16th Edition. (New York: Irvington Publishers, 1994).

Johnson, C., Johnson, B., Murray, J., Apgar, B. *Women's Health Care Handbook.* (Philadelphia, PA: Hanley & Belfus, 1996).

Kitzinger, Sheila. *The Experience of Childbirth, 6th Edition.* (New York: Penguin, 1987).

Kus, Robert J. *Keys to Caring: Assisting Your Gay and Lesbian Clients.* (Boston, MA: Alyson Publications, 1990).

Oxorn, Harry, and Foote, William. *Human Labor & Birth, 6th Edition.* (Norwalk, CT: Appleton-Century-Crofts, 1986).

Peterson, Gayle. *Birthing Normally.* (Berkeley, CA: Mind-body Press, 1981).

Resse, Robbins, Mahoney and Petrie. *Handbook of Medicine of the Fetus and Mother.* (Philadelphia, PA: J.B. Lippincott, 1995).

Silverton, Louise. *The Art and Science of Midwifery.* (Hertfordshire, England: Prentice Hall, 1993).

Varney, Helen. *Varney's Midwifery, 3rd Edition.* (Sudbury, MA: Jones and Bartlett Publishers, 1997).

Wagner, Marsden. *Pursuing the Birth Machine: The Search for Appropriate Birth Technology.* (Camperdown, Australia: Ace Graphics, 1994).

Weaver, Pam and Evans, Sharon. *Practical Skills Guide.* (Bend, OR: Morningstar Press, 1994).

Weed, Susun. *Wise Woman Herbal for the Childbearing Year.* (New York: Ash Tree Publishing, 1986).

Index

contraindication for home birth, 11
Ruptured cervical polyp, 59
Ruptured membranes
  artificial, 120–121
  infection prevention, 133
  prolonged, 132
  spontaneous, 87
Rural practice, 201–202

S

Sacral curve, 19
Sacral promontory, 20, 119
Sacrococcygeal joint, 22
Sacroiliac joint, 22
Sacrum, 20
Sage, tea/tincture for milk production, 173
Sagittal suture, 91–92, 119
Scalp (baby's)
  massage, 130
  sampling, 130
Scar tissue, 12
Sciatica, herbal remedy, 41
Screaming during second stage, 99
Screening
  for alpha-fetoprotein, 32
  genetic, 32
  for glucose, 32, 60
  HIV, 30
Screening out, 11
  on psychological basis, 84–85
Screw maneuver in delivery, 137
Secondary apnea, 154, 155
Second stage
  bradycardia, 129
  checking fetal heart tones during, 100
  difficulty of charting during, 211
  herbs in, 108
  hypoxia, 101
  and midpelvic disproportion, 129
  midwife duties during, 98–102
  normal length, 128
  oxygen therapy during, 101
  pelvic press, 129
  prolonged, 101, 128–30
  See also Labor

Self-Care in Pregnancy (test), 51–52
Sepsis, 174–75
Sequestered clots, 144
Sex/sexuality
  abuse, 122
  and circumcision, 176
  contraindicated with herpes, 39
  postpartum, 184–85
  problems, 81–82
  resuming after birth, 170
  in threatened abortion, 56
Sexual abuse and pelvic examination, 18
Sexually transmitted diseases (STD), 14
  issues for home birth, 11
SGA. *See* Small for gestational age
Shepherd's purse, tea/tincture for sleep problems, 109–10
Shoulder dystocia, 11, 61, 68, 136–39
Show, 87
Shultz mechanism of placenta separation, 110–12
Sibling participation, 45
Sickle-cell anemia, 32, 55
Simpkin, Penny, 83, 189
Sinciput, 91
Single mother, 74–75
Skin (baby's)
  checking color, 113
  color, 167
  consistency, 167
Skull, fetal, 91, 100–101
Skullcap, tea/tincture for hypertension, 37, 41, 62
Sleep difficulties, herbal remedies, 37, 41, 132
Sleepiness, baby's, 167
Sleeping arrangements postpartum, 169
Sleep problems, herbs for, 37, 41, 132
Slippery elm for heartburn, 41
Slow trickle bleeding, 144
Small for gestational age (SGA), 69–70
Smith, Trevor, 41
Smoking (heavy)
  contraindication for home birth, 11, 28
  dangers, 16
SOAP, SOAPIER charting, 211
Sonogram
  in biophysical profile, 72
  to detect breech presentation, 67

to detect twins, 65
to diagnose fibroids, 12
for placenta praevia diagnosis, 59
for polyhydramnios, 64–65
risks, 25
Sperm banks, 79
Spina bifida, 32, 64, 157
Spinal meningitis, baby, 30
Spine, checking baby's, 115
Spiritual Midwifery (Gaskin), 189
Spoiling baby, 169
Spontaneous abortion, 12, 56
Spontaneous rupture of the membranes
    (SROM), 87
Squatting in labor, advantage, 129
SROM. *See* Spontaneous rupture of the
    membranes
St. John's wort, tea/tincture for nerve pain, 41
Startle (Moro) reflex, 115
Station, 92
    checking for, 47–48
STD. See Sexually transmitted diseases, 9
Steam for lung congestion, 174
Stepping Stones to Labour Ward Diagnosis
    (Hamlin), 127
Steps to Successful Breastfeeding (list), 181
Stillbirth, 157–59
    grief of mother, 158
    and intrauterine growth retardation, 70
    unrelated to gestational diabetes, 60
Stimulants and hypertension, 62
Stitches. *See* Suture/suturing technique
Streptococcus infection and apnea, 175
Stress reduction, 34
Student Evaluation: Assessment and
    Management Abilities (checklist), 218–20
Study groups, midwifery, 195
Succenturiate lobe, 113, 141
Sugar, 55
    normal baby level, 174
    See also Hypoglycemia
Supplies
    for midwife, 255–56
    for parents, 256
    for suturing, 150
Support

cesarean birth, 184
organizations for parents, 156
postpartum system, 168
prenatal groups, 28
second week postpartum, 169
Suprapubic pressure, 138
Surprise breech, 139–40
Suture material, 150
Sutures (of baby's skull)
    checking during early labor, 91–92
    coronal, 91
    lamboidal, 91
    sagittal, 91, 119
    temporal, 91
Suture/suturing technique, 149–52
    contraindications, 147
    mother's follow-up, 153
    principles, 152
    pucker prevention, 152
    setup procedure, 150–51
    supply kit, 150
    suturing steps, 151
    triple-tie knot, 151
    types, 149
Swelling
    cervical, 120
    perineal, with delivery, 103
    perineal, immediate postpartum, 153
Swollen ankles, 37
Symphysis pubis, 20, 127
    joint, 22
    in pelvic press, 124
Syphilis screening, 29
Systolic pressure, 17
    See also Blood pressure

T

Tachycardia in fetal heart tones, 94
Tachypnea, 68
    transient, 174
TaySachs disease, 32
Tears (muscle)
    avoiding, 104
    checking for, 113
    from disproportion, 124

Vitamin B-12, 54
Vitamin C, 53, 54, 88, 133
   daily supplement, 25
Vitamin E, 37
   daily supplement, 25
Vitamin K, 114, 139–40
Vomiting, 34

W

Wagner, Marsden, 25, 190
Walking during active labor, 94
Walsh, John, 147, 149
Water birth, 95
Water for baby, 174
Weaning, 181–82
Weaver, Pam, 196
Weed, Susan, 190
Weight
   checking baby's, 115
   gain causes and problems, 55–56
   of mother, 16
Western Blot test for HIV, 30
Wharton's jelly, 111
What Every Pregnant Woman Should Know
   (Brewer and Brewer), 62

What to Do If the Baby Cries (list), 177
Whitson, June, 205
Williams Obstetrics, 59, 60, 71, 146, 190
Will It Hurt the Baby? (Abrams), 14, 156
Wise Woman Herbal for the Childbearing Year, The
   ß(Weed), 190
Witch hazel extract and hemorrhoids, 41
Women
   emotionally oriented, 73
   mentally oriented, 73
   physically oriented, 73
Working mothers, 75

Y

Yeast infection, 60
Yellow dock root, 41
Yoga, 27, 69
   postpartum, 171

Z

Zinc oxide, 39

"Emphasizes pregnancy as wellness ... this book parallels the family-centered approach that I advocate in established medical and nursing practices."

— Celeste R. Phillips, R.N., Ed.D.

"The elements of *caring for* and *caring about* women are so maturely thought out and articulated that I readily recommend the book to all midwifery students of any type of educational program, for any practice setting."

— Mary V. Widhalm, C.N.M., M.S.
Director of Midwifery
Lincoln Medical and Mental Health Center
Bronx, New York

"Elizabeth Davis has done her profession a very valuable service by providing a textbook that is eminently readable and which gives the aspiring midwife the benefit of having a *friend and mentor* in the form of a book—and that is no small accomplishment! She delves into the area of judgment, which is the acid test for any midwife. The is the Wise Woman speaking, the Sage Femme who can cut through the morass of information, the current standards, the new theories, and take us to the heart and kernel of what this work is all about."

— Tish Demmin, L.M.
Former President, The Midwives Alliance
of North America (MANA)